Communication and Communication Disorders

A Clinical Introduction

Elena Plante
Pelagie M. Beeson
The University of Arizona

Allyn and Bacon

Boston • London • Toronto • Sydney • Tokyo • Singapore

Executive Editor: Stephen D. Dragin
Editorial Assistant: Elizabeth McGuire
Editorial-Production Administrator: Joe Sweeney
Editorial-Production Service: Walsh & Associates, Inc.
Composition Buyer: Linda Cox
Manufacturing Buyer: Dave Repetto
Cover Administrator: Linda Knowles

Copyright © 1999 by Allyn & Bacon
A Viacom Company
160 Gould Street
Needham Heights, MA 02494
www.abacon.com

Library of Congress Cataloging-in-Publication Data

Plante, Elena, 1961–
    Communication and communication disorders : a clinical
introduction / Elena Plante, Pelagie M. Beeson.
      p.   cm.
    Derived in part from: Human communication and its disorders /
Daniel R. Boone, Elena Plante. 2nd ed. c1993.
    Includes bibliographical references and index.
    ISBN 0-205-28320-9
    1. Communicative disorders.   2. Communicative disorders in
children. I. Beeson, Pelagie. II. Boone, Daniel R. Human
communication and its disorders. III. Title.
    [DNLM: 1. Communication Disorders. 2. Communication. 3. Speech-
Language Pathology.   WL 340.2 P713c 1998]
RC423.P59   1998
616.85′5—dc21
DNLM/DLC
for library of Congress   98-28923
                                                            CIP

Printed in the United States of America
10 9 8 7 6 5 4 3 2 1   02 01 00 99 98

Photo Credits: p. 1, Elliott Smith/Silver Burdett Ginn; p. 17, David Young-Wolf/PhotoEdit; p. 41, Dwight Ellefsen/Omni-Photo Communications, Inc.; p. 61, PhotoEdit; p. 85, Will Faller; p. 117, Department of Speech and Hearing Sciences, The University of Arizona; p. 147, Laura Dwight; p. 175, Dennis MacDonald/PhotoEdit; p. 197, Will Faller; p. 229, Blair Seitz/Photo Researchers, Inc.; p. 255, PhotoDisk, Inc., p. 275, John Coletti

To our patients,
who continue to teach us.

Contents

Preface

We were blessed to have found our way to professional careers that have remained intellectually challenging, personally rewarding, and fun for many years. So when we sat down to write this book, we wanted to capture the essence of our experience. To that end, we strove to provide an introduction to speech, language, and hearing science that stimulates the reader's interest as it does ours. We also wanted the book to convey the reality of clinical practice in speech-language pathology and audiology, so we included many case studies to introduce and exemplify various communication disorders. We think that these clinical cases bring the book to life and give the reader an appreciation for the clinical and scientific endeavors embodied within the fields. We called upon our professional colleagues to share their thoughts about the challenges and rewards of their work, and they confirmed our thought that we are a diverse group of professionals who derive enjoyment from a wide range of experiences.

This book was derived in part from a earlier text, *Human Communication and Its Disorders*, 2nd edition, by Daniel Boone and Elena Plante. The current text retains the strong introduction to communication processes and communication disorders and is complemented by our focus on clinical illustration of normal and disordered speech, language, and hearing. Because we wanted the text to reflect insights gained from first-hand clinical, research, and teaching experience across a variety of clinical populations, we invited chapter contributions from three colleagues. We are pleased to include chapters on hearing disorders in children and adults by Anne Marie Tharpe and Linda Norrix, respectively, and a chapter on voice and swallowing by Julie Barkmeier. We worked together extensively to create a book that presents the range of content central to the professions, yet maintains a consistent introductory style throughout. We think that instructors will appreciate the breadth of content and consistency of style, and that readers will find the book interesting and fun to read. We had fun writing it.

We appreciate the editorial guidance of numerous friends and colleagues, including Carol Boliek, Richard Curlee, LouAnn Gerkin, Theodore Glattke, Jenny Hoit, Diane Ohala, Ralph Shelton, and Lyn Turkstra, who read various sections of this manuscript. We thank the reviewers for their time and input: Margaret Brooks, Assumption College; Edward C. Hebert, Springfield College; Robert D. Olsen, Marshall University. We also thank the 35 clinicians and 7 researchers who shared their professional experiences with us. We are also indebted to Decemna Chow, Jennifer Fisher, Molly Rewega, and Carmen Plante who assisted with the administrative tasks involved in producing this book. Finally, we thank our families for their immeasurable support in all our endeavors.

About the Authors

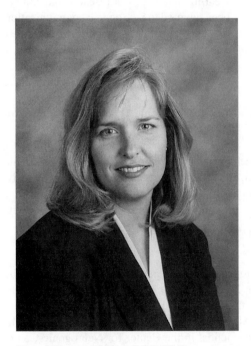

Elena Plante, Ph.D., CCC-SLP

Elena Plante completed bachelor's and master's degrees in speech-language pathology at Loyola College in Maryland. Before returning for a doctorate at the University of Arizona, she worked as a speech-language pathologist in the public schools. Since completing her doctorate and postdoctoral studies, she has been on the faculty at the University of Arizona. She also holds a research appointment with the National Center for Neurogenic Communication Disorders. Her research has focused on the behavioral and biological correlates of developmental language disorders. Her work was among the first to identify a neuroanatomic correlate of developmental language disorders using magnetic resonance imaging (MRI). Subsequent investigations have used electrophysiology and functional magnetic resonance imaging to examine the brain correlates of language processing. In addition, she has produced a series of studies that focus on identification of developmental language disorders in both children and adults through diagnostic testing. She has received support for her research from grants from the National Institutes of Health, National Institute on Deafness and Other Communication Disorders. Dr. Plante is a member of the American Speech-Language-Hearing Association and a member of two of its special interest divisions. She is on the editorial board of the *Journal of Communication Disorders* and has reviewed for several of ASHA's professional journals. She speaks regularly at national and international conferences on the topic of developmental language disorders.

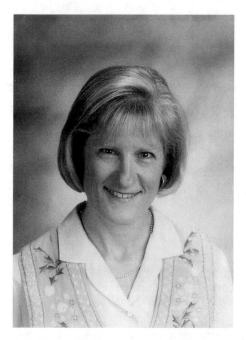

Pelagie M. Beeson, Ph.D., CCC-SLP

Pelagie Maritz Beeson received her bachelor's and master's degrees in speech-language pathology from the University of Kansas. She began her clinical career at a community speech and language center in Fairbanks, Alaska, where she provided service to a diverse clinical population. She later completed her doctoral work at the University of Arizona where she also served as the coordinator of the American Indian Professional Training Program in Speech-Language Pathology and Audiology. Currently, Dr. Beeson is a member of the faculty at the University of Arizona with the National Center for Neurogenic Communication Disorders and the Department of Speech and Hearing Sciences. Her research and clinical work has been devoted to neurogenic communication disorders in adults with a particular emphasis on the nature and treatment of aphasia, alexia, and agraphia. In Tucson, Dr. Beeson oversees the University of Arizona Aphasia Clinic where she remains active in clinical research and service delivery. She is board certified in Adult Neurogenic Communication Disorders by the Academy of Neurologic Communication Disorders and Sciences. She is currently serving as Chair of the Steering Committee for the American Speech-Language-Hearing Association Special Interest Division 2: Neurophysiology and Neurogenic Speech and Language Disorders and is an active member of the International Neuropsychological Society. She has contributed numerous publications to refereed journals, written several book chapters, and regularly speaks at professional meetings.

Linda Norrix, Ph.D.

Linda Norrix is a clinically certified audiologist who has experience assessing and treating individuals with hearing disorders. She worked at McFarland Clinic in Ames, Iowa for two and one-half years where she performed audiologic testing and provided rehabilitation services that included counseling and the fitting of hearing aids. After completing her doctoral studies at the University of Arizona in 1995, she worked as a research scientist in the Center for Neurogenic Communication Disorders at the University of Arizona. Her research involved examining the perception and integration of auditory and visual speech. During her doctoral and post-doctoral studies she has continued to assess and treat individuals with hearing disorders at several medical facilities in Tucson. Dr. Norrix currently is an Assistant Research Scientist in the Cognitive Sciences program at the University of Arizona.

Anne Marie Tharpe, Ph.D.

Anne Marie Tharpe is an Assistant Professor of Audiology in the Department of Hearing and Speech Sciences of the Vanderbilt Wilkerson Center for Otolaryngology and Communication Sciences. Dr. Tharpe has been involved in the provision of clinical audiology services to the pediatric population for almost twenty years. In addition to clinical service, her activities include research, writing, and teaching. Her clinical and research work has focused on assessment and management of children with hearing loss, normal auditory development in infants, and practitioner education. She has published numerous scientific articles and pediatric audiology textbook chapters and has co-authored a text on amplification in children.

Julie Barkmeier, Ph.D.

Julie Barkmeier has extensive experience with assessment and treatment of voice and swallowing problems. She worked in the Department of Otolaryngology-Head and Neck Surgery at the University of Iowa Hospitals and Clinics for seven years where she initiated assessment and treatment services for patients with dysphagia. In addition, she coordinated and participated in the assessment and treatment of individuals with voice problems in the University of Iowa Voice Clinic. After completing her doctoral studies in speech pathology at the University of Iowa in 1994, Dr. Barkmeier worked as a Research Scientist in the Voice and Speech Section of the National Institute on Deafness and Other Communication Disorders (NIDCD). Her research at the NIDCD focused on modulation of laryngeal reflexes during swallowing as well as studying long-term effects of botulinum toxin treatment on adductor-type spasmodic dysphonia. Her clinical work while at the NIDCD focused on assessment and treatment of neurogenic voice disorders. Dr. Barkmeier is presently a member of the faculty in the Department of Speech and Hearing Sciences at the University of Arizona.

Chapter *1*

Introduction to the Professions of Audiology and Speech-Language Pathology

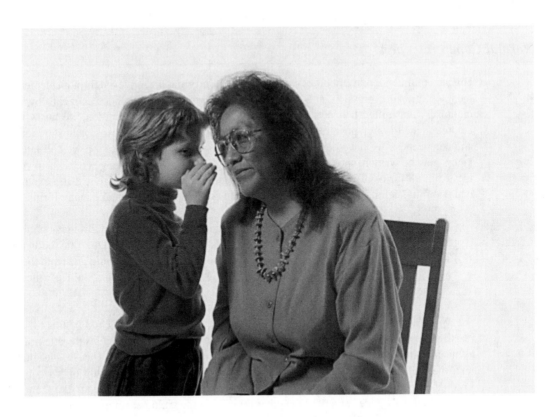

Preview

Communication is so pervasive in daily life that we often take it for granted. In this chapter, we introduce the field of communication disorders. We begin by examining normal communication in its various modalities. Then six individuals with communication disorders are introduced who are among the estimated 10 percent of the population for whom communication is impaired. We can begin to understand the bases of these disorders by briefly examining the components of normal communication, which are discussed in detail in later chapters. For individuals with communication impairments, the services of a speech-language pathologist or audiologist may improve the quality of daily life. We will meet some professionals who work in the field of communication disorders and hear their perspectives of this dynamic field.

Normal Communication

Human communication embodies a rich tapestry of information conveyed through elements of movement, emotional expression, and vocalizations. Communication includes all means by which information is transmitted between a sender and a receiver. By this definition, we know that animals communicate through posture, facial gestures, scent, and vocalizations. Humans are unique among animals because we have developed a system of symbolic communication we call language. Language may be written, spoken, or signed. Although all forms of language are used to communicate ideas, not all forms of communication involve language. A look at some real-life examples of normal communication illustrates that language and communication can take many forms.

A father carried his eighteen-month-old son in his arms as he walked through a public park. His son leaned over and excitedly extended his arms into the air. "Da?" the toddler asked. The father looked to see what had caught his son's attention. A young girl from the neighborhood was walking her dog. "Oh, it's the dog," the father replied. "Da! Da!" the son exclaimed while bouncing with excitement.

With the use of a single "word," tone of voice, and gestures, this child begins to use language to ask a question, make a statement, and indicate interest. The father accepts the attempt at language as meaningful, even though it only approximates a word in its adult form. He uses the situational context, the child's gestures and emotional tone to support his interpretation of his son's meaning. Through context, it becomes obvious that the child is using "da" to mean "dog" and not "dad," "man," "teddy," "juice" or any of the other things that the child has referred to in the past with those sounds. The father's response to his son turns an attempt at a word into a conversation, to the enjoyment of both. As we will see, not all attempts at communication are equally successful.

Sixty-four students sat in a lecture room, one without any windows, listening to their professor. The professor, who had taught the course nine times before, was lecturing: "One might question, uh, the relational meanings that best describe, uh, the language of young children. Remember, that Bloom said (as well as Sinclair or, uh, and Bowerman) that it is possible to put in a logical order the kind of language experiences that occur in a typical order of, uh, let us say, emergence."

Some of the poorest communication may exist in the lecture. This lecturer's poor word order and interruptions due to word-retrieval pauses interfered with effective communication. The meaning of the subject matter may be difficult for the student to comprehend even without the teacher's poor sentence formulation. The students may not be listening for many reasons, such as the instructor's poor narrative, fatigue from a previous activity, lack of ventilation in the closed room, and other real-world or imagined concerns.

Effective use of language for communication is not restricted to spoken words. Humans have developed additional modalities for the expression of language. One alternative developed because some individuals are unable to perceive spoken language.

A twenty-three-year-old student was hired as a classroom interpreter for a nineteen-year-old deaf engineering student. The interpreter had limited knowledge of the highly technical content of the engineering classes. To this was added the strain of translating the heavily accented and often broken English spoken by the foreign-born instructor into the completely different grammatical organization of American Sign Language. The engineering student, who had a pronounced playful streak in his personality, took advantage of these conditions for a little good-natured ribbing of the interpreter. At one point during the lecture, a fly was buzzing around the interpreter's nose and she swatted at it in mid-sentence. The student leaned forward, looked at her face, and repeated the gesture of swatting the fly, indicating he needed the gesture defined as if it were a word he did not know. When the interpreter ignored this obviously facetious request, he only repeated it with increasing elaborations on the gesture and facial expressions. This act finally caught the attention of the instructor, who stopped the class to see if there was a problem. Thoroughly embarrassed, the student and interpreter finished out the lecture without further interruption.

American Sign Language (ASL) uses a system of manual gestures instead of spoken words to convey information. In ASL, hand and arm movements, facial expressions, and locations in space are used to express vocabulary and a grammatical structure that is different from that of other spoken, written, and manual languages. Rather than hearing the message, signed languages are perceived through the visual modality. Like other languages, ASL has a normal developmental sequence when learned as a first language. Fluent users are able to express the full range of human ideas and emotions. No matter the mode, all languages can be used for a variety of purposes, such as communicating, thinking, creating, learning, and even teasing and humor.

ASL, and other manual forms of language, provide an alternate modality for expression. Like signed language, written language also uses the visual modality for communication. Like spoken or signed language, written language may be used to inform and to regulate behavior.

While traveling in the Southwest, we had occasion to visit the Ghost Ranch Living Museum in northern New Mexico. This center includes a small zoo of animals indigenous to the area.

Signs in front of each animal habitat warned, "Do not feed your fingers to the animals. Their diet is carefully monitored."

This clever sign conveyed at least two important pieces of information: The animals should not be fed by visitors, and the animals will bite. In this case, the sign's creator used a humorous approach and indirect language to convey the message. The tone of the written message was particularly appropriate to the setting as it contributed to, rather than detracted from, the visitor's enjoyment of the sights. The use of indirect language is interesting here, in that much more is communicated than the words actually denoted.

Normal communication encompasses verbal and nonverbal elements that, in combination, are used for a variety of purposes. Communication is successful when information is accurately transmitted from a sender to a receiver. Some aspects of communication, such as nonverbal elements, are not always intentional. Sometimes, our bodies "give us away." For example, posture, facial expression, and voice quality may combine to indicate fatigue, even when we may be very interested in the topic of a conversation. Other elements, such as proximity and gestures, are used to communicate the speaker's status, attitudes, and emotions.

Many of the nonverbal elements of communication are culturally regulated. For example, Anglo listeners tend to provide speakers with periodic feedback by nods and vocalized signals of affirmation. Navajo listeners provide less overt signs of attention; polite listeners attend unobtrusively. Some cultures maintain constant eye contact when listening; for others, "staring" at a speaker is rude. Even such aspects as the length of time one pauses between utterances is culturally determined. Although this may seem to be a minor component of communication, violations may have profound effects on the listener. A speaker who pauses too long may appear to be withholding and unsociable. One whose pauses are too short may appear to be impertinent and domineering. Most individuals are able to monitor and use an ongoing stream of nonverbal information for effective communication.

Six Individuals with Communication Impairment

Communciation is so pervasive in our lives that we sometimes take it for granted. However, those with a communication disorder feel the impact every day. There may be no better way for us to appreciate the diversity of these problems than to review a few cases of individuals with various forms of communication disorders. As we will see from these cases, communication disorders affect both children and adults, and they do not discriminate by ethnic background or economic status.

Beth Feldman[1] is a twenty-three-year-old student teacher who has developed bilateral vocal nodules, or bumps on both vocal folds. By noon every day, she loses her voice completely, making it impossible to control the twenty-six children in her fourth-grade class. She was warned by her supervising teacher that she will lose her student teacher status if she does not improve her voice. Seeking help in a voice clinic at a university hospital, she was told that she speaks at the very bottom of her pitch range, clears her throat excessively, speaks in a loud voice with a pronounced hard glottal attack and a vocal focus that is "in the bottom of

---

[1]We have changed the names of all individuals whose communication disorders are described in this book.

her throat." She consulted two ear-nose-throat physicians (otorhinolaryngologists), who each told her that she has two small nodules, one on each vocal fold, that are not big enough to explain the severe voice symptoms she is experiencing. Both recommended voice therapy. Subsequent voice therapy attempts were thwarted by school and teaching activities that leave her little time for either therapy or practice of voice techniques. Recent counseling efforts with Ms. Feldman were successful in making the point that her type of voice problem (hoarseness and loss of voice related to vocal nodules) could probably be well resolved with voice therapy. However, she has not yet made her first therapy appointment.

Jim Fields is a forty-three-year-old promoter who arranges concerts for rock and pop musicians. His wife convinced him to have his hearing checked when she noticed that he was no longer hearing his wristwatch alarm and that he had difficulty understanding her over the telephone. His evaluation by an audiologist revealed a moderate to severe hearing loss of the type associated with noise exposure. The audiologist learned that his history of noise exposure dated back to his teens, when he sang in a band that in his words "substituted volume for talent." Since that time, there had been many occasions when he remembered leaving a performance with "ringing ears" or "fuzzy hearing." The audiologist explained the connection between exposure to loud sound and the hearing loss Mr. Fields was experiencing. He now uses hearing protection when exposed to loud music (and other loud sounds) to slow further hearing loss. He has enrolled in a lipreading course to help compensate for the loss he already has. In addition, he returns for regular hearing checkups to monitor his hearing acuity. He has elected to forgo a hearing aid at this time but understands that one may become a necessity in the future.

Rudolpho Torres, age thirteen months, was evaluated by team members of a university orofacial-disorders clinic. He was born in Mexico with a bilateral cleft lip and palate. Although his cleft lip was surgically repaired within a few weeks of his birth, the roof of his mouth remained unrepaired. All of his attempts at speech (or when crying) appear to come out of his nose since there is open coupling of his oral and nasal cavities. He was examined by the plastic surgeon, who recommended immediate surgery to finish the repair of his cleft. Both the audiologist and otolaryngologist found that the boy had a middle-ear infection, which was producing a moderate hearing loss. The speech-language pathologist felt that Rudolpho exhibited normal language comprehension for Spanish and urged early surgical intervention in an attempt to minimize his severe hypernasality. The boy and his mother were going to live temporarily with his uncle in Tucson, so the first stage of surgery could be started. The social worker on the team met with the speech-language pathologist, the plastic surgeon, and the boy's mother to arrange the temporary move from Mexico to Tucson.

Karen Burghart, a thirty-three-year-old attorney, had stuttered all her life. She would repeat words over and over, and sometimes she would fix her mouth in a tight, twisted manner, unable to say anything. Although she received some speech therapy for her stuttering while in high school, she felt that it did not help her. While attending a university, she was the victim of a savage beating and sex crime. Her attacker was arrested and subsequently tried for his crime. Unfortunately, he was acquitted, in part because of her inability to speak during her attempts to testify against him during the trial. During counseling sessions with a psychologist, she was advised to receive speech therapy for her stuttering. She began receiving individual therapy twice weekly and participated in a young-adult stuttering group at the university speech clinic. She began to realize in therapy that most of her life had been spent trying not to stutter, and she found that she was beginning to do a lot of things to keep from speaking. The speech therapy taught her how to speak easily, prolonging the vowels in her speech. As the result of her courtroom experience and the injustice she witnessed, she became fascinated with law and the criminal justice system. Upon graduation from the university, she went to law school and became an attorney. She continues in speech therapy to maintain her controlled fluency, but her speech now permits her to function as an assistant district attorney.

Bruce Murrich, age sixty-nine, was a retired executive who suffered a stroke while sleeping, awakening with a right-sided paralysis (hemiplegia) and aphasia (loss of language and speech). His sudden symptoms transformed him from a golf-playing, fun-loving retiree in Arizona to a man unable to speak any words except occasional profanity and powerless to move his right arm and leg. He and his wife reacted initially to the severe disability with disbelief and denial, hoping that, with proper medical attention within the first few days of onset, his symptoms would go away. After several weeks of continued impairment, Mr. and Mrs. Murrich sought rehabilitation, which included speech-language pathology services. Mr. Murrich began receiving twice-weekly group therapy and daily individual speech therapy (plus physical and occupational therapies). His wife attended a weekly spouse group and received individual counseling with a social worker in the rehabilitation center. As his speech improved to the point that he could communicate many thoughts and needs in two-to-three word utterances with less profanity, his overall spirits improved dramatically. Now, about eighteen months after the stroke, both Mr. Murrich and his wife seem to accept the relative permanence of his disability.

Devon Douglas was seventeen when we first met him. His younger brother had been diagnosed with a rare genetic condition that could affect development. The family lived in a remote town and traveled two hours each way to reach our clinic where they participated in a research study to determine the language impact of the genetic disorder. When we first talked with Devon's mother, she had more concerns about him than her younger son, despite the fact that Devon did not have the genetic disorder. She reported that he had struggled his entire school history to maintain average grades. Over the years, she had asked the school system to evaluate Devon for a learning disability. The first time was when he was in second grade. Each time, the school staff indicated that they did not see Devon as having any educational handicaps, so he was never evaluated. Devon himself reported that teachers had told him that he was lazy and could do better if he tried. His mother was now worried that school was such a struggle that Devon might drop out. As part of our research program, we were able to evaluate his cognitive and linguistic skills. Testing revealed that his general cognitive abilities were in the high average range. However, he had great difficulty putting together grammatical sentences, following spoken directions, and understanding what he read. In fact, his overall language skills were quite weak. At age seventeen, we diagnosed a language-based learning disability for the first time in this young man's life.

These cases represent the challenges and diversity encountered by professionals in the field of communication disorders. Each of these people had been struggling to overcome a communication handicap. Ms. Feldman's vocal nodules had a direct impact on her effectiveness as a teacher. Mr. Murrich's stroke forever altered both his and his wife's plans for retired life. Devon's difficulty with language had a direct impact on his school success. Each case demonstrates how difficulty in just one aspect of communication can affect an individual's daily life.

Classification of Communication Disorders

Breakdowns in communication may be understood by looking at the components of normal communication. Communication requires the transmission of information from one person to another. Information can be conveyed through tone of voice, facial expressions, posture, and gestures. Language, however, is the medium of choice when we wish to communicate specific ideas. **Language** involves the coding of meaning into a system of arbitrary symbols that are recognized by members of the community. This system of symbols includes rules for how sounds are combined into words, how words are combined into sentences, and the conventions for how conversations are conducted and written language is organized. For example, in English, words may begin with a "st" combination, as in "stairs," but not with a "ts" combination. However, Navajo includes words that start with the "ts" combination (e.g., tseí). These conventions within each language are completely arbitrary; English speakers are capable of producing the "ts" combination (e.g., "its"), but do not use it at the beginning of words. Other rules govern how words are combined into sentences (the grammar of a language). These are also arbitrary and vary among languages. For example, English requires the use of nouns or pronouns to specify the subject of a sentence. In Italian, however, the pronoun can be dropped from the sentence without any resulting confusion. We will explore the nature of language in more detail in Chapter 4.

For most individuals, language is communicated from speaker to listener through an oral-to-auditory pathway. The vocal mechanism and oral structures are used to form the individual sounds of language that we recognize as **speech**. A change in tongue placement is sufficient to differentiate a "t" from a "k." The addition of vocal fold vibrations changes the "k" to a hard "g." In other languages, further manipulations of sound contribute to speech. For example, Chinese is considered a tonal language because changes in the pitch of the voice are also used to differentiate between sound elements. Our vocal mechanism also allows us to vary the pitch and loudness of speech to convey emotion and emphasis. For the average person, these aspects come together seamlessly to produce a fluent flow of words. We introduce the physical structures that support speech in Chapter 2 and follow with a discussion of the sounds of speech in Chapter 3.

Because of their knowledge of the anatomy and physiology of the oral structures, speech-language pathologists have become involved with treatment of certain disorders that do not strictly involve communication. These include such conditions as tongue thrust and swallowing disorders. As we will see in Chapter 9, tongue thrust can be associated with a lisped "s" sound. It also has an impact on eating and on dental alignment, as the tongue pushes forward on the front teeth during swallowing. Other, more severe forms of swallowing disorders are covered in Chapter 11. Swallowing disorders often result from the same types of disease processes and acquired damage that can affect communication. Swallowing evaluation and treatment has become a prominent component of many speech-language pathologists' work in health-related settings.

Spoken language is received by the listener through the aural modality. This requires an intact auditory system. **Hearing** includes such aspects as the awareness of sound, the ability to distinguish among sounds, and the ability to process sound that occurs at a rapid rate. These abilities are central to being able to decode speech. When language is presented in the auditory-oral modality, normal hearing is also important. By hearing language spoken around us, we learn the rules of our native language, the sounds of speech, and even the accent and intonation patterns that characterize our regional dialect. When we speak, we monitor our own production and modify or correct our speech as we talk. The mechanisms of hearing, on which all these skills rely, are addressed in Chapter 2.

When impairments in communication occur, they typically involve a breakdown in one or more of the elements involved in speech, language, or hearing. In Figure 1-1, we see these three aspects of normal communication and how they relate to classes of communication disorders. Language disorders may include conditions that emerge as a child develops. These *developmental* language disorders may first appear during childhood, but may persist into adulthood. This was the case for Devon, whose difficulties were apparent in grade school. In contrast to developmental language disorders, acquired language disorders occur when an individual suffers an injury or disease that causes a loss of language skills. Mr. Murrich's case presents one type of *acquired* language disorder called aphasia. Although acquired language disorders can occur at any time during life, the majority of individuals with acquired language disorders are adults. Disorders involving language skills in children and adults are discussed in Chapters 7 and 8.

Disorders of speech also may also occur in children and adults. These disorders may include aspects of **articulation**, or the way the sounds of words are produced. For Rudolpho, his cleft palate altered the oral structures needed for speech articulation. If left unrepaired, he would have little

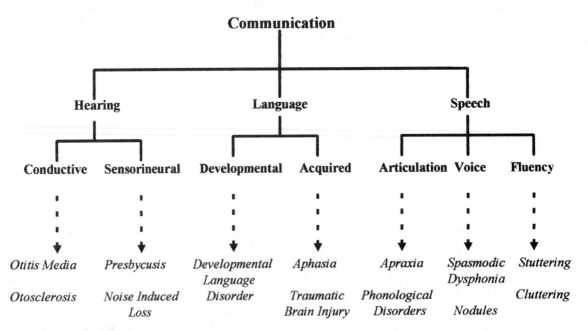

FIGURE 1-1   A conceptual representation of different types of communication impairments with examples of specific disorders (listed below the dashed arrows).

chance to develop normal speech. In other children, a developmental articulation disorder may appear without a known cause. As with language disorders, articulation disorders may be acquired following accident or disease. In other cases, difficulty with speech may involve the vocal mechanism. **Voice** disorders may alter the pitch, quality, or loudness of the voice. We saw in the case of Ms. Feldman that poor speaking practices may lead to physical changes of the vocal mechanism that interfere with speech over time. In her case, the voice disorder interfered with her professional life. In other cases, an overly breathy or harsh vocal quality, or a loss of voicing may signal a health concern that requires immediate medical intervention.

Finally, a disorder of speech may involve **fluency**. Fluency disorders occur when the normally smooth flow of speech becomes interrupted. The individual may struggle to produce sentences that come effortlessly for others. Ms. Burghart had first-hand experience with the most prevalent of fluency disorders: stuttering. For most individuals, stuttering begins during childhood. Many of those who stutter will eventually overcome this difficulty. A few, like Ms. Burghart, will have to monitor their fluency indefinitely. We will examine disorders of articulation, voice, and fluency in Chapters 9 through 11.

Disorders of hearing may arise from factors that prevent the conduction of sound into and through the hearing mechanism. These are referred to as a **conductive hearing loss**. Rodolpho had a conductive hearing loss due to fluid in the middle ear. Although children with cleft palate show high rates of this type of conductive loss, middle ear infection (otitis media) is also one of the most common afflictions of otherwise normal children. In contrast to conductive hearing loss, **sensorineural hearing loss** refers to a hearing loss caused by disease of the inner ear or the neural transmission of sound. In Mr. Field's case, exposure to loud sound over time produced a sensorineural hearing loss. In other cases, an individual may be born with a hearing loss or lose hearing after an illness. Although we classify hearing disorders as conductive or sensorineural, in some instances, hearing loss may involve a mix of both types. We will discuss disorders of hearing in Chapters 5 and 6.

Careers in Communication Disorders

As described in the cases at the beginning of this chapter, most individuals with speech, language, or hearing disorders can improve their communication. The professionals who provide front-line services for the remediation of communication disorders are **audiologists** and **speech-language pathologists**. The professional organization for audiologists and speech-language pathologists is the American Speech-Language-Hearing Association (ASHA). In 1989, ASHA passed a resolution that specified the fields of Audiology and Speech-Language Pathology as separate professions. Because of the common concern for human communication impairments and the historical association of these two professions, most individuals in either field have some knowledge and training in areas served primarily by the other. At the present time, for example, the undergraduate curriculum in most training institutes does not differ for the two fields. Instead, students specialize in one or the other profession as part of their graduate school training. Although there are some opportunities for individuals without graduate degrees (see Chapter 12 for a discussion of support personnel), a master's degree is required to become certified as an audiologist or speech-language pathologist. Following completion of all graduate courses for a master's degree (or its equivalent), the newly trained audiologist or speech-language pathologist spends a year in supervised clinical practice. Upon completion of the clinical fellowship year, and after passing a national certification examination, he or she becomes certified to work in a wide variety of clinical settings.

The individuals who have careers in communication disorders are a diverse group. The membership survey of the American Speech-Language-Hearing Association (ASHA, 1997) reveals the variety inherent to the field. According to the survey, there are over 11,000 thousand certified audiologists and over 73,000 certified speech-language pathologists. Like the American population, they represent all major ethnic groups, White, African American, Hispanic, Asian/Pacific Islander, and Native American. Although women are a majority within the professions, the Council of Graduate Programs reported that student enrollment by men has increased and was at a ten-year high in 1997. Most audiologists and speech-language pathologists (75.3 percent) are employed full time. For audiologists, the most common place of employment was in a healthcare facility (72 percent), which included hospitals, clinics, private practices, and as part of a physician's practice. Other employment settings included school systems (11 percent), industrial facilities (2 percent), and colleges or universities (8 percent). In contrast, 53 percent of the speech-language pathologists reported working in a school system. Other common employment settings for speech-language pathologists included healthcare facilities (39 percent) and colleges or universities (4 percent).

The results of the ASHA membership survey provide an overview of those who comprise the professions. To get a more personal view, we asked audiologists and speech-language pathologists from around the country to share their perceptions about their professions. Our informants included individuals who represent nearly all segments of the demographic groups that comprise the profession. We interviewed 35 individuals who had over 350 combined years of experience within the field.

Clinical Careers

We began by asking our colleagues why they chose to work in the field of Communication Disorders. As one might imagine, some were first introduced to the field because they knew someone with a communication disorder. That was the case for Nancy, who lives in Arizona and is a relative newcomer to the field with two years of experience. Nancy wrote, "I worked for a gentleman who had Parkinson's disease and he piqued my interest in the rehabilitation fields. He persuaded me to 'lose interest in the law' (a previous pursuit) and to become involved in a 'helping profession.' After doing some research, I found Speech-Language Pathology to be the most interesting." A few colleagues knew someone who was working in the field or had received clinical services themselves at some point. Kim, a speech-language pathologist from Colorado, reported that she received therapy for articulation as a young child. She "decided one day on my way to day care to be a 'Speech Therapist.' At the time, I only knew the 'r,' 'l,' 's,' part of the field." In her six years in the profession, Kim now has more extensive experience working in both school and hospital settings. Donna is an audiologist with 35 years experience who is employed as the director of a university clinic. She reported that a relative was a teacher of the deaf, whose experiences sparked her interest in deafness. As an undergraduate, she was in the enviable position of having three fellowships, in theatre, linguistics, and audiology, to choose among. She chose audiology and wrote "I have *never* regretted this decision."

Those with direct or indirect exposure to the field were in the minority. Others were attracted to the field because of a specific interest or desire that was encompassed by the field. Many of our colleagues noted a desire to enter a field where they could "make people's lives better." This sentiment was echoed by Jenifer, who wrote "I knew I always wanted to work with children, but I wasn't sure how until I watched some Speech Pathologists work with some language-impaired preschoolers at a local hospital. Watching them, I realized how much impact a person could have in a child's life." Jennifer has had many opportunities to rediscover this impact in her own hospital-based position as a pediatric speech-language pathologist. Paula reported that she had an initial interest in languages and language development. "Then I took an Audiology course and became fascinated with the process of hearing and what can happen when people—especially children—are unable to hear." She has combined these interests for fifteen years as an educational audiologist in Colorado.

We are also seeing increasing numbers of individuals who come into the profession after having worked in another field. Zarina was a bilingual second grade teacher before deciding to go back to school. "I wanted to get out of teaching and I noticed that there were a lot of Spanish-speaking kids with language difficulties. I decided to go into Speech-Language Pathology to help bilingual children. I also wanted the option of working in other settings in addition to schools." Erin was a public relations account executive before returning to school for a master's in speech-language pathology. "What it all came down to was more meaningful work. I wanted a job helping people instead of just helping a company make money." She picked Speech-Language Pathology because it allowed her to combine her interests in languages (she speaks English and French) and allied health. Bret wrote, "I've had a long-standing interest in how we communicate (my B.A. is in Speech Communication). I was advised by a family friend to investigate Speech-Language Pathology . . . and learned just how diverse our field is and that it could provide a lifelong, stable career." He now works in a rehabilitation center in Colorado.

There is also what we like to think of as "the luck factor" that led people to discover the field. Consider Anne, who has been practicing for two years in Missouri. "I didn't really know what I wanted to do," wrote Anne. "I had several friends who talked me into taking a Speech-Language Pathology class, and (after enrolling) I decided then and there that I was in the right field." Carol, an audiologist of ten years in California had a similar reaction to her initial academic exposure. "I found the coursework interesting and challenging. There didn't seem to be a single course in the program I wasn't interested in taking." For Ellen, who has now been practicing for eleven years in Tennessee, a problem with her own voice lead to a career in Speech-Language Pathology. "I wanted to work with voice disorders as I was a voice major in music and experiencing problems. I took a class in phonetics and loved the content."

We were impressed with the variety of reasons that our colleagues entered the professions. This may be because the professions can accommodate the wide range of personality traits and backgrounds that these individuals brought to it. We saw this when we asked our colleagues to tell us about the personality traits that they saw as important to their job. Here are a few of the recurring themes that our colleagues expressed. Lane's experience in hospitals and skilled nursing facilities in Arizona have taught him that a "speech-language pathologist needs to be flexible, adaptable, a team player, a good communicator, and very clear about personal and professional integrity. These characteristics are crucial for survival in a rapidly changing health care system." Angie, a speech-language pathologist from Tennessee, commented, "I believe that you must be assertive in this field. People's quality of life is at stake and you must do whatever you can to help." The complementary position was expressed by Mike, a Colorado resident who wrote, "I think patience may be the key to some of my success as an audiologist [of twenty-three years], especially when working with families with young hearing impaired infants who need the gift of *time* to accept their child's impairments and to implement the many recommendations we make." In fact, patience was mentioned as a personality trait by almost all our respondents. Another common characteristic of our colleagues was an orientation toward solving problems. Ellen commented that "task analysis is at the center of what we do;

identify problems then determine the best method of improving function." Not surprisingly, she feels traits like analytical skills and a questioning nature, mixed with enthusiasm and an action-oriented nature, apply to her. Rebecca, a speech-language pathologist of twenty-one years and the director of a hospital-based center for communication disorders in New York, adds qualities such as persistence, self-confidence, maturity, and a generous nature to the list.

Among the most frequently identified trait was independence. This trait characterized clinicians in private practice, university clinics, schools, hospitals, rehabilitation centers, and skilled nursing facilities. This is not surprising in that clinicians in most settings have a great deal of autonomy as to how they manage their caseload, develop programs, and provide quality service. Regardless of clinical setting or clientele, the field demands individuals with the motivation to identify areas of need and seek out information in this ever advancing field.

We were also curious about what keeps these professionals in the field year after year. Some cited specific aspects of their jobs, such as the experience of developing a new program for service delivery or working with cutting edge technology. Donna works with such new advances as programable hearing aids and cochlear implants. She wrote, "Patients who are realizing dramatic functional gains do keep me going!" "I love the diagnostic process," writes Shara, a speech-language pathologist of eleven years. "To be able to identify strengths and weaknesses and explanations for behavior is very challenging. Also, to be able to change those behaviors, to see them 'get it' is exciting." Shannon, a Michigan-based speech-language pathologist echoed several common themes: "It's the versatility of being able to work with children or adults. I also like having a solid base of knowledge in a variety of disorders. And there's always the advantage of always being able to find a job!" Angie expressed the sentiments of many of our colleagues. She wrote, "It's a fast-paced field. I am always encountering new situations that allow me to learn continuously." Lou, a speech-language pathologist of three years wrote, "The most exciting thing for me to experience is children's first words—the look in their eyes when they realize they are able to impact their environment using words." When asked what keeps her going, Jennifer put it succinctly, "Two words—the kids. Two more words—their smiles."

All clinicians have stories about particular clients that stand out, punctuating their careers like exclamation points along the way. This was the case for Angie who wrote about a difficult case involving a man who had had a stroke. "He once told me 'you remember those old movies where there are slaves rowing the boat and there is a man standing on deck cracking his whip. That is what you were for me. I never could have done it without you.' I never gave up on him, nor he on me." Ellen writes that one of her staff was able to identify an important medical issue for a patient that had been previously missed by several other professionals. "This speech-language pathologist referred the patient back to the Ear, Nose, and Throat physician and highlighted her findings. The ENT diagnosed the actual cause of the swallowing disorder and was able to surgically repair it. The patient resumed a regular diet." Sometimes the smallest gains are the most important to the clinician. Susan, a speech-language pathologist in Minnesota, wrote of a severely autistic child who for the first time communicated a specific desire by selecting a picture of an activity. "We were so excited for him and what this skill will do for him in the future." She is now working to expand this child's first step into skills that will allow him to communicate with others through the use of pictures. The impact of these cases is captured by Lane, who commented that "the emotional rewards and the opportunity to powerfully impact and connect with people during a difficult time in their lives" are primary advantages to a career in this field.

Research Careers

Audiologists and speech-language pathologists impact lives through direct clinical services. But this is not the only avenue to effect change within the professions. The desire to advance the field beyond its current boundaries attracts professionals to incorporate research as a component of their career. Although opportunities for research exist in almost all job settings, less than 1 percent of the professionals see themselves primarily as researchers. Another 3 percent are college or university professors, for whom research is a typical component of their careers (ASHA, 1997). For most of these individuals, their education included doctoral studies, which provide core training in research methods. The majority of these researchers work in university settings. We asked some of these individuals to tell us why they elected this career path and what it is like to be a researcher in the field of communication disorders.

Amy Skinder had just begun her doctoral studies at the University of Washington when we talked with her. Prior to her enrollment, she had worked as a speech-language pathologist for four years, part of which was spent as a traveling clinician in a variety of settings around the country. "I am the last person out of my graduating class . . . that I expected to be going back for a Ph.D.," she reported. "My goal when I finished my master's was to be able to work with a broad range of disorders. After a while, I decided that instead of knowing a little about a lot, it would be nice to focus on one area. At the same time, I was working with a client in the public school system who had severe developmental apraxia of speech as well as attention deficit disorder and other learning disabilities. I went to a seminar . . . and asked lots of questions. I found out there weren't a lot of answers. After talking with the speaker [a noted researcher], I felt encouraged to go on for my doctorate. Doctoral studies are an opportunity to indulge in trying to answer all your burning questions."

This motivation has been echoed by many researchers we have talked with over the years. Anne Cordes, Ph.D., is on the faculty at the University of Georgia, where she conducts research in the area of stuttering. She realized during her master's degree that she wanted to go on for a doctorate. "The things that were catching my interest during my coursework and with my practicum clients were the things that we as a field didn't know or didn't yet understand—it wasn't the answers that I thought were interesting, it was the QUESTIONS! And the Ph.D. is a research degree, which is about questions, so it became pretty obvious that this is where I belonged."

Nancy Helm-Estabrooks, Sci.D. wrote, "In many ways I think I was always an informal researcher—trying new approaches, developing new materials, regarding every case as a case study—even before my doctoral studies, which I pursued in my thirties. I decided to get a doctorate to further my knowledge and to write grant proposals as a Principal Investigator so I could explore and test some ideas I had for new treatment approaches."

Steven Camarata, Ph.D. has been on the faculty at Vanderbilt University for seven years. He wrote "I wanted to teach at a university and was interested in clinical research. Being able to follow my curiosity for research [is an exciting component of the job]. This freedom is a very precious gift. I knew that research would involve a lot of mundane work, but the discovery is worth it. Plus, I want to help children with speech and language problems and realized early on that I could best do this, not only by seeing patients (which I still do), but also by developing better treatments."

The efforts of getting a doctorate were definitely worth the time and effort for our colleagues. Barbara Lewis, Ph.D., of Rainbow Babies and Children's Hospital and Case Western Reserve University, has been conducting research for over ten years. Her work on the genetic basis of phonological disorders has drawn her into collaborations with psychologists, pediatricians, epidemiologists, and geneticists. She wrote to us, "I like the challenge of asking difficult research questions and finding results that do not always correspond to my prediction."

This is also apparent to Amy Skinder, who was just beginning her research career. "It's not so easy to answer those big, burning questions. It's surprising how small you have to start out with your research. It's a lot more complicated than you anticipate." Those results, however unanticipated they may be, advance the state of professional knowledge.

Dr. Cordes wrote, "I love to pick up a new journal and read the report of a new study that flowed from a creative idea or from a creative way of approaching an old problem. If the method is good and sound so the results are believable, then it is such fun to enjoy the new findings and enjoy that sense of 'Well, of COURSE! Why hadn't anybody ever thought of that?' For the same reason, I love seeing a reference to my own published work in something that's almost unrelated, because somebody else saw some connection that I never even thought of." But the final impact of research is on clinical practice. We are one of the few therapeutic professions for which research advances are provided by its own membership, a situation that adds to the strength and autonomy of the professions as a whole.

Audiologist Theodore Glattke, Ph.D., expressed the importance of researchers within the profession, "If we fail to develop new knowledge, we will face extinction as service providers." Leslie Gonzalez Rothi, Ph.D., added, "We are the professionals best suited to perform this applied research; a bridge between basic research and clinical application."

Many of the most active researchers in our field are in academic positions. This brings with it the opportunity to interact with students. Anne Cordes relates some of her favorite aspects of an academic position. "I like being able to sit with one student and figure out where she is and what the student's needs are and being able to point her in the right direction. I get a kick out of phrasing something just right in class so that I can see twenty light bulbs come on over the students' heads. And every so often, I get a kick out of the sudden realization that I DO know how to solve some problem after all." Dr. Glattke is on the faculty of the University of Arizona and has been in a faculty position for twenty-seven years. He has extensive experience mentoring students in research experiences. "It is a pleasure to witness the genuine excitement that the students express when they share their work. . . . Sometimes they discover something about themselves as a result of the effort they put into writing about their research or synthesizing the literature base." He also had this to say about teaching in a university setting: "Contributing to the development of new knowledge, integrating the new knowledge into the curriculum, and adapting mentoring styles to respond to the needs of the students are invigorating activities. It is a privilege to be allowed to teach in a university setting."

Others conduct research within health care settings. Among the leading non-university research sites are some of the Veteran's Administration (VA) Medical Centers. Dr. Gonzalez Rothi is employed at the Gainesville Veteran's Administration Medical Center where she combines clinical practice with cutting edge research. She wrote that "my research background offers me a willingness to open doors that are not yet available to most. Second, no day is ever the same. Each time I come into the hospital, I find that new challenges are facing me, testing the limits of my abilities and always inspiring me to know more." Dr. Helm-Estabrooks has also worked in the VA system and has extensive experience conducting research in clinical settings. "Research appeals to my detective instincts, developing new assessment and treatment methods appeals to my creative instincts, and clinical research allows me to work directly with patients. Also, there are many aspects to my work—

patient evaluations and therapy sessions, writing, teaching, mentoring, etc.—so that I'm always challenged and never bored."

Research careers present their own unique challenges. "One of the main challenges has been to remain focused on my primary interest—genetics of speech and language disorders," Dr. Lewis expressed. "There are many temptations to digress into related but very interesting areas. You have to realize that you can't do it all." Dr. Cordes agrees. "Balance and organization [are challenges]. My job gives me at least twice as many options as any one human being could reasonably keep track of. . . . An academic position is described as 'teaching, research, and service,' but what that really means is that the challenge is to find time for good teaching, good research, and a reasonable amount of service when it often seems that each day has about two days' worth of little stuff that has to get done. The challenge is to keep track of what's really important for the long term."

What advice do these individuals have to new generations of potential researchers? Dr. Lewis advises that "a student interested in research should learn as much as possible about research methodology and statistics while keeping a strong tie to the clinic. Most important is to identify an area of interest and explore related disciplines." Our research colleagues do not recommend so narrow a focus that outside studies and collaborations are ignored, however. Dr. Gonzalez Rothi urges students to "look for a program where you have an opportunity to look at a wide variety of perspectives. Set up an advisory committee that reflects this diversity. Take courses outside of your [major area of focus] that might be able to contribute to your knowledge base." Finally, Dr. Camarata provides this perspective: "Look in your heart and mind to determine whether satisfying your curiosity will sustain you. The key requirement for research is not 'intelligence' per se, but an interest in problem solving (with a large dose of persistence thrown in). If you like asking questions, a research career might be the most satisfying option."

Clinical Problem Solving

We have introduced some of the types of communication disorders that concern the professions of audiology and speech-language pathology and have allowed some practicing professionals to share their insights about the field. In the ensuing chapters will lay the groundwork necessary to understand normal and disordered communication processes in children and adults. We will consistently introduce the reader to clinical cases who bring to life the realities of the communication disorders. These individuals will help the reader appreciate the diagnostic and treatment processes that are at the heart of the professions.

Audiology and speech-language pathology are, by nature, fields in which memorization of facts is not enough for success. It requires the application of knowledge to real-life problems. For this reason, we will end each chapter with a section on clinical problem solving. This is an opportunity to take the information covered in a chapter and apply it to a case. We saw in this chapter how individual components of communication can break down in cases of disorder. Many communication disorders involve a combination of difficulties within the areas of speech, language, and hearing. Consider the following case:

Bonnie, age eight, was born with a severe hearing loss. Her loss was first diagnosed at age eighteen months. She has some usable hearing for low frequency sound and was fitted with hearing aids to help her capitalize on the little hearing she does have. Bonnie was placed in a preschool program that combined the use of hearing aid amplification with sign language and speech. Despite this early help, her spoken language skills were two years behind other children her age and her speech was grossly unintelligible when she entered first grade. Since then, she has made gains, but still struggles with grammar in both spoken and written language. Her speech is still difficult to understand, as she makes many articulation errors involving sounds that are out of her hearing range. Her voice has an effortful quality and sounds as if she is speaking from the back of her throat. Bonnie continues to receive academic tutoring and speech training. Her ability to communicate with spoken and written language lags far behind her ability to communicate through sign language.

1. Using Figure 1-1, identify which areas of communication (i.e., speech, language, hearing) are involved in Bonnie's case.
2. Identify the components of speech, language, or hearing that appear to be involved in this case.
3. Would Bonnie's communication disorder be classified as developmental or acquired?
4. Which professionals are likely to be involved with Bonnie to maximize her communication potential?

References

American Speech-Language-Hearing Association (1997). Semiannual counts of the ASHA Membership and Affiliation. Rockville, MD: American Speech-Language-Hearing Association.

Council of Graduate Programs in Communication Sciences and Disorders (1997). National Survey. Author.

Chapter 2

The Biological Foundations
of Communication

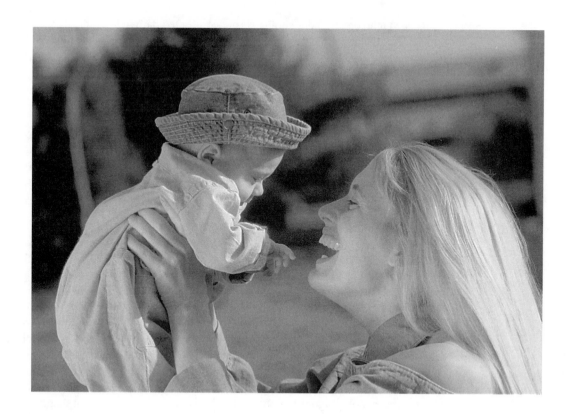

Preview

A knowledge of the biological underpinnings of normal hearing, speech, and language is central to understanding the many ways in which communication can be disrupted. We will examine the vocal mechanism, which is responsible for sound production. The articulatory mechanisms shape the sound into the individual consonants and vowels that form words. Those words are perceived by the listener through the auditory system. Finally, they are comprehended by the brain, which then may store that information or formulate a response. The physical mechanisms normally do not function independently, but work together to support communication. When communication is disrupted by developmental disorder or acquired pathology, the disruption can often can be traced to one or more of these basic biological systems.

Speech-language pathologists and audiologists are confronted daily with clinical cases that require an understanding of the physical and neurological underpinnings of communication and how break-downs in these systems lead to communication disorders. Consider the following scenarios:

Mr. Blades, age 71. In an acute-care hospital, a speech-language pathologist is asked to evaluate the speech and language of a seventy-one-year-old man named Mr. Blades. He had been admitted to the hospital the day before, following a car accident in which he was a passenger. In addition to other injuries to his body, he had hit his head and lost consciousness for almost an hour. Although alert, he seemed to have difficulty understanding what was said to him. The clinician was concerned that the blow to the head may have damaged the parts of his brain that support language. Could the accident have caused difficulties in understanding language? Or could there be another cause for Mr. Blades' poor comprehension?

Alicia, age 3. Alicia was born with Down syndrome. This developmental disorder can be traced to a genetic abnormality that results in an extra copy of chromosome 21. For this engaging three-year-old girl, the occurrence of this genetic abnormality could impact her communication skills in various ways. Low muscle tone associated with the disorder might interfere with her ability to move and explore her world. The changes to her oral-facial structure could interfere with speech articulation to some extent. Changes in the structure of the ear make children with Down syndrome prone to hearing loss. Her brain development has also been altered by the genetic abnormality, which has resulted in some degree of mental retardation. It might also have affected her capabilities for normal language development. An assessment team, consisting of a speech-language pathologist, an audiologist, a special educator, a psychologist, a physical therapist, and an occupational therapist, must determine how the effects of Down syndrome appear in this child. The team will then determine how she can be assisted to maximize her overall development, including development of communication skills.

In both of these cases, the clinicians must have a thorough understanding of the physical mechanisms that support communication in order to determine the most likely sources of the communication problems these two individuals face. In the following sections, we will explore the biological systems that support normal communication and consider how they might be affected in clinical cases.

The Vocal Mechanism

It is said that communication is an "overlaid function" that makes use of structures that have other primary functions. The same muscles and organs that allow us to breathe also provide the driving force behind sound production. The larynx, which keeps us from choking on food or liquid that might otherwise be misdirected into the airway, also contributes to sound production. The structures of the mouth and throat that allow us to eat and drink also permit us to change the vocal tract in ways that result in the sounds that make up words and sentences.

The Respiratory System

The main function of the respiratory system is to sustain life through the continuous exchange of gases, primarily the exchange of carbon dioxide for oxygen. Since the body cannot store oxygen, it requires a continuous renewal of its oxygen supply, usually from twelve to eighteen inspirations-expirations (breath cycles) per minute. For the majority of persons without some kind of respiratory disease, the breath cycle continues almost unnoticed and without conscious effort.

Humans as a species demonstrate far more control of the breathing mechanism than any other mammal. When singing or talking, we have the capability of taking in a quick inspiration followed by a prolonged expiration, which activates phonation for singing or talking. The musculo-skeletal **thorax**, as seen in Figure 2-1, can expand its size by muscle contraction. For example, on inspiration, the **diaphragm** (a composite of many muscle fibers and tendons) contracts, it descends, increasing the vertical dimension of the lungs and expanding the dimension of the lower rib cage; lifting the shoulders also increases the vertical dimension of the thorax, but not as efficiently as diaphragmatic movement. The horizontal dimension of the thorax can be increased by action of the **intercostals** and other chest wall muscles. The outside of the lung adheres to the inside of the chest wall. Therefore, when the rib cage expands by active muscular contraction, the lungs and airways are stretched, which increases their size and results in a decrease in density of the air within the lungs (intrapulmonary air). With the reduction of intrapulmonary air density, the air outside the body rushes in. On expiration, the thorax becomes smaller as the muscles relax. The abdominal muscles can also contract, assisting in expiration by applying force from below on the ascending (relaxing) diaphragm. The lungs become smaller. Normal lung tissue is highly elastic and recoils back to a smaller size when no longer stretched. As the lungs collapse, the air within them develops a greater density than atmospheric air, and the pulmonary air rushes out of them until intrapulmonary and atmospheric pressures are the same. At this point, the inspiration phase begins again. In summary, inspiration is related to thoracic expansion (greater lung area produces lower intrapulmonary pressures), whereas expiration is related to a decrease in thoracic size (less lung area produces denser air). The movement of air into and out of the lungs is achieved, then, by differential air pressures created by active muscular contraction (and relaxation) of thoracic and abdominal muscles.

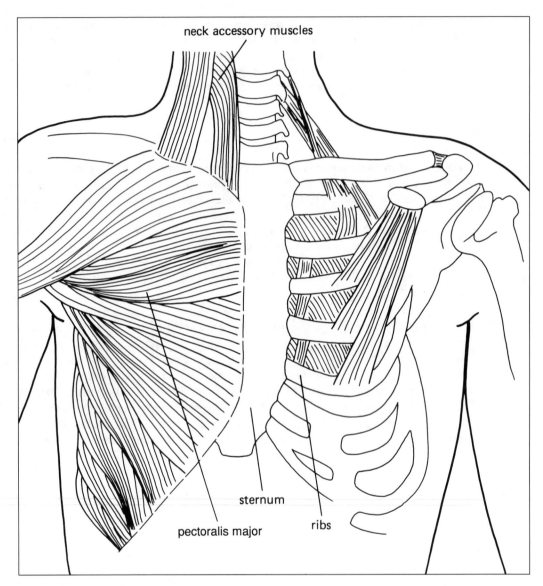

FIGURE 2-1   The musculo-skeletal components of the thorax include the ribs and sternum as well as muscle groups that allow for movement of these structures.

The inherent forces and active muscular contraction work, for example, during sleep in a natural, synergistic way. Our "in" breath is about as long as our "out" breath. When we sing or talk however, volitional forces are able to change the normal in-and-out pattern enabling us to take a quick inspiration and follow it with a prolonged expiration, which we use for phonation. For a detailed understanding of aerodynamics of speech and voice, see Hixon and Abbs (1980), Kent, (1997), or Zemlin (1998).

Many disorders can disrupt the musculo-skeletal system that underlies control of speech breathing. Let us refer back to Alicia's case from the perspective of the respiratory system. When the evaluation team works with Alicia, several professionals will look at her musculo-skeletal system. The physical therapist will examine postural support and gross motor movements. The occupational therapist will examine fine motor control, particularly in relation to age-appropriate play activities. The speech-language pathologist's primary concern will be whether Alicia has sufficient control over the muscles that support posture and respiration to permit connected speech. Alicia's muscle tone, although less than normal, is adequate to support spoken communication. However, there are concerns about her ability to support her body and her motor skills.

The Phonatory System

Voice (or phonation) is produced by the vibration of the two vocal folds within the larynx. Although phonation is a vital part of communication, the primary function of the larynx is to guard the airway against aspiration, the inhalation of fluids or other matter into the airway. The larynx sits at the top of the trachea, where it plays this primary "watchdog" role, guarding the airway. To prevent aspiration there are three valve sites within the larynx (vocal folds, false folds, and aryepiglottic folds). When we swallow, the larynx elevates as the three muscle valves constrict to protect the airway. In some individuals with structural damage to the vocal folds (a result of cancer, for example) or with muscular impairment of laryngeal function (perhaps part of a degenerative neuromuscular disease), the valving mechanism can be compromised and the patient may experience life-threatening choking spells.

The human voice represents perhaps the highest function of the larynx in the mammal. To appreciate the perspective that the human voice may well not be an evolutionary accident, one has only to listen to the sheer beauty and control of the voice as heard in an operatic aria or popular ballad or vocal interpretations of an accomplished actor. The communicative and artistic functions of the larynx take it well beyond its basic valving responsibilities. The average person, for example, is unaware of the valving role of the larynx and when asked what the larynx (or "voice box") does, may answer, "We make sound with it."

The front and back view of the larynx can be seen in Figure 2-2. The **cricoid cartilage** forms the base of this structure and the **thyroid cartilage** sits above the cricoid. The thyroid cartilage is shield-shaped and forms the prominent anterior wall of the larynx. In many young men, we can see the prominent thyroid cartilage (Adam's apple). The vocal folds originate just below the thyroid notch (the notch one can feel with the fingertips just above the middle of the thyroid cartilage). From the thyroid cartilage, the vocal folds extend posteriorly to the anterior base of two pyramid-shaped cartilages called the arytenoids. The vocal folds can be seen by looking down on the larynx from above, as seen in Figure 2-3. In this figure, we can see the open vocal folds and the arytenoid cartilages. The view of the thyroid cartilage is blocked by the epiglottis.

In Figure 2-2, the **arytenoid cartilages** sit on top of the posterior cricoid cartilage. The arytenoid cartilages move and rotate on their mounts atop the cricoid cartilage by the action of several intrinsic muscles in the larynx. For example, when the posterior cricoarytenoid muscles contract, they

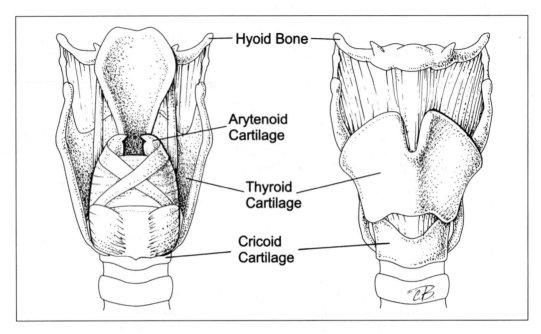

FIGURE 2-2   Structures of the larynx.

move the arytenoid cartilages in such a way that they pull the vocal folds apart; the posterior cricoarytenoid muscles, therefore, are known as laryngeal abductors (they separate the vocal folds). The lateral cricoarytenoids are laryngeal adductors, which rotate the arytenoids together in such a way that the folds come together. This muscle action is extremely quick, permitting the speaker to produce in milliseconds the voiced and voiceless sounds in a word by rapid vocal-fold adduction followed by an equally rapid abduction.

Another intrinsic muscle function is to lengthen (by stretching and tensing) or to shorten (by relaxing and thickening) the folds. Either action has some effect on pitch level. Thinner folds vibrate more quickly, producing higher frequencies (pitches); thicker folds vibrate more slowly, producing lower frequencies. The area between the vocal folds is known as the **glottis**. When the vocal folds are brought together (adduction), they are in the phonation position. The outgoing air builds up below the vocal folds, causing increased subglottal air pressure. When this subglottal pressure is greater than the pressure holding the folds together at the midline, it blows the vocal folds apart. A puff of air is released between the open folds, which then return to the midline. The closure results from the elastic recoil of the vocal fold tissues and is assisted by the movement of air across the surface of the folds. The movement of air between the folds causes the folds to move inward, just as the movement of air across the wings of a plane creates the upward lift during takeoff. This aerodynamic principle is known as the Bernoulli effect. This opening and closing produces what is known as one cycle of phonation. Repeated cycles produces sound, or phonation.

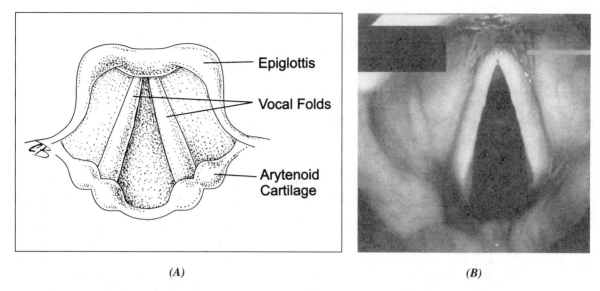

(A)   (B)

FIGURE 2-3 **The vocal folds can be viewed by looking down on the larynx from above. (A) Diagram of the vocal folds, arytenoid cartilages, and epiglottis. (B) Normal vocal folds.**

The speed of the vibratory cycle is dependent on the mass, elasticity, and length of the vocal folds. The tiny vocal folds in babies produce high voices because their vocal folds vibrate quickly. Nine-year-old children, for whom puberty has not begun, produce speaking voices very near middle C on the musical scale, or about 260 vibrations or cycles per second (260 **Hertz**). The speaking voice of an adult male, whose vocal folds have increased in size since puberty, is about an octave lower than it was when he was nine years old. Its pitch is near one octave below middle C, or about 125 cycles per second. The adult female, whose larynx is usually half again as big as it was when she was nine, typically speaks near G below middle C, which is close to 200 cycles per second. The normal pitch of the speaking voice is primarily determined by the size and mass of the vocal folds.

Frequency changes (which can be measured on frequency-analyzing equipment) or pitch changes (a perceptual change) are produced by the action of several of the intrinsic muscles of the larynx. When the **cricothyroid muscles** at the anterior-lateral borders of the larynx contract, they produce an elongation of the vocal folds, which has the effect of tensing the folds. The thinner, tenser folds produce higher frequency vocalization (perceived as a higher pitch). A lowering of pitch is produced by the relaxation of the cricothyroid muscles and the shortening of the **thyroarytenoid muscles** (vocal folds). When the vocal folds themselves contract by action of the thyroarytenoids, they in effect become thicker, producing a slower rate of vibratory cycle. For a more detailed and graphic look at laryngeal functions of phonation, including frequency and intensity, see Weismer (1988), Kent, (1997), and Zemlin (1998).

Remembering that voice is basically the product of an aerodynamic event—that is, outgoing airflow causes the vocal folds to vibrate—changes in intensity or loudness of the voice are produced by changes in **subglottal pressure**. Subglottal pressure can be raised by increasing the force that holds the vocal folds together or by increasing the pressure of the suglottal air. When the airflow finally breaks through the vocal folds, they are blown apart with greater force. This, in turn, produces a greater lateral excursion of the vocal folds resulting in greater air displacement. In this way, a speaker can increase the loudness of the phonation without any change in the frequency or pitch. Although people tend to elevate their pitch when speaking louder, it is the case that an increase in vocal intensity can be produced solely by increasing the expiratory volume of air used to produce the vocal utterance.

The Resonance System

Although the source of the voice is the larynx, sound waves are modified by the other structures within the throat, mouth, and nasal cavities. The eventual outflow of sound waves that are recognized as the human voice is the result of the filtering of that sound by the resonance system. The first area of the vocal tract through which the sound waves travel is immediately adjacent to and above the larynx. This cavity is called the pharynx. The pharynx is divided into two sections, the lower *hypopharynx* and the upper *oropharynx* (see Figure 2-4). The height of the pharynx changes as the larynx rises (shortens the pharynx) or lowers (lengthens the pharynx). The overall shape and width of the pharynx changes as the tongue comes back and the posterior and lateral pharyngeal walls move. The hypo- and oropharynx can be studied via **videoendoscopy**, which involves placement of an illuminated lens behind the velum to look down toward the larynx. The images of these structures can then be viewed on a video monitor. By doing this, we would find that the hypopharynx and the oropharynx are constantly changing shape during speech. In a fascinating videoendoscopic tape distributed by the Voice Foundation (1985) of two famous impersonators, Rich Little and Mel Blanc, we can see that much of the muscle action used to produce many different voice impersonations takes place in the pharyngeal cavities. Although the pharynx plays an important role in shaping vocal resonance, it obviously plays two other vital roles, as a conduit for the passage of air and food.

In addition to the pharynx, the oral cavity also shapes the resonance characteristics of the voice. The opening within the mouth is constantly changing size and shape during speech. The overall size of the oral opening is primarily determined by the position of the **mandible**, or lower jaw, which is continually lowering and elevating during speech. As the jaw drops for saying a low vowel, such as "ah," the tongue drops with it. However, the tongue has the greatest flexibility of any muscle group in the body, constantly changing its shape and position. When the tongue rides high, as in producing the "i" vowel, it occupies much of the anterior oral cavity. Vocal resonance is heavily influenced by the posture of the mouth, which is determined by the position of the mandible *and* the position of the tongue within the oral cavity (Boone & McFarlane, 1988).

Anyone who has been in a choir or taken a singing lesson remembers the teacher's reminder: "Open your mouth." An open mouth will often improve the perceived quality of vocal resonance. Laver (1980) described as "settings" the overall configurations that an individual uses for resonance, such as the amount of lip action, the opening of the jaw, the height of the tongue, and so forth. We all have our own habitual setting of the vocal tract, which determines how we sound. The pitch and resonance of our voices are what contribute to our unique sound, so individualized that a few words on a telephone will usually allow the listener to recognize a familiar voice.

The roof of the oral cavity is formed anteriorly by the bony hard palate and posteriorly by the muscular soft palate (also known as **velum**). The velum is a muscular structure, noticible for its dangling appendage, the *uvula*. It hangs down during normal breathing and connects the nasal cavity with the oral cavity. The point at which the velum meets the pharynx is the beginning of the nasal

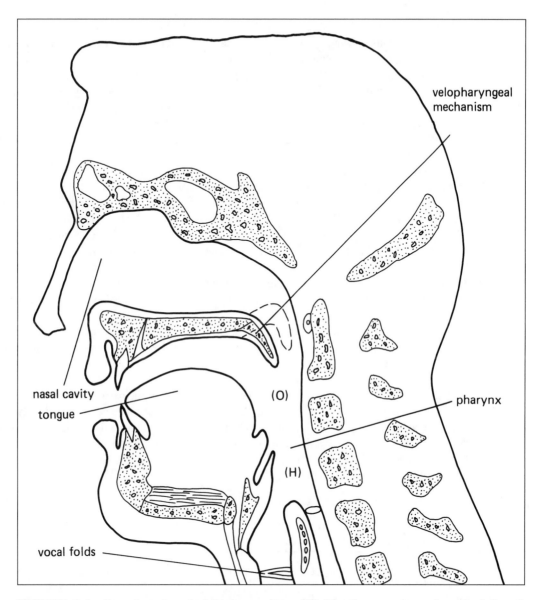

FIGURE 2-4 **Sound produced at the larynx is modified by the resonance characteristics of the vocal tract. The pharynx, which consists of the hypopharynx (H) and oropharynx (O) and nasal cavities, modifies sound as it travels through the oral and nasal cavities.**

cavity. The airway between the oropharynx and nasal cavity is typically open. However, during certain activities, such as drinking and eating, the pathway between these two cavities is closed as the velum raises and the pharyngeal walls constrict around it. The site of this closure is known as the **velopharyngeal port**. During speech, the closed position is required for the oral resonance of all the vowels and consonants in the English language except the three nasal sounds. When nasal sounds are produced, sound waves enter the nasal cavity through an open velopharyngeal port. This nasal-oral coupling is the position required for the nasal resonance of the three nasal consonants in English "m," "n," and "ng." When the velum lifts itself by muscular action (sometimes assisted by the lateral and posterior pharyngeal wall moving inward a bit), the velopharyngeal port is closed. If we were to say *banana*, for example, the initial "ba" would require a raised velum, closing the velopharyngeal port. The "n" would require a rapid drop of the velum, with the next vowel, "a," requiring closure again, only to be followed by another rapid drop for the next "n," ending with an elevated velum again for the vowel "a."

Failure to move the velum rapidly enough to match the demands of the particular utterance can result in excessively nasal speech, called **hypernasality**. Many problems that involve hypernasality are related to faulty velopharyngeal closure, which could be related to a number of factors, such as cleft palate, short velum, injured palate, or paralysis or weakness of the velopharyngeal muscles (such disorders are discussed in several subsequent chapters). A less common resonance disorder is **denasality**, which is insufficient nasal resonance often related to excessive velopharyngeal closure. The *nasal cavity* may become blocked with swollen tissues (perhaps due to allergies and colds) that dampen sound waves and block the airflow through the nasal cavities. Excessive tonsil and adenoid tissue in the nasal cavity will sometimes create enough obstruction to give the voice a denasal vocal quality.

The resonance system gives each voice its distinctive quality. Changes in the quality of the voice can signal vocal pathology, as we will see in Chapter 11. Let us now look at the resonance system in the case of Alicia, the child with Down syndrome.

> Down syndrome can involve congenital malformations of the naso- and oropharynx. These can result in altered voice quality. For Alicia, the speech-language pathologist notes some instances of hypernasality. This can result from poor control of the velopharyngeal mechanisms, or from a defect in the articulatory mechanisms, explained below. To differentiate between these two possible causes, the speech-language pathologist evaluated both the oral structures and velopharyngeal functioning.

The Articulatory Mechanisms

The Tongue

Looking at Figure 2-4, we can see that the tongue occupies most of the space of the oral cavity. The tongue body is a composite of intrinsic muscles that run both the length and width of the structure and enable us to change its shape easily (curled, pointed, and so on). Other muscles of the tongue originate outside the tongue from various sites, such as the hyoid bone. These extrinsic muscles allow the tongue to be elevated, lowered, protruded, and retracted. How our tongue is postured influences the overall sound and resonance of the voice and is critical for the production of individual speech sounds. The vowels and diphthongs of our speech are produced primarily through changes in the shape and movement of the tongue (and elevation of the mandible). Most consonants are produced by vocal tract constriction, which results in some airflow restriction, more often than not caused by some precise movement of the tongue. Without the precision of tongue movements, there could be no articulate speech.

The Facial Muscles

The lips are made up primarily of facial muscles (such as the **orbicularis oris**), which make it possible for them to pucker, spread, or make a circle. The lips are the most visible structures of the mouth and are easily shaped and altered to produce various facial expressions. They also play a vital role in such oral behaviors as sucking, kissing, chewing, and smiling. The lips represent the beginning (or the end) of the oral vocal tract and also contribute to the resonance of the voice. For example, if one were to say an extended *"eee"* for five seconds and alternately pucker and then relax the lips while prolonging the sound, one would hear distinct changes in the vocal resonance with each pucker. This is because the lips extend or shorten the length of the oral cavity with each movement. The lips also play a primary function in the production of many consonants. Sounds such as "m," "p," "b," and "w" are produced by movements of the lip; "f" and "v" are produced with the upper teeth on or against the lower lip.

The Teeth

The hard palate is circled on three sides by the alveolar process, or bony ridge, that houses the teeth sockets on the upper jaw, or maxilla. The maxillary and mandibulary teeth play a primary role in the chewing of food. Their contribution to speech articulation is somewhat secondary. However, a few English sounds, such as "f" and "v," are made by labial-dental contact, the lower lip being tucked under the upper central incisors. The alveolar ridge behind the base of the maxillary teeth is an important contact point for the tongue for the production of such sounds as "n," "s," "z," "t," and "d." The tongue also extends out between the upper and lower central incisors for the production of "th" sounds.

The Mandible

The movement of the mandible allows for the quick opening or closing of the mouth. Some mandibular movement contributes to change in the shape and size of the oral cavity needed for the production of different vowels. The normal speaker moves the mandible in quick synergistic movements with the lips and tongue during normal speech. If, however, a speaker were to talk with a pipe in his mouth, the mandible would stay closed to trap the pipe stem, which would require an immediate compensatory adjustment of the tongue and lips to maintain speech articulation. Optimal speech production and vocal resonance require continuous mandibular movement. Occasionally, we see patients with voice problems who speak with a clenched jaw most of the time, requiring the tongue to make all the muscle movements needed for vowel differentiation. Speaking this way is inefficient and often results in a muffled voice and sloppy articulation.

The Palate

The bony hard palate and the muscular soft palate make up the structures of the roof of the mouth, or **palate**. The hard palate extends from the alveolar ridge and tooth sockets of the maxillary dentition. It is an arched structure with a vaulted ceiling that contributes greatly to oral resonance. The tongue moves freely, making various articulatory contacts with the palate. Attached posteriorly to the hard palate just beyond the last molar tooth is the muscular soft palate. The soft palate comprises four extrinsic muscles (paired) attached to the skull and the pharynx that lift the soft palate for production of most speech sounds and lower it for breathing and for the production of nasal consonants. Usually, the entire soft palate, including the four paired muscles and the dangling uvula, is called the velum. We discussed under The Resonance System the importance of the velum in its contact with the pharynx (at the site of the velopharyngeal port) in separating the oral cavity from the nasal cavity for oral vocal resonance.

When speech is slow to develop or the quality of spoken words is poor, it is important to rule out possible contributions by the oral and facial structures. In Alicia's case, the speech-language pathologist performed what is known as an **oral-peripheral examination**. This is an evaluation of the structure and function of the articulatory mechanisms.

Alicia's oral-peripheral exam revealed several factors that could be important for communication. Some of her front teeth are quite crooked, which may interfere with sounds made against the teeth, such as "th" or "s." Her hard palate is highly arched, but does not contain any clefts or holes that would allow air to flow into the nasal cavity to produce hypernasality. Although her tongue appears large for her mouth and tends to protrude a bit, it is not actually too large, but lacks the muscle tone to rest within the mouth. Alicia's face has a soft, rounded appearance, which also suggests low muscle tone in the facial muscles. Low tone in the oral and facial muscles can interfere with the movements needed to produce the sounds of speech. All these factors may account for the perception that Alicia's words sound "thick" and imprecise.

The Nervous System

The remarkable ability of human beings to communicate so efficiently is related primarily to a most complex nervous system that permits (and even facilitates) communication between a person and the environment, other creatures, and other people. The nervous systems of other animals may have features that permit them to perform a particular behavior "better" than human beings. For example, predator birds have more acute eyesight than humans, and the porpoise has a more advanced auditory system. However, it is the complex human brain that allows human beings to master the complexities and subtleties of human language. When the nervous system is compromised due to developmental anomalies, acquired damage, or illness, communication is often compromised as well. The nervous system can be grossly divided into two parts, the **central nervous system** (CNS), and the **peripheral nervous system** (PNS). We will consider each separately.

Central Nervous System

The brain and the spinal cord, seen in Figure 2-5, are considered the two primary CNS structures. The brain enables humans to engage in high-level functions, such as learning from the environment and synthesizing information. Because of its critical role in such functions, factors that alter brain development or damage the brain underlie many types of communication disorders. Between the

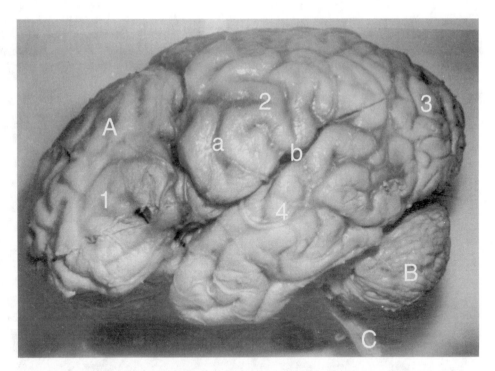

FIGURE 2-5   **Structures of the human nervous system include (A) the cerebrum, (B) the cerebellum, and (C) spinal cord. The cerebrum is divided into hemispheres (the left is seen here), which are further divided into (1) frontal, (2) parietal, (3) occiptial, and (4) temporal lobes. Dividing the frontal and parietal lobe is the (a) Rolandic fissure; dividing the temporal lobe and parietal lobe is the (b) Sylvian fissure. (Used with permission of the University of Nevada School of Medicine, Reno)**

brain and spinal cord is the brainstem (seen in Figure 2-6). The brainstem and spinal cord comprise the primary pathway for much of the sensory information that comes from the body. Conversely, the brain sends motor commands through the brain stem to the spinal cord that result in our ability to support and move our bodies. Therefore, damage to the brainstem or spinal cord, with the resulting loss of muscular control, can disrupt the biological support necessary for speech.

The vast range of human abilities is supported by various, specialized regions within the brain that act synergistically. Breakdowns in communication can be attributable to disorders that affect one or more of the regions of the brain. The brain consists of the **cerebrum** and the **cerebellum** (see Figure 2-5). The cerebrum occupies the majority of the brain cavity within the head. The cerebellum sits below the cerebrum and behind the brainstem. Both the cerebrum and the cerebellum can be further divided into right and left **hemispheres**. The hemispheres of the cerebrum are joined at the midline by the **corpus callosum**, which is a large band of fibers that carries information between the cerebral hemispheres (see Figure 2-6). The surface of the brain appears as a series of ridges, called *gyri*,

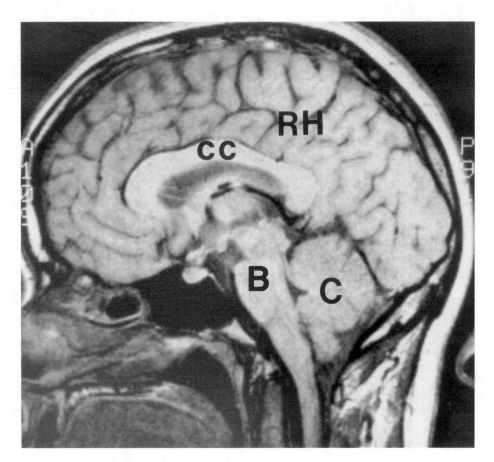

FIGURE 2-6   A midline view of the brain, obtained with magnetic resonance imaging (MRI), reveals the right hemisphere (RH), corpus callosum (CC), brainstem (B), and cerebellum (C).

and grooves, called *sulci*. All gyri and sulci can be individually identified by name, so that the location of both normal and pathological features of cortex can be described in specific terms.

The cerebral hemispheres can be further divided into four lobes (see Figure 2-5, each of which contains regions that are highly associated with particular functions. The **frontal lobe** contains the primary motor cortex and other regions that have to do with attention, impulse control, and judgment. The **parietal lobe** contains the primary sensory cortex, which receives sensory information from the body, as well as other regions that support a number of cognitive functions. The **occipital lobe**, at the back of the brain, receives and processes visual information. The **temporal lobe** contains the primary auditory cortex as well as regions important for language comprehension and memory.

The specialized functions of each of the hemisphere's lobes are attributed to differences in cells found within these regions. If we examine a cross section of the cerebrum (see Figure 2-7), we can see the surface layer, or **cortex**. The cortex contains layers of **neurons**, which are cells that support different types of brain activity. Because the bodies of these neurons appear gray, the cortex is also

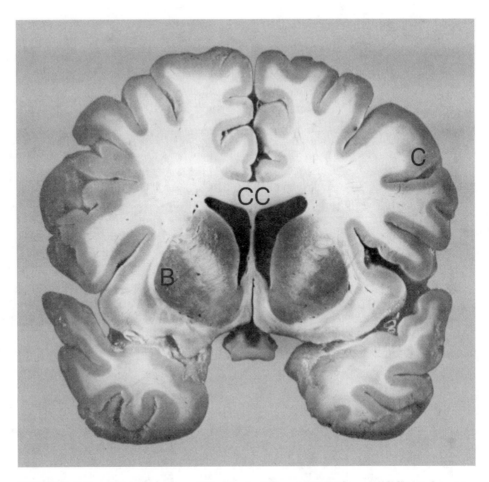

FIGURE 2-7   A cross section of the brain. The corpus callosum (CC) can be seen bridging the right and left hemispheres. The gray matter of the cortex (C) and white matter can be clearly distinguished. The basal ganglia (B) can viewed in the central portion of the brain.

called *gray matter*. The layers of the cortex within the primary motor area of the frontal lobe, for example, contain many neurons that send signals to the body for the control of movement, whereas the primary sensory cortex contains many cells that receive incoming signals from the body. Neurons contain one **axon**, which is a fiber that sends impulses away from the neuron. Those impulses are received by other neurons through another set of fibers, called **dendrites**. Axons and dendrites can connect neurons over short distances within the lobes, or over long distances between lobes, between hemispheres, or between the brain and spinal cord. If we look at the cross section of the cerebrum (Figure 2-7), the lighter gray tissue beneath the cortex consists of these cell fibers. This area of fibers is commonly called *white matter*, so called because the fatty myelin cells that surround the fibers appear white.

In addition to cortical neurons, the brain also contains several collections of subcortical neurons. In the front half of the brain is a collection of subcortical bodies known as the **basal ganglia** (see Figure 2-7). These neural bodies are highly connected to the cerebellum and to cortical regions involved in movement. Disorders of the basal ganglia often result in impaired movements. In the posterior half of the brain, behind the basal ganglia, is another collection of subcortical neurons known as the **thalamus**. This highly complex region receives all types of sensory information that is relayed to all regions of the brain.

Several regions of the brain are particularly important to communication in the oral-aural modalities and are frequently involved when communication disorders occur. Neural impulses that occur in response to sound first reach the level of the cortex at the *primary auditory cortex* within the temporal lobes of both the right and left hemispheres. This region is on the superior surface of the temporal lobe inside the Sylvian fissure and is sometimes called *Heschl's gyrus*. Within the left hemisphere, the primary auditory cortex is surrounded by cortical tissue that supports higher level auditory functions, including the comprehension of spoken language. Areas particularly important to this skill occupy the posterior regions of the superior temporal lobe and parts of the parietal lobe. Sections of the left inferior frontal lobe, on the other hand, appear particularly important to aspects of language expression. Finally, the motor movements of speech are supported by the *primary motor area*, which is located in the frontal lobe of each hemisphere. This area works in conjunction with subcortical structures and the cerebellum to produce the movements needed for speech.

In a normal, healthy brain, these various regions work in concert to support normal communication in all its complexity. However, when a brain is compromised during development or due to disease or injury, communication breakdowns can occur. For Alicia the effects that brought her to the developmental center began long before the day of her birth. The genetic anomaly that leads to Down syndrome affects the development of the brain. Research with this population has revealed certain brain characteristics that co-occur with this disorder. In Down syndrome, changes in fetal brain development can be detected by ultrasound between 16 and 21 weeks gestation (Bahado-Singh, Wyse, Dorr, Copel, O'Connor, & Hobbins, 1992). These changes reflect neurobiologic features such as reduced brain size, particularly reduced frontal lobe size, fewer cells within specific layers of the cortex, and smaller cerebellar size (see Schmidt-Sidor, Wisniewski, Shepard, & Seren, 1990 for a review of the brain correlates of Down syndrome). After birth, these neuroanatomic differences can have functional correlates of concern for communication. For example, neuroimaging research has demonstrated reduced metabolic activity in the brain's language areas associated with Down syndrome (Azari, Horowitz, Pettigrew, Grady, Haxby, Giacometti, & Schapiro, 1994).

Even for a baby like Alicia, brain development is not complete at birth. Normal brain development is characterized by overproduction of neurons and of connections between cells. After birth, the brain normally begins a lifetime of refining itself by pruning back excess cells and connections and strengthening those connections that are most functional. What determines which cells and connections are most functional? A large determinant of "functionality" is the experience the young child receives. In other words, Alicia's brain has been shaped by the things she has seen, heard, and explored. Although experience continues to shape the brain throughout life, a child's early experiences are critical for realizing that child's full potential throughout life. This is one reason that professionals advocate for early intervention for children with communication disorders and those at risk for these problems.

In other instances of communication disorders, the brain may have developed normally, only to be damaged later by illness or injury. In fact, much of what we know about the brain's organization was learned by observing the behavior of individuals who suffered damage to localized regions of the brain. This work began in the 1800s with two landmark cases. Paul Broca described a case of a man who lost his ability to express himself through spoken language, but retained much of his ability to understand language and his general cognitive functioning. When this man died, Broca described the area of damage within the left frontal lobe, which has come to be known as Broca's area. Since that time, this area has been closely associated with processes important for expressive language. Conversely, Carl Wernicke described a case of a man who lost the ability to comprehend spoken language whose brain lesion was in the posterior part of the left temporal lobe. This general area, associated with language comprehension, has come to be called Wernicke's area.

The early work of Broca and Wernicke, which continues today with advanced imaging techniques, has given rise to the *localization* perspective on brain functioning. The premise of a localization perspective is that certain locations within the brain that appear necessary for a particular skill or function. We now know that, for most people, the left hemisphere is specialized for language. In particular, the regions of the left hemisphere that surround the Sylvian fissure are critical language areas. This so-called **perisylvian region** includes the primary auditory cortex and the primary sensory and motor regions for the face that are located on either bank of the **Rolandic fissure**, just superior to the Sylvian fissure. It also includes both Broca's and Wernicke's areas and additional areas of association cortex in the region. Damage within this broadly defined perisylvian region can lead to various types of language disorders, as we will see in Chapters 7 and 8.

The localization perspective focuses on regions that contribute to particular functions. However, we have become increasingly aware that brain areas do not act in isolation. Rather, systems comprised of various brain structures and the connections between them act together to support behavior. This insight has given rise to the *connectionist* perspective, which emphasizes the interconnectedness of functionally related brain regions. For example, Geschwind described a connectionist model of language functioning that involved the sequential transfer of information through various left hemisphere regions in support of activities like reading aloud or repeating words (Geschwind, 1977). These types of models of brain functioning provide a basis for understanding the behavioral deficits that occur after brain damage.

For most individuals, language is a left hemisphere function; however, effective communication relies on many regions within both hemispheres of the brain. For example, listening to a lecture can involve all lobes simultaneously. As each person concentrates on the speaker, he or she tries to ignore other distractions (frontal lobe), take in the auditory and visual speech signal (temporal and occipital lobes), interpret its content (left temporal lobe), and visually monitor the facial expressions and affect of the speaker (occipital and right parietal lobes). It is the integrated function of all these brain regions that allows the listener to receive the verbal and nonverbal information and comprehend its meaning.

Peripheral Nervous System

To be functional, the brain must be connected to the outside world. This connection is made through the peripheral nervous system. The upper section of the peripheral nervous system includes twelve pairs of nerves that enter or exit the CNS within the cranial space occupied by the brain and brainstem. These are known as the **cranial nerves**.

    I. Olfactory, sense of smell
   II. Optic, vision
  III. Oculomotor, eye movements
  IV. Trochlear, eye movements
   V. Trigeminal, motor: jaw movements; sensory: face
  VI. Abducens, eye movements
 VII. Facial, motor: facial muscles; sensory: anterior two-thirds of tongue, soft palate
VIII. Auditory, sensory for hearing and vestibular system
  IX. Glossopharyngeal, motor: pharynx; sensory: posterior one-third of tongue, pharynx
   X. Vagus, motor: larynx, pharynx, soft palate, diaphragm, heart, abdominal viscera; sensory: heart, lungs, larynx, throat, GI tract, external ear
  XI. Accessory, motor: large muscles of head, neck, shoulders
 XII. Hypoglossal, motor: many muscles of tongue, supra laryngeal muscles

Below the level of the cranial nerves are thirty-one pairs of nerves that enter or exit the spinal cord, known as the **spinal nerves**. The **spinal cord** is made up of ascending and descending nerve tracts. There are anterior and posterior nuclei at thirty-one levels of the spinal cord. From the anterior nuclei exit the thirty-one paired motor nerves (right and left) that innervate (depending on their level and site) the muscles of the chest, the abdomen, the anal-genital area, and the four extremities. The posterior nuclei in the spinal cord have sensory functions. Sensory nerves come into the posterior spinal nuclei from various peripheral sites, such as glands, tissues, joints, and muscles. Much of the peripheral sensory information is "handled" at the spinal level, where various sensorimotor reflexes may occur. In other cases, the sensory information may be passed up into the central nervous system through the medulla into the cerebellum, where sensorimotor adjustments may be made. The sensory information may also travel to the thalamus, where it may be processed further. Some sensory impulses from the spinal nerves probably project directly (with little filtering or adjustment along the way) to the sensory cortex.

The Hearing Mechanism

The Outer Ear

The outer ear consists of the visible portion, called the **auricle**, that funnels sound waves into the ear canal. In some animals, the auricle is very large and movable (e.g., horse, rabbit), enabling the animal to locate a sound without any movement of the head. The human external ear is smaller and fixed on the sides of the head. The many shapes and sizes of human ears appear to have no particular relevance to an individual's hearing sensitivity. Sound waves that reach the auricle are funneled into the **ear canal**, or *auditory meatus* (see Figure 2-8). The ear canal originates at the auricle and extends about 2.5 cm (in the adult), terminating at the *eardrum* or *tympanic membrane*. The walls of the canal, or meatus, contain many hair follicles and cells that secrete *cerumen*, a wax-like substance that apparently protects the outer ear from foreign objects and insects. For a detailed look at the au-

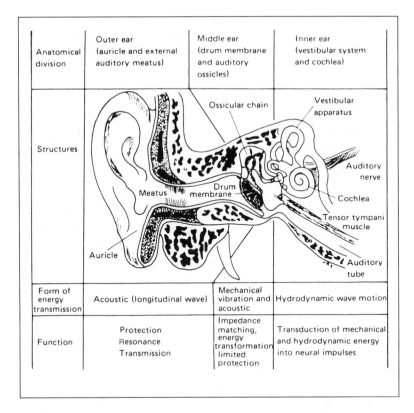

Anatomical division	Outer ear (auricle and external auditory meatus)	Middle ear (drum membrane and auditory ossicles)	Inner ear (vestibular system and cochlea)
Structures			
Form of energy transmission	Acoustic (longitudinal wave)	Mechanical vibration and acoustic	Hydrodynamic wave motion
Function	Protection Resonance Transmission	Impedance matching, energy transformation limited protection	Transduction of mechanical and hydrodynamic energy into neural impulses

FIGURE 2-8 **A schematic drawing of the anatomical divisions of the hearing mechanisms and their functional roles. Used with permission of W.R. Zemlin,** *Speech and Hearing Science* **(3rd ed.) (Englewood Cliffs, NJ: Prentice Hall, 1988).**

ditory mechanism and its function, a number of basic texts provide detailed pictures and sketches of the various sites within the auditory system, including Martin (1986), Perkins and Kent (1985), and Zemlin (1998).

The Middle Ear

The sound waves that travel through the ear canal eventually hit the tympanic membrane, setting it in vibration. In effect, the tympanic membrane separates the outer ear from the **middle ear**. The tympanic membrane is the outer, lateral wall of the small middle ear, "which is about the size of a garden pea with a ceiling, a floor and walls" (Van Riper & Emerick, 1984, p. 405). There are three tiny bones within the middle ear, known as the **ossicles**, that articulate with one another. These bones, the smallest in the human body, are the *malleus, incus,* and *stapes.* The malleus (a hammer-shaped bone) is attached to the inner side of the tympanic membrane. When the tympanic membrane vibrates, it sets the malleus into vibration. Because the malleus is attached to the incus, it makes the incus vibrate, which in turn causes the stapes to vibrate.

The transduction process (changing energy from one form to another) begins in the middle ear. The displacements of the tympanic membrane in response to the sound-wave variations produce a mechanical motion. This motion in turn sets up vibratory patterns in the ossicular chain. The vibrations move across the ossicular chain because of the tensions provided by the small muscles in the middle ear (the *stapedius* and the *tensor tympani*) and their supporting ligaments and tendons. Finally, the vibrating stapes is attached to a tiny footplate that fits on the *oval window* of the inner ear. The footplate of the stapes has a much smaller area than the inner surface of the tympanic membrane. This reduction in size from one end of the ossicular chain to the other increases the amount of energy allowed to pass through the ossicles into the inner ear, which has the effect of increasing the pressure or force on the fluid in the inner ear. As the footplate vibration moves the fluid in the inner ear, hydraulic movement becomes the energy source.

The middle-ear cavity is air filled. It is ventilated by the **eustachian tube**, which originates in the nasal cavity and terminates medial to the tympanic membrane. Middle-ear ventilation is essential for maintaining a cavity atmosphere that permits free vibration of the ossicles by maintaining the same air pressure within the middle ear and outer ear and by keeping fluids out of the middle ear. Fluid in the middle ear (such as might be experienced when one has a cold) and negative pressure (such as one might feel when the eustachian tube remains closed when changing altitudes while flying) can produce impaired hearing.

The Inner Ear

The cochlea is the organ of hearing within the inner ear. It is a fluid-filled, snail-shaped structure that coils around itself (see Figure 2-8). The footplate of the stapes, from the middle ear, connects to the side of the cochlea at the **oval window**, at the cochlear base. When the footplate vibrates, it creates motion within the fluid of the cochlea. With each inward movement by the stapes in the oval window comes a corresponding outward movement at the **round window** on the opposite side of the cochlea.

This fluid movement produces a corresponding movement of the **basilar membrane**, which runs the length of the cochlea (see Figure 2-9). The distance over which the motion of the basilar membrane travels is related to the frequency of the sound. Sounds that are high in frequency produce motion that is maximal at short distances along the length of the basilar membrane; sounds with lower frequencies reach their maximum amplitude further along the basilar membrane. As a result, sounds heard as different pitches are segregated in different regions of the cochlea due to the physical distance along the basilar membrane where movement associated with the corresponding frequencies occurs. Thus, the basal end of the cochlea responds to sounds that we perceive as high pitched, and the apical end responds best to sounds low in pitch. This is known as *tonotopic* organization because changes in sensitivity to tones can be mapped sequentially over the length of the cochlea.

Movement of the basilar membrane disturbs hair cells that sit in rows on the basilar membrane. These hair cells rest below the *tectorial membrane*. This membrane and the underlying hair cells are part of the **organ of Corti**. There are two sets of hair cells, a single row of inner hair cells, and three rows of outer hair cells. These hairs are delicate and can be easily damaged through aging, disease, exposure to certain drugs, or by prolonged exposure to loud noise. Once damaged, they do not naturally self-repair or regenerate like other cells of the body. The inner and outer hair cells are not only different in number, but also in structure, suggesting they play different roles in hearing. The outer hair cells seem particularly sensitive to displacement of the basilar membrane. The movement of the basilar membrane sets off a shearing motion of the hair cells. This motion is translated by the inner

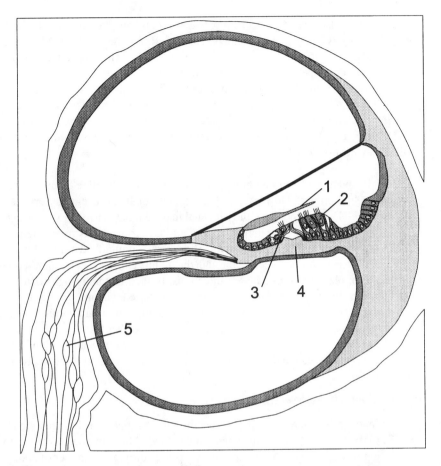

FIGURE 2-9   Components of the inner ear and organ of Corti: (1) tectorial membrane; (2) outer hair cells; (3) inner hair cells; (4) basilar membrane; (5) cell body within the acoustic nerve.

hair cells into a chemical-electrical signal that then exits the cochlea via the nerve fibers that make up the acoustic nerve. In this way, information about sound is transmitted to the brain.

Not only does the inner ear receive sound, it can also be the source of sound. Sounds that are produced by the inner ear are called **otoacoustic emissions**. These were first described by Kemp (1978) who discovered that low-level sound could be picked up in the ear canal after presentation of a click to that ear. This phenomenon was referred to as a "Kemp echo" because the resulting sound lagged in time behind the original stimulus, much like an echo off a canyon wall. However, unlike echoes, which are a passive reflection of sound, otoacoustic emissions reflect active processes within the cochlea. Although the physiological basis of these emissions is not yet completely understood, it appears that the outer hair cells, and the associated nerve fibers that descend from the brain, play a critical role in the production of emissions (Probst, Lonsbury-Martin, & Martin, 1991). In many people, spontaneous otoacoustic emissions occur in the absence of sound stimulation to the ear.

Emissions can also be *evoked*, as Kemp discovered, by presenting sound to the ear and recording the resulting sound (Glattke & Kujawa, 1991; Martin, Probst, & Lonsbury-Martin, 1990). As we will see in Chapter 5, emissions can be recorded via a small microphone inserted into the ear canal and serve as a basis for one type of audiological evaluation.

Audiologic evaluations are often of central importance to understanding the reasons for poor communication. Structural problems of the ear can produce a hearing loss, as we will see in Chapters 5 and 6. Passing illnesses can produce fluctuating hearing loss. Either condition may interfere with the development of oral communication skills. For this reason, an audiologist was included on Alicia's evaluation team.

> Alicia underwent a full audiological evaluation to determine hearing function. Like most other children with Down syndrome, she has small and irregular auricles. For some children with Down syndrome, the ear canal may be much narrower than usual. However, Alicia's ear canals are open and clear. The middle ear mechanisms are frequently affected by Down syndrome. These children have a high rate of middle ear infections, which interferes with the transmission of sound through the middle ear. Alicia's mother reports that her child has been plagued by middle ear infections. In fact, the audiologist determines that Alicia had some fluid in the middle ear, which was producing a mild degree of hearing loss on the day she came in for testing. Such infections are common in all children, but children with Down syndrome are particularly prone to them. Further testing, which focused on the central auditory system, established that Alicia's inner ear and auditory pathways appeared to be functioning adequately for the support of auditory-oral communication.

Central Auditory System

It is not enough for sound energy to move through the inner ear. Information about sounds must be passed to the brain to be recognized and understood. Along the way from ear to brain, the auditory signal, initially carried by the acoustic nerve, passes through a number of auditory nuclei that shape our perception. From the cochlea, the nerve fibers of the acoustic nerve (cranial nerve VIII) run toward the brainstem (see Figure 2-9). The first stopover in the ascending pathway is within the *cochlear nucleus*. There are two cochlear nuclei, one on each side of the brainstem. Fibers coming from each cochlear nucleus connect with the *superior olivary complex*, which is another nuclear group. Some of the fibers from the cochlear nucleus cross the midline so that each ear sends fibers to each superior olivary complex. Therefore, there is a mechanism for mixing the auditory signal from each ear early on in the auditory pathway. This is why people who have had damage to one side of the central auditory system are not completely deaf in the corresponding ear. This dual representation of sound coming from each ear also aids our ability to localize sound sources around us.

From the superior olivary complex, fibers move up both sides of the brainstem, through the medial lemniscus to the nuclei of the inferior colliculus and on to a section of the thalamus called the *medial geniculate body*. The medial geniculate body is the last stop prior to the arrival of impulses from sound at the primary auditory cortex of the brain. Like the cochlea, the brain's response to sounds of different pitches is also laid out in tonotopic fashion within the nuclei along the auditory pathway and within the primary auditory cortex. At the cortical level, for example, cells found more medially along the cortical surface respond best to higher pitches, and cells that lay more laterally respond best to lower pitches.

Not only do neural signals pass from the organ of Corti into the brainstem and up to the brain, but signals also pass from the brain and brainstem back to the organ of Corti. This *feedback* mechanism may help regulate the function of the organ of Corti. The pathway for fibers traveling from the brainstem to the cochlea is called the *olivocochlear bundle*. As the name implies, fibers originate at the olivary complex and terminate at the cochlea, in the organ of Corti. Like the ascending fibers, some fibers run uncrossed to the cochlea and some cross the midline to the opposite cochlea. These fibers may connect either directly with outer hair cells or with the fibers that receive signals from the inner hair cells in the organ of Corti. The presence of these descending, or *efferent*, fibers may function to regulate the activity of the neurons or hair cells within the cochlea.

Clinical Problem Solving

We opened this chapter with a case description of Mr. Blades, the man who had been in a serious car accident. The speech-language pathologist was asked to help determine why his comprehension may be poor.

1. Why would the clinician suspect that the car accident may have produced the language comprehension problem?
2. What other biological system(s) could also be the source of poor comprehension? Why?
3. If Mr. Blades also had difficulty speaking, what other biological system(s) could be involved? Why?

References

Azari, N.P., Horowitz, B., Pettigrew, K.D., Grady, C.L., Haxby, J.V., Giacometti, K.R., & Schapiro, M.B. (1994). Abnormal pattern of cerebral glucose metabolic rates involving language areas in young adults with Down syndrome. *Brain and Language, 46*: 1–20.

Bahado-Singh, R.O., Wyse, L., Dorr, M.A., Copel, J.A., O'Connor T., & Hobbins J.C. (1992). Fetuses with Down syndrome have disproportionately shortened frontal lobe dimensions on ultrasonographic examination. *American Journal of Obstetrics and Gynecology, 167*, 1009–1014.

Boone, D.R., & McFarlane, S.C. (1988). *The Voice and Voice Therapy* (4th ed.). Englewood Cliffs, NJ: Prentice Hall.

Geschwind, N. (1977). Specialization of the human brain. *Scientific American, 241*: 180–201.

Glattke, T.J., & Kujawa, S.G. (1991). Otoacoustic emissions. *American Journal of Audiology, 1*, 29–40.

Hixon, T.J., & Abbs, J. H. (1980). Normal speech production. In T.J. Hixon, L.D. Shriberg, & J.H. Saxman (Eds.), *Introduction to Communication Disorders*. Englewood Cliffs, NJ: Prentice Hall.

Kemp, D.T. (1978). Stimulated acoustic emissions from within the human auditory system. *Journal of the Acoustical Society of America, 64*, 1386–1391.

Kent, R.D. (1997). *The Speech Sciences*. San Diego, CA: Singular Publishing Group, Inc.

Laver, J. (1980). *The Phonetic Description of Quality*. London: Cambridge University Press.

Martin, F.N. (1986). *Introduction to Audiology* (3rd ed.). Englewood Cliffs, NJ: Prentice Hall.

Martin, G.K., Probst, R., & Lonsbury-Martin, B.L. (1990). Otoacoustic emissions in human ears: Normative findings. *Ear and Hearing, 11*, 106–120.

Perkins,W.H., & Kent, R.D. (1985). *Functional Anatomy of Speech, Language, and Hearing: A Primer*. Waltham, MA: College Hill Press/Little, Brown.

Probst, R., Lonsbury-Martin, B.L., & Martin, G.K. (1991). A review of otoacoustic emissions. *Journal of the Acoustic Society of America, 89*, 2027–2067.

Schmidt-Sidor, B., Wisniewski, K.E., Shepard, T.H., & Seren, E.A. (1990). Brain growth in Down syndrome subjects 15-22 weeks gestational age and birth to 60 months. *Clinical Neuropathology, 9*, 181–190.

Van Riper, C., & Emerick, L. (1984). *Speech Correction: An Introduction to Speech Pathology and Audiology* (7th ed.). Englewood Cliffs, NJ: Prentice Hall

Voice Foundation. (1985). *The Voice of the Impersonator.* (Videocassette developed by R. Feder.) New York: Author.

Weismer, C. (1988). Speech production. In N.J. Lass, L.V. McReynolds, J.L. Northern, & D.E. Yoder (Eds.), *Handbook of Speech-Language Pathology and Audiology*. Philadelphia: B. C. Decker.

Zemlin, W.R. (1998). *Speech and Hearing Science Anatomy and Physiology* (4rd ed.). Boston: Allyn & Bacon.

Chapter 3

Sounds in Communication

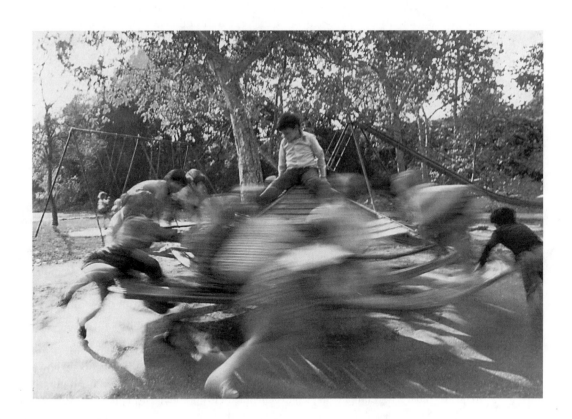

Preview

*Sounds are the currency of auditory-oral communication. Both speech-language patholo-
gists and audiologists are concerned with acoustic elements of sound as they are heard or
produced. Because of this, they need a firm grasp of the basic physical nature of sound, how
it is produced by humans, and how it can be described in spoken language. Furthermore,
the sounds of language must be acquired as an individual learns language. We will examine
this process in a young child who is in the process of acquiring English as his native
language.*

Auditory functioning supports communication at many levels. A short bark at the back door lets us
know that the dog wants to come inside. The phone's ring tells us someone is trying to reach us. With
speech, humans are able to use sound to express an infinite variety of ideas, moods, and attitudes.
We will examine the sound system first at its most basic level as an acoustic signal, and then as the
signal is modified to form the sounds of human speech.

Acoustic Aspects of Sound

Sounds are described in terms of intensity and frequency. What we perceive as the loudness of a
sound can be given a relative measurement of **intensity** by using the **decibel** (dB) scale. The faintest
sound that most humans can detect is a sound pressure of .0002 dynes/cm^2. This level is the reference point for the decibel scale. A sound of .0002 dynes/cm^2 corresponds to zero decibel sound pressure level (0 dB SPL). The decibel scale is a logarithmic scale that gives us an intensity level (relative
to the reference for 0 dB) for any particular sound. The logarithmic scale is such that the loudness
of sounds increases faster than the decibel values assigned to them. To illustrate, Kelly (1985) wrote
that "the loudest sound that can be heard without physical discomfort is 1 million times louder than
the faintest sound that the ear can detect" (p. 397), but on the logarithmic scale the difference between these two sounds is only about 120 dB. Some possible intensity levels of common sounds (borrowed in part from the work of Northern and Downs, 1978) are seen in Table 3-1. Of interest to us
at this point is the relative loudness of the human voice compared to many of the environmental sounds
around us. Yet we will see that the developing infant seems to give priority to the human voice, seeking it out from a background of varied intensities and frequencies.

Frequency is the measurement of what we hear as the pitch of a sound. Most sounds that we
hear in the environment are a combination of several frequencies. A musical note, however, such as
middle C (or C4) on the musical scale, is more likely to represent a pure or single frequency. On
frequency-analyzing equipment, the musical note of C4 produced by a piano would yield a frequency
value of approximately 256 cycles per second. That is, the piano string (C4) when struck by the piano
hammer would vibrate 256 times in one second. The vibrating movements of the piano string would
alternately increase and decrease the density of the air molecules surrounding it, setting up a sound
wave. Our ears perceive the sound wave as a pitch at middle C; our measuring devices give us the
value of 256 cycles per second. The number of complete cycles representing frequency is expressed
in Hertz (Hz); therefore the middle-C value would be expressed as 256 Hz. For those of us who sing

TABLE 3-1   Possible Intensity Levels of Common Sounds

10-20 dB	Whispering heard from over five feet away
30 dB	A ticking watch
40 dB	Birds chirping out the window
50-70 dB	Conversational speech
70 dB	A baby crying over 10 feet away
80 dB	Inside a 76 Ford Falcon parked on a highway
80 dB	A dog barking in the same room
81 dB	A telephone ringing on an office desk
90 dB	Yelling at the referee at a ball game
100 dB	An outboard motor on a boat
120 dB	Dancing in front of an amplified band at a bar

or play musical instruments and inadvertently produce a flat tone (lower than the target model), our Hz value would be less than 256 Hz. In contrast, the soprano who sings most of her notes sharp could be producing C4 at values near 270 Hz or higher.

We might better understand the concepts of intensity and frequency if we take a brief look at how we measure the intensity-frequency responses of the human ear. By testing a person in a quiet room, as we will discuss in greater detail in Chapters 5 and 6, we are able to plot how well the person hears each frequency tested and at each intensity level. An electronic instrument, an **audiometer**, generates pure-tone frequencies with increasing or decreasing levels of intensity. The goal of hearing testing is to determine the lowest intensity level at which various pure tones are detected. The person's responses are plotted on an **audiogram**. A sample audiogram of a person with normal hearing can be seen in Figure 3-1. It shows the test frequencies marked along the horizontal row at the top of the audiogram, with the lowest pure tone representing 125 cycles per second or 125 Hz and the highest 8000 Hz. The intensity is represented in decibels and is marked in the column on the left margin. A typical normal threshold is zero, and the most intense signal that can be produced by most audiometers is 120 dB. The typical audiometric examination uses an airborne signal, with the person listening to the signal through earphones. The right-ear response is plotted with a circle (red, if color is used), and the left-ear response is plotted with an X (blue, if in color). If a hearing loss is found, the examiner may test also by **bone conduction audiometry**, obtained by putting a sound vibrator on the mastoid bone behind the ear. Bone conduction symbols are plotted by using a blue > for the left ear and a red < for the right ear. In this sample audiogram, only air-conduction thresholds were plotted, as the person demonstrated normal hearing.

The sounds of speech are transmitted to the ear by complex sound waves. The auditory system receives these patterns of vibration and is able to decode them into recognizable **phonetic** units and words to which meanings are attached. Examples of speech sound waves corresponding to three different words are provided in Figure 3-2. The complex waves corresponding to these words have been analyzed so that their component energies at different frequencies (in kilohertz) can be seen graphically. This visual display of the speech signal is called a speech sound **spectrogram** (see Figure 3-2). Using the spectrogram, we can see the difference among the words *bit*, *bat*, and *bait*, which is readily apparent to our ears. These three words differ along two of the parameters of sound we have already discussed: frequency and intensity. For each of the vowel sounds in these words, we can see a different distribution of the sound energy at different frequencies. This appears as dark bands on the spectrogram that signal higher intensity at particular frequencies. The spectrogram also reveals

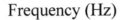

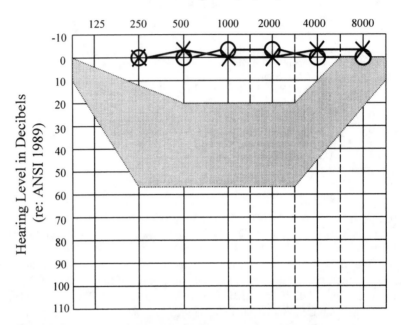

FIGURE 3-1   An audiogram displays results of hearing testing. An individual's responses to pure tones of varying frequencies (labeled across the top of the audiogram) are plotted according to the lowest intensity level at which they heard those tones (labeled along the vertical axis). Round symbols correspond to responses to tones in the right ear; the x's correspond to responses to tones in the left ear. The gray region represents the range frequencies and intensities over which most speech sounds occur.

a third parameter that differentiates the sounds of speech: time. It is the combination of the distribution of sound energy over certain frequencies and the particular timing patterns that lead to the perception of three different vowels, and thus, three different words. For other words, changes in the spectral energy and timing differentiate consonants as well as vowel production.

Within each of the words in Figure 3-2, we see additional differences in the relative intensity and duration of each sound that makes up the word. The portion of speech corresponding to vowel sounds contains regions of strong acoustic energy, which appear as dark bands on the spectrogram. When we listen to words, we pick up information about the speaker's voice primarily from vowels, because of the relatively long duration of voiced sound production. In contrast to the vowels, the unvoiced consonant "t" produces a short and relatively weak burst of energy, which is represented by a much lighter shade of gray on the spectrogram. These differences in the frequency and intensity of speech sounds may seem subtle when examined visually. However, they are adequate to distinguish between words, even under difficult listening conditions, for those with normal hearing.

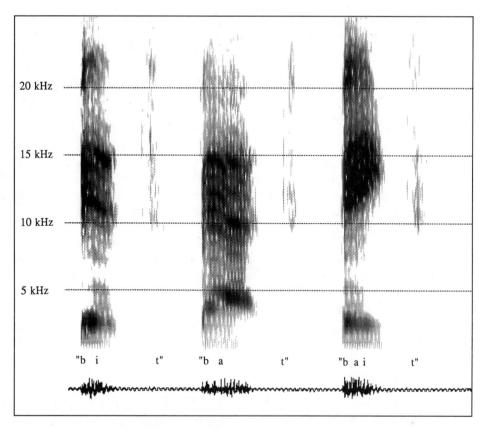

FIGURE 3-2   Complex speech sounds can be analyzed to show the component frequencies that we hear as different speech sounds.

We can see how the energy within the speech signal corresponds with normal hearing by returning again to Figure 3-1. In this figure, the gray area within the audiogram represents the frequencies and intensities over which much of the speech sounds are concentrated. As the audiogram indicates, the intensity of speech sounds at conversational levels is relatively low. One can appreciate how easy it is to interfere with speech sound discrimination, either with background noise or a relatively mild degree of hearing loss.

The Spoken Sounds of Communication

Vocalization

As we learned in Chapter 2, the production of speech sounds relies on the coordinated action of many physical elements, including muscles of the throat, neck, larynx, face, and oral structures. **Vocal-**

ization requires a sound generator—the larynx—and a force to drive this generator—air. During normal breathing, the vocal folds of the larynx are open, allowing air to flow in and out unobstructed. For speech, the vocal folds are open during the production of voiceless sounds and are closed to produce voiced sounds. When exhaled air hits the closed (or closing) vocal folds with sufficient force, the folds blow open and the exhaled air hits the stationary air above the folds, setting off a sound wave. We can make this sound louder by increasing the air pressure at the larynx, either by increasing muscle tension at the larynx or by driving more air through it.

The frequency of the sound created by the vibrating vocal folds depends on the size and elasticity of the folds. Larger vocal folds tend to vibrate fewer times per second and therefore produce sounds at a lower frequency. Thus, men's voices tend to be lower than women's, and women's voices are lower than children's. Table 3-2 shows some frequencies of different voices for comparison. The fundamental frequency of the voice is carried by the vowel sounds in speech. The frequency of air rushing through narrowed oral cavities to produce consonant sounds is much higher than the fundamental frequency of the voice.

The frequency of the voice during conversational speech changes to convey intentions and emotions. The pattern of frequency changes are part of the **prosody** of speech. Prosodic patterns are produced by alterations of the larynx that affect the length and tension of the vocal folds. One can feel these changes by placing the thumb and index fingers on each side of the larynx while producing sounds of different pitches. In conversational speech, we automatically produce these changes to emphasize words, ask questions, declare an opinion, and the like. We will discuss other aspects of prosody below.

Speech Sounds

As clinicians, we need a precise system for differentiating among the sounds that people produce. The written word, as produced with the English alphabet, is inadequate for this task because one letter can correspond to more than one sound. Consider the "o" in *off* versus in *over*, or the "c" in *cat*

TABLE 3-2.   The Fundamental Frequency of the Human Voice

Source	Frequency Level of the Voice in Hz
Fundamental Frequencies	
An infant cooing	380
Boys and girls, age 9, talking	260
An adult woman saying "hat"	210
An adult man saying "hat"	125
Consonant Sounds	
[s] or [z]	4000–8000
[t] or [v]	6000–7000
[θ]	7000–8000

versus in *certain*. For other consonants, more than one letter represents the sound (e.g., "th," "sh," "ng"), and the same sound can be represented in more than one way (e.g., "f" and "ph"). Further complicating matters is the occurrence of "silent letters" (e.g., "p" in *ptomaine*, "gh" in *weight*) in English orthography. For these reasons, clinicians use the *International Phonetic Alphabet* (IPA). The IPA symbols appear in Table 3-3, along with their corresponding sounds. As this table shows, 41 different symbols are needed to specify the sounds of English, compared with the 26 letters of the English alphabet. These 41 symbols allow us to specify the different sounds, or **phonemes**, of the English language. When writing phonemes, clinicians place the phonetic IPA symbol within parallel lines (e.g., /bɛt/ for *bet*). The actual production of a sound by a speaker is referred to as a **phone**, which is designated by the use of the IPA symbol placed within brackets (e.g., [bɛt] for *bet*). The term

TABLE 3-3   The International Phonetic Alphabet (IPA)

Phonetic Symbol	Word Examples	Phonetic Symbol	Word Examples
	Consonants		
m	mama, come	r	rain, arrow
p	papa, cop	l	lamp, pillow
b	baby, bob	ʃ	she, fish
t	total, tot	tʃ	chip, pitch
d	daddy, bad	ʤ	jet, fudge
k	cake, book	θ	thin, with
g	got, tag	ð	those, bathe
n	none, bun	w	won, swim
f	fife, wife	ʍ	when, white
v	vote, love	j	yes, yuppie
ŋ	wing, bring	ʒ	treasure, version
s	sin, bliss		
z	zoo, booze	h	ham, behind
	Vowels		
i	each, see	ɒ	paw, song
ɛ	head, bet	ɝ	bird, curls
ɪ	itch, bit	ɚ	percent, soldier
æ	sack, bad	u	you, booboo
e	bake, aching	ʊ	cooker, book
ɑ	bother, mockery	ʌ	money, hug
a	class, banned	ə	upon, banana
o	phone, comb	ɔ	ball, fog
	Diphthongs		
ai	bye, sigh	ur	sure, lure
au	house, wow	ɔr	bore, Capricorn
ɔɪ	boy, boil	ir	fear, beard
ɛr	bear, fair	aɪr	sire, tired
ɑr	yarn, car	aʊr	our, bower

allophone refers to the variations in phones that are still categorized as the same phoneme. For example, we say the "t" in *tap* slightly differently than in *setting*, although both are considered versions of /t/.

Vowels

The vowel system (vowels and **diphthongs**) requires 26 symbols and combinations of symbols in the IPA alphabet. Diphthongs are distinguished from vowels in that they are a combination of two vowel sounds. Vowels and diphthongs are produced with vocal fold vibration, or voicing. The sound generated by the vocal fold vibration is then modified in the vocal tract through movements of the soft palate, tongue, jaw, and lips. These modifications of the initial voicing allow for production of the distinct vowels that characterize any given language. For each vowel, there is a distinctive configuration of the vocal tract. For example, in the production of the /i/ ("ee" as in *beet*) vowel, the vocal tract is shaped by the tongue positioned as high and forward as possible, with the jaws relatively close together and the lips slightly withdrawn. The differences in the acoustic characteristics of vowels are dependent upon the position and height of the tongue in the oral cavity as well as the configuration of the lips. As shown in Figure 3-3, for example, we can see that the /i/ vowel is produced with the tongue high and anterior in the mouth. Conversely, we see that the /ɑ/ ("o" as in *bop*) vowel is produced lowest in the oral cavity, with the jaw dropped and the back of the tongue held low. None of the 16 vowels listed requires any kind of vocal-tract constriction as is necessary for consonant production. Diphthongs, such as /aɪ/ or /ɔɪ/, are assimilated blends of two separate vowels, producing a two-vowel glide. Production of a diphthong requires a quick sequence of vocal-tract adjustments, usually requiring rapid movements of the tongue from low to high (or vice versa) and back to front (or vice versa).

The vowel chart in Figure 3-3 generally reflects the contour of the tongue from front to back as it raises or lowers to produce the vowel. The tongue tip is highest and most forward for /i/ ("ee" as in *beet*). It is slightly lower and back for /ɪ/ ("i" as in *bit*). The mid-anterior position is used for /e/ ("a" as in *bait*) and slightly lower and back for /ɛ/ ("e" as in *bet*). Both /æ/ ("a" as in *bat*) and /a/ ("a" as in *bad*) require the lowest anterior positioning of the tongue. The /r/ consonant basically exists only in the initial or medial positions in words. Although we write the orthographic "r" in words like *bird* or *water*, we represent these sounds with the phonemes /ɝ/ and /ɚ/. In speech, /ɝ/ and /ɚ/ are actually r-colored vowels produced with the tongue in a high, central position, as shown in Figure 3-3. The unstressed vowel at the end of a word like *polka* is represented by the phoneme /ə/, produced with the tongue with a medium height with a central anterior-posterior positioning. The /ʌ/ ("u" as in *but*) vowel has the same central positioning, slightly lower in height than /ə/. There are five back vowels produced with the tongue withdrawn posteriorly; each vowel is differentiated by a change in the vertical height of the tongue. In order from high to low, the back vowels are /u/, /ʊ/, /o/, /ɔ/, /ɑ/.

As mentioned earlier in this chapter, it is the vowels that allow us to hear the voice of the speaker. The sound of one's voice, for example, whether it is hoarse or hypernasal, is determined by listening to vowel production. Although consonants play a primary role in how well speech is understood, or its *intelligibility*, the vowels we utter also contribute to how well someone can understand us. Each vowel found in a particular language has its own distinctive production characteristics. For example, listening to an Australian speaker and an American speaker, one will perceive the same English language with the same consonants embedded in markedly different vowels and diphthongs. These differences may cause difficulties for the listeners as they try to understand one another.

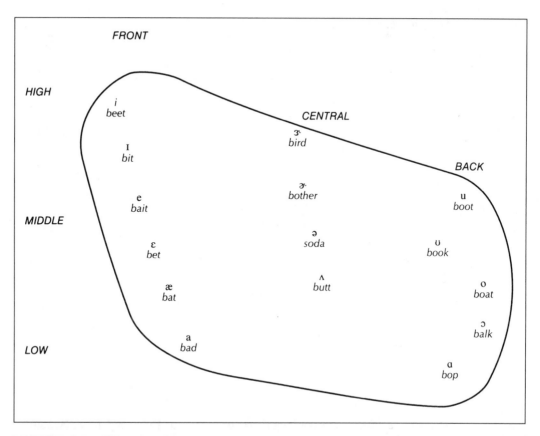

FIGURE 3-3   This schematic shows the place of production within the oral cavity for each vowel in the English language.

Consonants

As discussed above, vowels are distinguished primarily by their place of production. Consonants, in contrast, can be characterized by three general parameters: their *place* of articulation, the *manner* in which the sound is produced, and the *voicing* characteristic of the consonant. The place-manner-voicing system can be used for specifying the production of specific sounds. It can also be used to highlight differences in the consonant systems of different languages. For example, English contains only one glottal sound (a place distinction), the glottal continuant /h/, whereas other languages, like Navajo, include glottal stops. On the other hand, English contains certain consonants (e.g., /l/ and /r/) not found in some other languages, like Chinese. Sometimes, what we perceive as the "accent" of a nonnative speaker of English relates to a subtle alteration in either the place, manner, or voicing aspects of the consonants. Likewise, as we will see in Chapter 9, the ability to characterize sounds by place, manner, and voicing can help reveal common patterns when articulation disorders occur.

In Table 3-4, the consonants in English are listed to show how each phoneme is distinguished by its place, manner, and voicing characteristics. The anatomical sites of production, or the *place of*

Table 3-4   The Consonants in English

Manner of Articulation	Place of Production						
	Bilabial	Labiodental	Interdental	Alveolar	Palatal	Velar	Glottal
Stop or Plosive	p (pa)			t (toe)		k (kick)	ʔ (bottle)
	b̊ (bat)			d̊ (doe)		g̊ (gap)	
Fricative		f (fat)	θ (thin)	s (sip)	(shoe)		h (hip)
		v̊ (vat)	ð̊ (that)	z̊ (zip)	ʒ̊ (azure)		
Affricate				tʃ (chop)			
				d̊ʒ (job)			
Nasal	m̊ (mom)			n̊ (nun)		ŋ̊ (sing)	
Lateral				l̊ (lap)			
				r̊ (rare)			
Glide	ẘ (wall)				j (yes)		
	ʍ (when)						

*Consonant is voiced.

production, are listed from front (bilabial) to back (glottal), indicating the various structures of articulation: lips, teeth, tongue, hard palate, velum, and glottis. If the consonant is voiced, an asterisk is placed above it. We see the manner of production in the left-hand margin. There are seven consonants (/p/, /b/, /t/, /d/, /k/, /g/ /ʔ/) that are classified as stops or **plosives**, produced by a brief cessation of airflow, followed by a sudden release of the sound. The consonants that are paired in Table 3-4 (e.g., /p/ and /b/; /t/ and /d/) are called **cognates**. These sounds have the same manner and place of production, differing only on the dimension of voicing. The **fricative** consonants (/f/, /v/, /θ/, /ð/, /s/, /z/, /ʃ/, /ʒ/, and /h/) are created by having an articulator form a tight constriction that produces some audible noise from the airflow (voiced or unvoiced). All of the nine fricatives are also **continuants**, as they can be continued as long as the airflow is present. The **affricate** consonants (/tʃ/, /dʒ/) are combinations of a stop and a fricative. Only three consonants in the English language (/m/, /n/,and /ŋ/) are produced with the velopharyngeal port open, allowing their production to be nasalized. There are two commonly recognized liquids, or lateral, consonants: first, the lateral (/l/), produced by the tongue tip raised to contact the central alveolar ridge with openings along the sides of the tongue where the air stream passes during sound production; second, the consonant /r/, produced by two points of lingual constriction on the anterior hard palate (just posterior to the alveolar ridge) and on the anterior velum. The last consonant grouping in Table 3-4 is the glide sounds (/w/, /ʍ/, /j/), which are often classified as semivowels that become consonants because of added constriction.

The flow of articulatory movements used for the series of phones produced in running speech is continuous and constantly changing. Any one sound in isolation has a specific series of requirements or "targets, ideal places of contact, forces of contact, particular shapes, particular airflows, and particular patterns of movement necessary for a given speech sound" (Daniloff, 1973, p. 198). Speech articulation is a motor behavior that requires muscular specificity (one has to be on-target or listeners will hear another phone) with a continuously variable rate and rhythm. The sounds that precede or follow a particular sound influence the production of that sound, a process often called sound **assimilation**. For example, if we said, "Tea, too," the production of the /t/ phone in each word will be slightly different; the high vowel /i/ in tea will bring the tongue tip slightly more forward than for the production of /t/ followed by /u/. Assimilation provides some evidence that speech production is organized by the nervous system in larger units than the single phone. Production of a phone in running speech is often simultaneous with the production of an adjacent phone preceding or following the target phone, a process known as **coarticulation**. If we said the word "tram," the production of the phonemes /t/ and /r/ would be said sequentially, with the vowel /ae/ influencing their production and coarticulated (said at the same time) with the production of the final consonant /m/.

Prosody

So far, we have discussed those constituents of speech that make up the individual sounds within words (i.e., the consonants and vowels). However, additional aspects of sound are critical in conveying meaning in conversation. These aspects include the tempo, rhythm, and intonation with which the sounds and words are spoken. These elements make up the prosody of speech.

In conversational speech, there are two distinct types of prosodic information. One differentiates between classes of sentences. For example, the words "You liked rhubarb pie" can be expressed as a statement (as in, "You had it before and you liked it.") or as a question (as in, "You really liked it?"). What conveys the difference between a statement and a question in English is the steady or falling intonation in the statement form and the rising intonation in the question form. In other sentences, prosodic cues include short pauses that set off the phrase embedded within the sentence (separated by commas in written text) as in "The report, which appeared to be composed by monkeys typing at random, received a failing grade." These types of prosodic cues are referred to as *linguistic prosody* and they provide information concerning the grammatical structure of the spoken sentence.

Emotional prosody is different from linguistic prosody. Whereas linguistic prosody is used purposefully to differentiate sentences of different grammatical forms, emotional prosody is often unintentional. This is why those who know us well can detect, from the tone of our voice, whether we are upset or secretly pleased, even when the words we use are relatively neutral. In other cases, we purposefully mismatch the content of our words with the emotional tone of our speech to express sarcasm or irony. Most individuals are exquisitely sensitive to the myriad of overtones that can be added to speech via emotional prosody. In fact, when there is a mismatch between what we say (i.e., the words used) and how we say it (i.e., the emotional prosody), our listener is likely to feel that the prosodic information conveyed our true meaning. For this reason, we hear comments like "She said it was OK, but she didn't seem too happy about it."

Development of the Sound System

When a child is born with a normally functioning hearing mechanism and is raised by people who speak to him or her, the child will systematically acquire the perceptual capabilities needed to understand the language he or she hears. As the baby develops, we see a corresponding development

TABLE 3-5   Approximate Ages for Milestones in the Comprehension and Production of Sound

Age	Milestone
0 weeks	Startles to loud sound
	Prefers mother's voice to strangers'
	Produces reflexive, vegetative sounds
4 months	Responds to household sounds
	Can discriminate among many speech sounds
	Produces differentiated cries
	Produces vowel-like sounds
7 months	Produces canonical babbling
	Uses sound with communicative intent
10 months	Produces "protowords"
	Repeats sounds made by others
	Produces jargon
	Understands some words
12 months	Produces words with simplified forms

of the sound system (see Table 3-5). In order to understand the development of the child's auditory and early sound production capabilities, let us look at the experiences of a single child.

Birth

Abraham was born in the early morning of May 15. He was the first child in his family. Within days of Abraham's birth, his hearing mechanism was screened for the first time in his life. Neonatal hearing screenings have become widely used as part of a well-baby checkup. The relative cost of widespread screenings is minor compared with the advantages gained by early intervention with children who have hearing loss at birth. In Abraham's case, the results confirm a normally functioning hearing mechanism.

The development of Abraham's sound system actually began while he was still in the womb. A developing fetus responds to sound by the third trimester of gestation (Birnholz & Benacerraf, 1983). The fetus will change positions and increase heart rate in response to sound. If the sound persists, these behavioral signs of hearing will wane, only to return if the characteristics of the sounds change (Leader, Baillie, Martin, & Vermeulen, 1982). However, the sounds that reached Abraham in utero were probably more limited in scope than what he can now hear. First of all, his mother's body tissues attenuated, or dampened sounds, particularly at the higher frequencies (Walker, Grimwade, & Wood, 1971). Because the voice of Abraham's father had to travel from the air into his wife's body to reach his developing child, Abraham probably heard only a muffled version of his father's voice in the womb. The lower frequencies carried by vowel sounds, and the pitch, rhythms, and intonation of the father's voice, were probably more clearly heard than the higher frequency sounds that distinguished the consonants of his speech. In contrast, his mother's voice had a direct route to her fetus, via internal sound vibrations that traveled through her body to the womb. This advantage makes maternal speech more intelligible when recorded within the womb than the speech of others (Armitage, Baldwin, & Vince, 1980; Bench, 1968).

The influence of prenatal auditory experience can be measured in babies soon after birth. Researchers use techniques such as "high amplitude sucking" in which infants suck on a pacifier that is wired to data-recording instruments. Infant abilities are explored by conditioning babies to change their rate of sucking in response to what they hear. DeCasper and colleagues conducted a series of studies that show infant preference for sounds available in the prenatal environment; infants show preferences for hearing recordings of the sound of an intrauterine heartbeat (DeCasper & Sigafoos, 1983) and the voice of their own mother (DeCasper & Fifer, 1980). Therefore, it is no surprise that Abraham is comforted by being held against his mother's body as she speaks gently to him. The warmth of her body and the sounds of her heartbeat and voice are already familiar to him.

At home, Abraham is already a beginning communicator. However, much of this is unintentional on his part. As his uncle holds him, Abraham makes a series of lip smacks. In response, his uncle responds playfully as if the baby had just related a shocking secret about his parents. Later, as his mother gives him a sponge bath, Abraham is fussy and emits a series of cries. His mother "explains" to him that she is bathing him and that she is trying to do this as fast as she can. She then picks him up in a towel to rock him, telling him he is okay. While dressing him, she "trades" sounds with him by repeating his short cries and other vocalizations. Soon, his parents begin to recognize the different types of cries he is now making. For example, Abraham's father recognizes a cry of protest as he removes a bottle of formula from Abraham's mouth in order to reposition him. These early interactions provide the infant with important information about communication. The infant learns that his or her vocalizations have the positive effect of parental attention and response. The close proximity of the parent's face allows the infant to see his or her parent's facial expressions. The give-and-take interchanges lay the ground work for conversational turn-taking.

Six Weeks

Abraham awakened from his nap. His legs and arms stretch and move about as he makes a series of sounds. His mouth is open and he emits a series of short [a] (as in "bad") and [ɛ] sounds as well as lip and tongue smacks. Sometimes these sound like exclamations, comments, or complaints. Early on, infants' cries and other vocalizations often occur with the velopharyngeal port open, giving sounds a nasal quality (Oller, 1980). Infants may produce sounds on both expirations and inspirations. Each infant is quite variable in how he or she produces sounds from one time to the next. It may be that the infant is "trying out" the many combinations of positions and movements that can be used to produce grunts, cries, and other vocalizations (Boliek, Hixon, Watson, & Morgan, 1996).

Abraham's father enters the nursery and gets down on eye level with his son. When he calls his son's name, Abraham lifts his head and looks at his father's face. His father asks "Are you waking up? Are you waking up now?" Abraham gives his father a big smile. These types of interactions demonstrate the infant's early interest in and preference for familiar faces and voices. In return, Abraham's interest in his father's voice is rewarded by more verbal attention from his father. In fact, Abraham's parents speak to him quite a lot. They name his body parts as they wash him. They tell him about his fashion options while dressing him for the day. They recite nursery rhymes while changing his diaper. Although all this language stimulation may seem beyond his level of comprehension, it provides him with an ongoing stream of information from which he is already beginning to gain knowledge about his native language.

Like parents around the world, Abraham's parents talk to him with exaggerated stress and pitch variations, slower rate, and liberal use of repetitions. This type of speech is often called *child-directed speech*, or sometimes *motherese*. Adults and older children often use child-directed speech when speaking to infants and toddlers, and babies seem to prefer this type of speech. Researchers feel that the exaggerations of child directed-speech may also play an important role in assisting the young child in cracking the code of communication by helping to segment the ongoing sound stream into units of phrases, words, and individual sounds (Jusczyk, 1997; Kuhl & Iverson, 1995).

Four to Six Months

At four months, Abraham's major activity for the day is putting things in his mouth, with a secondary emphasis on drooling. He tries putting his hand, his feet, his toys, and leaves on the ground into his mouth, then makes a grab for his grandmother's earrings. This is the typical infant's favored mode for exploring the world at this age. Whether or not his mouth is full, he makes a variety of vowel sounds. Sometimes, these vowels are prolonged while pitch is varied (e.g., "aaaaaah"), and other times they are staccato-like exclamations (e.g., "eh!"). These sounds are not necessarily directed toward anyone, although they stop when his mother approaches. His mother gets down on the ground with him and exclaims "How's my big boy?! How's my big boy?!" He looks at her intently and then squeals in response. Although Abraham does not yet understand just what was said to him, he has already begun the job of recognizing the sounds and patterns that comprise his native language.

We know that very early on infants have perceptual capabilities that allow them to begin to segment the ongoing sounds within running speech. As we saw in our discussion of consonant production, the production of individual sounds varies from one word to the next due to coarticulation effects. Nonetheless, we perceive all the variations of sounds like [b] as /b/, and all the variations of [p] as /p/. The auditory systems of mammals, including humans, appear equipped to handle such variation among sounds by accomplishing what is known as *categorical perception*. This trait of the auditory system allows us to perceive a range of acoustic signals whose voicing characteristics actually lie midway between a [b] or [p] as one or the other of these sounds. For the infant, this provides the advantage of delimiting the infinite variation in acoustic speech signals into a relatively small set of consonants (and vowels) that repeat over and over again in their own native language. An early study by Eimas, Siqueland, Jusczyk, and Vigorito (1971) showed that infants could distinguish between such acoustic contrasts at four weeks after birth. Subsequent work (e.g., Burnham, Earnshaw, & Clark, 1991; Streeter, 1976; Werker & Lalonde, 1988) has shown that infants initially perceive contrasts that include sounds not found in their native language. Over time, however, these nonnative contrasts appear to lose salience for the developing child. Thus, children's experience with the language (or languages) of their community shapes their perception of the sounds of speech.

A parallel situation occurs for the processing of vowel sounds. Like consonants, a specific vowel can be pronounced with a range of acoustic variation, depending on the speaker, the word, and the context. However, by six months of age, infants show that they consider variants of the same vowel as perceptually similar, whereas variants of different vowels are considered distinct. This phenomenon has been called the *perceptual magnet effect* (Kuhl, 1994; Kuhl & Iverson, 1995) because the perceived difference between vowel variants appears to be less than the actual acoustic difference would otherwise suggest. In other words, when we hear variants of a particular vowel, our perceptions of those variants is drawn, like a magnet, towards the prototypical vowel of that type. In contrast, variants that correspond to different vowels seem more perceptually distinct than the acoustic differences between vowels would suggest. Cross-linguistic work indicates that infants show a perceptual magnet effect for prototypical vowels that occur only in their native language (Kuhl, Williams, Lacerda, Stevens, & Lindblom, 1992). This work suggests that the perceptual change reflects a developmental effect that requires exposure to spoken language.

Seven to Nine Months

At seven months of age, Abraham celebrated his first Christmas. Wearing his pajamas and a red Santa's hat, he sat on the couch and reached for the small gifts that fell out of his Christmas stocking. His parents began to rip the wrapping paper for him, but once started, he was able tear the remaining paper off his gifts. He mouthed each individual piece of wrapping paper, before tossing it aside. In all, handling wrapping paper appeared to be the most interesting part of the process to him. He patted the box with his open hand. Each gift held his interest and he looked at each while his parents named and commented about it. This "joint reference" between parent and child provided Abraham with the opportunity to observe objects and actions at the same time that he heard the words that related to them. His breathing was rapid and heavy, and he waved his arms with excitement.

During this period, Abraham reached a new milestone in the development of the speech sound system. His production of sounds no longer consisted solely of vowels. The first consonants were added to his repertoire. Abraham exclaimed "Da!" as he reached for an as-of-yet untasted piece of wrapping paper. These first consonant-vowel (CV) and consonant-vowel-consonant-vowel (CVCV) utterances are referred to as **canonical babbling**. This type of babbling is nonspecific, in that babies Abraham's age do not use these CV or CVCV combinations to refer to specific objects or intentions. However, Abraham, like other babies, produced these sound combinations with the prosody of speech, so that it seemed as though he was speaking, even though no true words were produced.

Abraham's initial production of canonical babbling at seven months was about average for developing infants. Eilers and Oller reported that normally hearing infants may enter the stage of canonical babbling as early as three months or as late as ten months (1994). Auditory experience seems critical for the development of this milestone. Hearing impaired infants are delayed in developing this milestone, with the onset of canonical babbling occurring after eleven months of age. In contrast, infants with other developmental problems that do not involve hearing loss may show little or no delay in obtaining this milestone (Eilers & Oller, 1994).

The vocalizations of babies at six and seven months of age include elements seen at earlier ages. They continue to make vowel-like sounds in addition to CV combinations. They make sounds regardless of whether another person is interacting with them. However, there are qualitative changes in sound production at this stage as well. For example, Abraham often seemed fascinated with his own babbling. He seemed to play with variations of his own babbling. He tried out one string of sounds and repeated the sounds with a slight change in the overall pattern. For example, while playing, he produced "di da . . . di . . da . . . daaaaaah . . da." As at earlier ages, these sounds appeared to be a form of vocal play, without reference to any one thing in particular.

Another change is the emergence of communicative intent behind Abraham's use of sound. This preverbal use of sound is typical among babies at this age. Parents recognize their baby's use of sounds to direct their attention to an object, to request actions ("give me"), or just as a social interaction. At this age, Abraham used sounds to signal refusal, for example. His mother offered him a spoon full of strained peas, which appeared to be out of favor at the time. He exclaimed his disgust and turned his cheek away from the offending food. These first intentional vocalizations are quite probably true precursors of linguistic behaviors yet to come. In fact, babies at this stage begin to comprehend a few spoken words, signaling the onset of the first true linguistic stage of development.

Ten to Fourteen Months

Abraham learned to walk before his first birthday. Initially, he used a coffee table or the couch to lift himself up and then "cruised" around the room holding onto the edges of the furniture. Then he walked without support. But often, he was only able to take a few steps before landing on his seat. His most efficient mode of locomotion was still crawling at that point.

Abraham also expanded his sound repertoire. In addition to the single syllables that were heard at seven to nine months, he learned to produce consonants in combination. As he stood ready to walk to his mother's outstretched arms, we heard "yee yeah adee di hee." Then Abraham's father, holding a VCR camera, caught his attention. His mother asked "Do you want to walk to Daddy?" Abraham piped in with an enthusiastic "da! dee!" Although this approximated the word "daddy," it was not yet a true word for Abraham. In fact, a few minutes later, we heard Abraham utter a chorus of "da dees" when attempting to walk toward his mother but also when attending to neither his mother or father. In this particular case, "da dee" reflected a different milestone in the development of speech sounds: the ability to repeat sound strings produced by others. We saw this new ability to repeat more explicitly when Abraham's mother was encouraging him to show off for the camera. She told him "Wave to the camera. Wave! Wave!" He echoed back "ey . . . ey" as a shortened form of "wave." Then he waved his hands, first with one hand and then with both hands. Next, his mother told him "Say 'Hey!' You know how to say 'Hey!' Say hey!" And he repeated "Hey!"

At this age, we often heard a chain of syllables with sentence-like inflectional patterns, such as "ba to aa aa na ?" We refer to these speech-like sound strings as *jargon*. Such an utterance is directed toward a listener, with the baby often searching to make eye contact, causing the listener to feel almost obligated to answer the jargon question with "yes" or "no." Abraham appeared to demand an object from the listener, give it back, and then demand it again. He changed his role within the communicative exchange, first becoming the asker, than the giver, and then the asker again. The sound of his voice carried as much of the message as the reaching gestures or looking at the object.

Jargon displays many combinations of consonants and vowels, and there does not appear to be a one-to-one representation for a particular object or desire. That is, the baby is not using the same combination of sounds to represent particular words. Although many of the consonant-vowel combinations are repeated, many are unique. The intention of the utterance is carried more in the inflection and prosody than in the consonant-vowel combination. At earlier ages, vocalizations flowed easily and there was no demand that babies produce any specific sounds. When they use vocalized jargons as intentional communication, however, babies begin to use the inflectional patterns that have been heard in their native language that represent particular needs and wants. At this stage, we hear front, middle, and back vowels sandwiched between many different consonants. Many of the consonants will drop out of babies' speaking repertoire as they get older and attempt to say words, which require exact specificity of production to be understood by others as true words.

Like other babies at this stage, Abraham was fun to play with. He enjoyed playing sound games, often reacting to his parents' model with exact or altered vocalization patterns of his own. Babies at this age may amaze their parents with novel, innovative jargon not previously heard. How well babies this age interact with others and the quality of their vocalizations may each have clinical implications for future communicative competence. Normal babies nine to ten months of age enjoy vocal play with others and seem to enjoy the human interaction both in play and during various caregiving tasks (feeding, bathing, diapering). Early parent-child interactions provide the baby with experiences that reinforce the positive aspects of communication. Such comfort and success in communication may go a long way in giving the baby the confidence needed for future attempts at communication. The absence of such enjoyment in babies this age may be symptomatic of future communicative interaction problems. As Van Riper and Emerick (1984) wrote, " . . . in this socialized babbling or vocal play of the baby we find the basic pattern of communication, of sending and receiving, although it is only sounds, not meaningful messages, that are batted back and forth" (p. 93). Perhaps the baby whose play attempts and reaching out toward others go unheeded does not experience the give-and-take of **dyadic** (two-people) **communication** required for successful communication skills development. Some future language problems may have their genesis in the first year if babies receive little satisfaction or reinforcement from their early attempts to communicate. Other babies seem to lack the interest in others that would lead to vocal play with another person. Such children are at risk for continued social and communicative problems as they grow.

Around the age of eleven months, Abraham entered a stage characterized by "nonreduplicated or variegated babbling" (Schwartz, 1984), meaning the jargon sounds were individualized and not often repeated. The infant begins to show real control over the stress and intonation of vocalization with the jargon pattern closely resembling the language the baby has been hearing. Ingram (1976) presented a number of diary studies that described particular babies at eleven to twelve months who were beginning to repeat the same vocalization pattern in a give situational context. There was still enough phonetic variability to prevent the utterance from being classified as true words. Most of the vocalization utterances at this age often sound more like phrases in that they are longer than that which would be perceived as single words.

The baby this age produces the immediate precursor to true words, in what Schwartz (1984) describes as vocalizations that are characterized by phonetically consistent forms known as **protowords** (primitive, early forms of an actual word). Whereas jargon vocalization appears to be more related to the affective, emotional state of the infant and is therefore rather free-flowing and without tight structure, the protowords have much greater specificity and appear to be more object- or action-specific. Sometimes, babies this age embed a protoword in the prosodic jargon. At other times, we observe a combination of prosodic jargon, then a slight pause, followed by the production of a protoword. It would seem that the first true words that often appear at twelve to thirteen months do not come suddenly but have developed gradually, from babble to jargon to protowords and then finally to a true word with relative phonetic stability.

Despite the arrival of the first few words, typical one-year-olds seem to attempt most of their communication by continuing differentiated jargon. The first words are not said very often. The jargon pattern becomes longer, sounding more like real language and occasionally containing a real word. Much of the intended message, when understood by the listener, is communicated not by the occasional word but by the general intonational pattern of the utterance and by the situational context.

Leonard and colleagues pointed out that children this age may comprehend the meaning of words that are beyond their phonologic capability to produce (Leonard, Schwartz, Folger, & Wilcox, 1978). It would appear that the selectivity process for production is basically related to the child's ability to produce the sounds of a particular word. However, before the first word is spoken, toddlers at this age produce many of the speech sounds that are used in their language community in the form of jargon. From about ten months onward, their sound repertoire expands to include at least approximations of all the phonemes of their language. Although a wide variety of sounds may be heard in the babbling of children, relatively few are heard in their first words.

When imitating the sounds of others, there is some selectivity regarding the kinds of sounds chosen for play. We also see this pattern as babies begin to produce their first words (Ferguson, 1978). Babies imitate the sounds they can physiologically produce; if the sounds are too complex to make, the babies will usually simplify the utterance, perhaps changing the consonant to one they can produce and preserving the vowel that was in the model. Abraham was heard doing just this when he produced "tita" when looking at a tiger in a picture book. As the first words are produced, there is some phonologic selectivity; the first words are those that are less motorically complex. Many of the first words may involve similar sounds, often voiced, front consonants. Sounds such as /m/ and /b/ appear in early speech in most languages. Babies often use the same consonant-vowel combination for several different words. For example, /ba/ may be used for words as different as "ball" or "car." Over time, as children add to their repertoire of speech sounds, the pronunciation of these two words becomes distinct.

Fifteen Months and Older

At this age, Abraham entered the true verbal stage of communication development. We will look in some detail at his development from single words to sentences in Chapter 4. However, development of the sound system continues to occur at this age. The developmental sequence of speech sounds in young children is somewhat predictable. Table 3-6 provides a listing of speech sounds that were produced by three groups of children of increasing ages. Over time, children begin to use the sounds they have acquired in different position within words (Dyson, 1988). As we saw with Abraham's speech development, vowel sounds are generally acquired early. Consonants emerge over a longer period of time. There may be months or years between the time a child first uses a sound in a word and the time when it is used correctly in all words. For example, consonants such as /r/ and /l/ may be inconsistently produced by normal five-year-olds (Kenney & Prather, 1986), although these sounds begin to emerge much earlier. Children's production of both consonants and vowels within words are heavily influenced by the other sounds within a given word. As children mature, the articulation of individual sounds becomes less affected by coarticulation and sounds become more distinct. Nittrouer and her colleagues demonstrated that children's speech shows decreased coarticulatory effects with increasing age (Nittrouer, Studdert-Kennedy, & McGowan, 1989). Articulation of individual speech sounds in conversational speech becomes increasingly refined until adult-like skills are acquired. By age three or four, most children can be readily understood, even by those who do not know them well.

Clinical Problem Solving

Kim was born with a severe hearing loss affecting both of his ears. He responded reliably to sounds of 500 Hz to 1000 Hz at 40 dB HL; sounds at 2000 to 4000 Hz were heard at 50 to 60 dB HL; and sounds above 4000 Hz required even greater intensities (up to 80 dB HL).

1. What does this mean for Kim in terms of everyday hearing experiences? What types of environmental sounds will he hear and what will he miss?

TABLE 3-6   Speech Sounds Produced by Children of Different Ages

Percentage Correct Use

	80% or Better	*60–79%*
Sounds Heard from Eighteen-Month-Olds		
Vowels	/ɑ/	/ʊ/ /i/ /ɪ/ /ʌ/ /ə/ /aʊ/ /ɔɪ/
Consonants	/b/ /m/ /j/	/h/ /f/ /d/ /n/ /w/
Additional Sounds from Two-Year-Olds		
Vowels	/u/ /ʌ/ /ɑ/ /i/ /æ/ /ʊ/ /o/ /e/ /ɛ/ /ɔ/ /ɪ/ /ɪʊ/ /aʊ/ /aɪ/ /ɪ/	
Consonants	/w/	/n/ /ŋ/ /k/ /g/ /p/ /f/ /d/
Additional Sounds from Three-Year-Olds		
Vowels	/ɝ/ /ɜ/ /ɚ/	
Consonants	/ʒ/ /n/ /h/ /d/ /p/ /ʃ/ /j/ /k/ /t/ /s/ /z/ /f/ /tʃ/ /dʒ/ /n/ /v/ /g/ /l/ /r/	

Adapted from Irwin and Wong (1983).

2. Give examples of how his experience with the sounds of speech might affect development of this aspect of communication?
3. Which components of speech (i.e., vowels, consonants, prosodics) will be most difficult for him to hear?
4. Some children (and adults) who experience a hearing loss become proficient lip readers. Which aspects of speech sound production can be best discriminated by this method and why? What aspects of conversational speech make lip reading difficult?

References

Armatage, S.E., Baldwin, B.A., & Vince, M.A. (1980). The fetal sound environment of sheep. *Science, 206,* 1173–1174.

Bench, J. (1968). Sound transmission to the human fetus through the maternal abdominal wall. *Journal of Genetic Psychology, 113,* 85–87.

Birnholz, J.C., & Benacerraf, B.R. (1983). The development of human fetal hearing. *Science, 222,* 516–518.

Boliek, C.A., Hixon, T.J., Watson, P.J., & Morgan, W.J. (1996). Vocalization and breathing during the first year of life. *Journal of Voice, 10,* 1–22.

Burnham, D.K., Earnshaw, L.J., & Clark, J.E. (1991). Development of categorical identification of native and non-native bilabial stops: infants, children, and adults. *Journal of Child Language, 18,* 321–260.

Daniloff, R.G. (1973). Normal articulation processes. In

F.D. Minifie, T.J. Hixon, & F. Williams (Eds.), *Normal Aspects of Speech, Hearing, and Language*. Englewood Cliffs, NJ: Prentice Hall.

DeCasper, A.J., & Fifer, W.P. (1980). Of human bonding: Newborns prefer their mother's voices. *Science, 208(1)*, 1741–1776.

DeCasper A.J., & Sigafoos, D. (1983). The intrauterine heartbeat: A potential reinforcer for newborns. *Infant Behavior and Development, 6*, 19–25.

Dyson, A.T. (1988). Phonetic inventories of 2- and 3-year old children. *Journal of Speech and Hearing Disorders, 53*, 89–93

Eilers, R.E., & Oller, D.K. (1994). Infant vocalizations and the early diagnosis of severe hearing impairment. *Journal of Pediatrics, 124*, 199–203.

Eimas, P.D., Siqueland, E.R., Jusczyk, P.W., & Vigorito, J. (1971). Speech perception in infants. *Science, 171*, 303–306.

Ferguson, C. (1978). Learning to pronounce: The earliest stages of phonological development in the child. In F. Minifie & L. Lloyd (Eds.), *Communicative and Cognitive Abilities: Early Behavioral Assessment*. Baltimore: University Park Press.

Fry, D.B. (1978). The role and primacy of the auditory channel in speech and language development. In M. Ross & T.C. Giolas (Eds.), *Auditory Management of Hearing Impaired Children*. Baltimore: University Park Press.

Ingram, D. (1976). *Phonological Disability in Children*. New York: Elsevier North Holland.

Irwin, J. V., & Wong, S. P. (1983). *Phonological Development in Children 18 to 72 Months*. Carbondale: Southern Illinois University Press.

Jusczyk, P.W. (1997). *The Discovery of Spoken Language*. Cambridge, MA: MIT Press/Bradford Books.

Kelly, J.P. (1985). Auditory system. In E.R. Kandel & J.H. Schwartz (Eds.), *Principles of Neural Science*. New York: Elsevier

Kenney, K.W., & Prather, E.M. (1986). Articulation development in preschool children: Consistency of production. *Journal of Speech and Hearing Research, 29*, 29–36.

Kuhl, P.K. (1994). Learning and representation in speech and language. *Current Opinion in Neurobiology, 4*, 812–822.

Kuhl, P.K., & Iverson, P. (1995). Linguistic experience and the perceptual magnet effect. In W. Strange (Ed.), *Speech Perception and Linguistic Experience*. Baltimore, MD: York Press.

Kuhl, P.K., Williams, K.A., Lacerda, F., Stevens, K.N., & Lindblom, B. (1992). Linguistic experience alters phonetic perception in infants by 6 months of age. *Science, 255*, 606–608.

Leader, L.R., Baillie, P., Martin, B., & Vermeulen, E. (1982). The assessment and significance of habituation to a repeated stimulus by the human fetus. *Early Human Development, 7*, 211–219.

Leonard, L., Schwartz, R., Folger, M., & Wilcox, M. (1978). Some aspects of children's imitative and spontaneous speech. *Journal of Child Language, 5*, 403–416.

Nittrouer, S., Studdert-Kennedy Y.M., & McGowan, R.S. (1989). The emergence of phonetic segments: Evidence from the spectral structure fricative-vowel syllables spoken by children and adults. *Journal of Speech and Hearing Research, 32*, 120–132.

Northern, J., & Downs, M. (1978). *Hearing in Children* (2nd ed.). Baltimore: Williams & Wilkins.

Oller, D. (1980). The emergence of speech sounds in infancy. In G. Yeni-Kamshian, J. Kavanaugh, & C. Ferguson (Eds.), *Child Phonology. Vol. 1: Production*. New York: Academic Press.

Schwartz, R. (1984). The phonologic system: Normal acquisition. In J. Costello (Ed.), *Speech Disorders in Children*. San Diego: College-Hill Press.

Streeter, L.A. (1976). Language perception of two-month-old infants shows effects of both innate mechanisms and experience. *Nature, 259*, 39–40.

Van Riper, C., & Emerick, L. (1984). *Speech Correction: An Introduction to Speech Pathology and Audiology* (7th ed.). Englewood Cliffs, NJ: Prentice Hall.

Walker, D., Grimwade, J, & Wood, C. (1971). Intrauterine noise: A component of the fetal environment. *American Journal of Obstetrics and Gynecology, 109*, 91–95.

Werker, J.F., & Lelond, C.E. (1988). Cross-language speech perception: Initial capabilities and developmental change. *Developmental Psychology, 24*, 672–683.

C h a p t e r *4*

Language

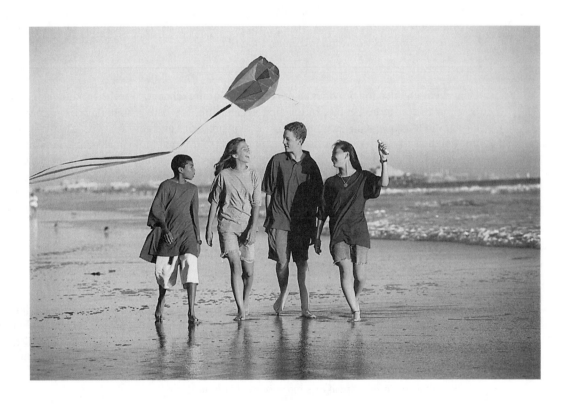

Preview

Human communication includes a wide range of activities. Much of it is nonverbal: A pointed stare or a strategic clearing of the throat is often sufficient to convey an emotion or prompt the recipient to action. A speaker's body posture and hand gestures convey aspects of attitude, emphasis, and emotion. Often, these nonverbal forms of communication are unintentional and nonspecific. When a specific message must be conveyed, people typically employ language. Language, whether spoken, written, or signed, involves a system of symbols that conveys meaning. Language involves the interaction of many skills, which combine for effective communication. A speaker must know the rules for combining sounds into words and words into sentences. The speaker uses both sentence structure and word meanings to convey the content of the message. Finally, the speaker must appreciate the rules of social discourse to use language effectively for communication. We will present some approaches used to study language acquisition that highlight various aspects of language in children. To illustrate normal acquisition, we will summarize the progression of language skills in a normally developing preschool child.

Human communication provides an opportunity for the exchange of feelings, knowledge, and wants between two or more people. In the first year of life, the baby communicates primarily through changes in the voice with accompanying facial expressions and gestures. These nonverbal vocalizations in the early part of life, primarily expressions of internal biological states, are affective in nature, and are interpreted by those around the baby as communicating emotion. The vocalizations soon begin to take on the melody of speech. When we left our discussion of infant vocalization in Chapter 3, Abraham, a child whose development we have been following, was just beginning to say his first words. At this point, the child's knowledge of the language (language competence) begins to show by the actual use of the language (language performance).

The Components of Language

As effortless as language appears to be for most people, effective use involves the interaction of many skills. To understand language better, it is sometimes useful to examine the skills that contribute to overall language functioning. Bloom (1988) suggested that language skills can be described in terms of form, content, and use. **Form** includes phonology, syntax, and morphology. **Content** includes the meaning, or **semantics**, of words and utterances. **Use** includes pragmatic skills such as the rules of social discourse and the speaker's purpose for communication.

Form

Phonology
Phonology is the study of the sounds of speech. Linguists have been studying the phonological development of children since the early 1900s (Ingram, 1981). Much of current phonological investi-

gation focuses on uncovering the rules required for speech sounds or phonemes as used in combination in syllables and words. In the phonological literature, four terms (phone, allophone, phoneme, and phonetics) are often confusing; let us define each and distinguish them from one another. A phone is the actual speech sound produced by a speaker, whether accurate or not. Allophones are groups of phones that are variations of a speech sound but to the listener may be heard as a single phoneme. A phoneme is the smallest speech sound that can be identified by a listener and makes a semantic difference when combined with other phonemes. For example, in the word *hat*, written phonetically as [hæt], by changing one phoneme, the vowel /æ/ to /ɪ/, we change the word to *hit* ([hɪt]). In this text, we indicate phonemes (speech sounds) when we place slash marks around the sounds, such as /a/ or /k/. In Chapter 3, we presented 52 individual phonemes listed as part of the International Phonetic Alphabet, which included consonants, vowels, and dipthongs.

Phonetics is the study of the physiology or motor production of speech sounds and their acoustic output. Vowels are produced with vocal fold vibration (i.e., voicing). Consonants may be either voiced or unvoiced. Phonological rules may dictate sound production in a given word. As we saw in Chapter 1, any given language contains only a subset of the possible sound combinations that can be produced. For example, the phonology of English permits the /st/ blend at either the beginning or end of words, but /str/ can only appear at word beginnings. Likewise, there are specific rules for voicing or unvoicing in pluralization. If we were to pluralize the words *hat* and *hit*, we would add the unvoiced consonant /s/. Pluralization of a noun ending in a voiced consonant requires the use of the voiced cognate of /s/, the phoneme /z/. So, if we were to pluralize the word bed, we would add the /z/ phoneme, writing the word in phonetics as [bɛdz]. Such rules for how sound is used are part of the phonology of the language.

Syntax

Syntax refers to the structure of sentences. The structure can be described in terms of hierarchically ordered components, as illustrated in Figure 4-1. A syntactic theory describes the rules by which words may be combined into grammatically acceptable sentences. For example, in English, the subject of

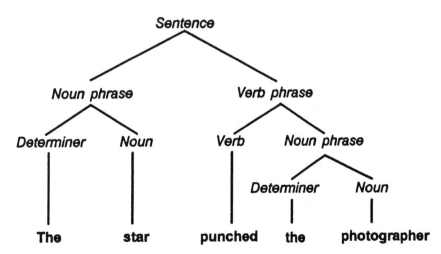

FIGURE 4-1 **The syntactic structure of a sentence.**

a declarative sentence (a noun or noun phrase) must precede the predicate of a sentence (a verb or verb phrase). Therefore, a sentence such as "He is swinging" is acceptable, whereas "Is swinging he" is not. Syntactic rules also describe the constraints in combining words and phrases of particular types. For example, for the predicate "is swinging," there are a limited number of phrases that might follow it in a sentence. We might say, "He is swinging wildly" or "He is swinging on the porch swing" or "He is swinging the baby." The predicate "is swinging" belongs to a class of verbs that can be followed by an adverbial phrase, prepositional phrase, or noun phrase. Other verbs do not allow all these combinations. We would not say, "He is wildly" because this form of the verb "is" cannot be followed directly by an adverb in standard English.

For most people, the rules for combining words into sentences are unconscious and automatic. Knowledge of these syntactic rules allows a speaker to produce grammatical utterances effortlessly. Syntactic knowledge also helps listeners to comprehend the utterances they hear. In any language there is a limited number of acceptable syntactic structures. Therefore, knowledge of these structures allows listeners to anticipate the words they will hear and draw conclusions about how the words relate to one another to convey meaning. For example, in "Jamie asked Adelida . . . " there is a high probability that the sentence will continue with either a prepositional phrase (e.g., "about . . . ") or a verb infinitive (for example, "to go . . . " or "to call . . . "). The listener, from the conversational context, may even be able to anticipate the precise phrase. Given the complete sentence "Jamie asked Adelida to go," the syntactic rules tell the listener that Jamie is doing the asking and that Adelida is being asked to go. In this way, the syntax has represented the general meaning of the utterance in a structured, rule-governed way. This phenomenon is referred to as mapping a deep structure (meaning) to a surface structure (syntax).

We will talk more about syntax in the next section of this chapter when we discuss language acquisition. Problems in syntactic comprehension and production in language-impaired children and adults will be presented in Chapters 7 and 8.

Morphology

Morphology refers to how meaning is represented by the use of words, affixes, various grammar tenses (such as past tense), and plurality. A **morpheme** is the smallest unit of a language that has meaning. It can be a whole word, one of several parts of a word, the beginning of a word (i.e., a prefix, such as *un-*), or a word ending (i.e., a suffix, such as *-ing*). The following words contain one morpheme; they cannot be divided into any smaller units and still carry meaning:

quick	(one morpheme)
build	(one morpheme)
structure	(one morpheme)

Words that can stand alone are called free morphemes. A second class of morphemes is called bound morphemes because they must be attached to other words. Bound morphemes include the suffixes in:

quickly	(two morphemes)
builder	(two morphemes)
structured	(two morphemes)

Each of these words contains two morphemes, one free and one bound. Notice that the bound morpheme changes the meaning of the word in each case. In some cases the addition of a morpheme actually changes the syntactic classification of the word. The addition of *-ly* changes *quick* from an adjective to an adverb. The addition of *-er* changes *build* from a verb to a noun. Conversely, the addition of *-ed* to *structure* changes it from a noun to an adjective. In other cases, morphemes add meaning without changing the class of the word. For example, English uses several combinations of morphemes to express different verb tenses:

opens	(present action; two morphemes)
is opening	(present ongoing action; three morphemes)
will open	(future action; two morphemes)
opened	(past action; two morphemes)

Other morphemes add meaning without changing the syntactic class or tense of the word. These include pluralization and many prefixes:

dogs	(two morphemes)
reignite	(two morphemes)

Note that *re-* is a morpheme in the word *reignite*. It is not a morpheme in the word *religion* because neither *re-* nor *-ligion* carries any unique meaning in that word. Therefore, it is not always the case that multisyllable words contain multiple morphemes.

Children's acquisition of morphology seems to follow predictable stages. After analyzing the utterances of children over time, Brown (1973) developed five stages of sentence construction that seem to parallel (or mirror) overall language development. The five stages were developed according to the number of morphemes a child said per utterance, known as the MLU, or mean length of utterance, in morphemes:

Stage I (1.75 morphemes). The child is using single words and is starting to put noun-verb sequences together, such as "Car go."

Stage II (2.25 morphemes). The child starts to change word endings to portray grammar, as in "Cars going."

Stage III (2.75 morphemes). The child begins to use questions and imperatives, for instance, "That a car?"

Stage IV (3.5 morphemes). The child begins to use complex sentences, for example, "Where's car going now?"

Stage V (4 morphemes). The child may use connectors and more functions, as in "Mom's in the car."

Although there is obvious overlap between successive stages, Brown and his colleagues conducted a number of studies over time that showed a progression from saying a single word to the two-word utterance, to the telegraphic sentence, with the gradual refinement of grammar leading to complete sentences compatible with the adult model.

Content

Content includes the meanings of individual words and words in combination. The study of word meanings is sometimes referred to as semantics. Our basic use of language as a tool for communication is to transmit meaning to someone else. Hubbell (1985) noted, "Meaning is the bridge between the thoughts and experiences of individuals and the sequences of sounds they produce to symbolize those thoughts and experiences. Words symbolize concepts, and concepts represent experiences or reality" (p. 33).

Of interest here is how young children attach meaning to a particular phonological sequence they have been hearing and how their meaning for a word develops into the adult-like meaning. As children hear words associated with particular actions and behaviors in social contexts, they begin to assign meaning to those words. Eventually, a word stands for those actions and feelings, without the need for the original context. As the child develops cognitively through various experiences, there is greater coupling of words with meaning. The child begins to use "words to refer to or represent external objects and events" (Clark, 1979, p. 193). Two kinds of meaning may develop for words, denotative and connotative. Denotative meaning is the literal meaning of the word. For example, for the word *milk*, we can use the dictionary definition of "a whitish fluid that is secreted by the mammary glands of female mammals for the nourishment of their young" as a literal, denotative meaning. (Few of us have thought of this meaning very often.)

Besides the literal, denotative meanings, words carry connotative meanings, which include the subtle overtones that distinguish words of very similar meanings. Thus, we would probably prefer to be called "unique" or even "unusual" rather than "atypical" or "abnormal." Connotative meanings often set the emotional tone of what is said. For example, "She requested it" has a more formal tone than "She asked for it." Connotative meanings also reflect concepts associated with particular words. For example, if we associate the concept of physical nourishment with milk, we can make the connection to spiritual nourishment to understand an alternate meaning of milk in the metaphorical "milk of human kindness." Speakers learn the rules of the semantic system by hearing and using words in ways appropriate to both their connotative and denotative meanings.

The sentence context influences the specific meanings that we attach to individual words. The meanings of nouns and verbs are modified by the use of adjectives and adverbs. The listener's expectations about the meaning of a sentence may change as later words cause its meaning to shift. For example, the noun *shoe* typically produces in the mind of the listener a picture of a leather covering of the foot mounted on a thicker sole. We can see how the sentence context is used to produce many different meanings for this word:

If the shoe fits, wear it.	(a nonliteral, proverbial meaning)
It fits like an old shoe.	(proverb, or from experience, old shoes feel good on the foot)
Make a ringer with a horseshoe.	(*horse* morpheme changes meaning, and *ringer* requires specialized knowledge of horseshoe game)
You can't stop with worn shoes.	(a brake shoe is ineffective when worn)

In the preceding examples, we see that the noun *shoe* (which we may first think of as the object we wear on a foot) can have many other meanings. We understand the particular meaning in the context in which the utterance was made. Disagreements in interpreting what someone intended to say may sometimes be related to different interpretations of word meaning. Someone speaks to a gathering of people in the hope that everyone assembled will make the same interpretation of the words; however, the literal meanings of the words may compete with their connotative meanings, often resulting in many different interpretations than that intended by the speaker.

Use

How we use words, and in what situations, is the focus of language use, or pragmatics. This is the study of the use of language in context. After the first six months of life, spontaneous vocalization begins to be replaced with intentional vocalization accompanied by expression and gesture (Oller, 1980). Bates (1976) and Bruner (1975) pointed out that the human interaction the baby experiences in the first year of life establishes various pragmatic roles long before the baby is using actual language. The preverbal behaviors described in Chapter 3 are basically employed to control and manipulate the environment. From about the age of nine months, the baby enjoys interaction with the caregiver, using vocalization appropriately for such games as pat-a-cake and peek-a-boo. In these early games, the child is using vocalization to interact with others, which Bates (1976, p. 426) calls "preverbal performatives." Even between twelve and eighteen months, the baby uses single-word responses like "bye-bye" more as part of a physical interaction with the caregiver than as true words that represent concepts. These utterances are called "performative acts" by Bates. The performative act serves a communicative purpose for the child, such as declaring, promising, asking questions, and so forth (Bates, Benigni, Bretherton, Camaioni, & Volterra, 1977).

The speech acts theory, developed by Searle (1969), focuses on the speaker's intention rather than on the words one uses. Searle described three types of intents: *asserting*, *requesting*, and *ordering*. These categories focus on how the speaker is using language rather than on the specifics of what was said. Assertions are almost as varied as topics of communication, whereas requests are usually for some kind of action or information. Others have elaborated on this focus with additional functions that language serves. Halliday (1975) listed seven human needs or functions that can be served by language:

1. Instrumental ("I need . . . ")
2. Regulatory ("Take the . . .")
3. Interactional ("How are you?")
4. Personal ("I'm hungry . . . ")
5. Heuristic ("Where . . . ?")
6. Imaginative ("Why don't we . . . ?")
7. Informational ("You know that . . . ")

As young children grow, so does their verbal repertoire, enabling the use of language forms that meet the demands of a particular situation. Children learn to communicate (verbally and nonverbally) one way to their peers, another way to their parents, and another way to the teacher or the doctor. The child learns that the situation or context of the communication has much to do with how things are phrased. The specific decision about what to say and how and when to say it is shaped by the success the child experiences in conversation. For example, the child soon learns that you can call your cousins by their first name but you better use "Aunt" or "Uncle" with their parents, even though the adults address each other by first name alone. Furthermore, the child soon understands that Grandmother likes to use baby talk and that Grandfather uses a very adult language form. In Chapter 3, we saw the use of "child-directed-speech" by Abraham's parents when addressing their infant son. However, it is unlikely that these parents speak to their bosses or co-workers in this style of speech. Instead, they adjust the register of their speech to match the age and social status of their listener.

Approaches to the Study of Language Acquisition

During the first year of life, infants all over the world hear the languages spoken around them and eventually organize what they hear into some kind of meaning. Toward the end of the first year, babies respond to their name. They are able to respond to simple verbal commands and make simple motor responses using the objects in their immediate environment. As we saw in Chapter 3, their vocalizations toward the end of the first year have become a complex vocal pattern that resembles the patterns of the spoken languages they have been hearing. The first spoken words are followed by the orderly acquisition of one- and two-word utterances; these first words have primary value to the baby, such as *ma* and *mi(lk)*. These first words are also relatively easy to say and phonetically simple. As language is acquired during the second year, children are able to produce (and understand) longer and increasingly complex language constructions. Children acquire a grammar (rules of structure and sequence) of the language through its everyday use. As children put two or three words together, they use the rules of the grammar to keep the words in the form and sequence needed to facilitate comprehension by the listener. Children learn that to be understood by the listener, the verbal message must be said in a way that is reasonably similar to the language code of the listener.

There appears to be some uniformity across cultures regarding the acquisition and form of language. In contrast, there is great diversity in theories of language acquisition. In addition to speech-language pathologists and audiologists, many scholars from different backgrounds have studied language over the years. The philosopher and the psychologist have examined the relationship between language and thought. The linguist has studied the origins and forms of language. The psychologist and biologist have viewed language from its neurogenic origins. The neurologist and psychologist have studied the neurological foundations of both normal and disordered language. The child development specialist, the linguist, and psychologist have looked at cognition and language. Although some of the diversity of opinion about language is related to the particular discipline, some of it is related to the chronology or history of studying language. Over the years there have been major shifts in focus and viewpoint. The historical time at which language acquisition was studied (such as in 1950, as opposed to 1970 or 1990) has a influential role in one's approach to the topic. It would be convenient and encouraging to identify a sequential and progressive theme in the study of language over the years, but it appears that there is some randomness, perhaps even circularity in our study of normal language. Among the many theoretical approaches to the acquisition of language that are available, let us select four (listed in Table 4-1) and cite a few of the theorists who have advocated each point of view.

It must be recognized that any selection or listing of theoretical approaches to language acquisition is an oversimplification. Further, there is considerable overlap of view between particular approaches, as well as single proponents advocating several theories. Cruttenden (1979) advocated a "balanced viewpoint" in consideration of various approaches to language acquisition, recognizing

TABLE 4-1   Four Approaches to Language Acquisition

Approach	Proponents
Behavioral	Bandura, 1969; Skinner, 1957; Staats, 1968
Nativist	Chomsky, 1965; McNeill, 1970; Pinker, 1984
Cognitive	Bates & MacWhinney, 1987; Crommer, 1988; Piaget, 1963
Biological	Geschwind, 1977; Lenneberg, 1967

that there is some truth in each. In this introductory work, our intent is to present each approach briefly, with no attempt to advocate any one theory of language acquisition.

The Behavioral Approach

According to the behavioral approach, language is a learned, conditioned behavior. This approach to language acquisition stresses the influence of environment rather than any innate abilities of the child. The origins of behavioral therapy perhaps started with the classical conditioning study of Pavlov, who conditioned dogs to salivate (Watson, 1970). Observing that dogs salivated when looking at meat, Pavlov presented a tuning-fork sound when the meat was presented. The dogs were soon *conditioned* to salivate when they heard the tuning fork (whether the meat was present or not). Like most automatic reflexes (such as salivation), many forms of human behavior, including language (Skinner, 1957), can be conditioned.

Behavioralists assert that language can be taught as well. For example, the nine-month-old baby learns to attend to the voice of her caregivers; when she hears these voices and looks closely at these people, she discovers that she can derive various forms of comfort. She then repeats the comfort-producing behavior. The twelve-month-old baby says "ma" when his mother is about to feed him. His *ma* production is followed by feeding, accompanied by many animated expressions of love from his mother. The positive response he received makes *ma* an attractive word to say. Every time he sees his mother (if there is enough positive reinforcement), he is likely to repeat it. He may also generalize the use of *ma* for all feeding situations regardless of who the caregiver may be. Such inappropriate stimulus generalization will eventually be extinguished through the reactions and feeding situations the baby experiences.

Skinner (1957) developed a behavioral theory of verbal learning. Language is conditioned as a child's early vocal behaviors receive positive reinforcement. As the child develops, correctly pronounced words and combinations of words are rewarded by approval or sometimes by the basic pleasure of verbalization (Cruttenden, 1979). Incorrect utterances are met with no approval and are subsequently replaced by correct (good) verbalizations. In this way, the caregiver becomes the teacher, providing reinforcements for the child's utterances, in effect *shaping* the child's productions to approximate those of the adult language model.

A behavioral approach to language learning strongly emphasizes shaping and reinforcement of speech attempts in the child's acquisition of language. In the first two years of life, when the child is in close proximity to a caregiver, one can appreciate that the latter has a primary role in reinforcing the child's utterances. However, the caregiver role may be as much modeling and interacting as it is reinforcing, per se. Once the child reaches the age of two, it is difficult to see how a heterogeneous society can provide a consistent model for shaping verbalizations. Young children encounter a great variety of linguistic models (baby talk, fragmented sentences, and sentences spoken in a way they do not understand) and varied reactions to their utterances (anger, annoyance, laughter, ignoring, and friendliness).

Despite its limitations for fully explaining normal language acquisition, the behavioral theory has been applied to teaching language in cases of language disorders. The behavioral approach to language acquisition was much utilized in the 1960s and 1970s as a clinical training model for children with deficient language. These approaches often involved repeated practice with reinforcement for correct productions. Although therapy approaches have become more naturalistic over the years, operant principles continue to be used for stimulating language in children with language disabilities of various kinds.

The Nativist (Innateness) Approach

The nativist approach, sometimes called the innateness approach, asserts that the infant is born with the basic physical equipment (neural and structural) required to be able to understand and express spoken language—the only necessity being that the infant be around other people who speak the language. The theory was originally formulated to account for children's seemingly rapid and effortless acquisition of language, which does not appear to be the result of explicit instruction by adults. Proponents of the nativist hypothesis (e.g., Chomsky, 1988; Pinker, 1984) point to the fact that children rarely receive correction for their ungrammatical sentences as they acquire language. This lack of "negative evidence" (correction) available to the child is taken as support for the proposition that the rules (or sensitivity to the rules) of language are part of the child's biological endowment. This endowment gives the child innate knowledge about the rules of language: "The child learning Spanish or any other human language knows, in advance of experience, that the rules will be structure dependent" (Chomsky, 1988, p. 45). Thus, children are presumed to have an innate knowledge of how words are organized into sentences, even before hearing the many types of sentences that comprise a language.

Both Chomsky (1965) and McNeill (1970) discussed a Language Acquisition Device (LAD), which provides an acquisition model consistent with the innateness theory. The LAD is often referred to as "the black box" because its inner workings are hidden and poorly understood. In the LAD model, the utterances the children hear (the language "corpus") pass through a central mechanism that contributes to the learning of a language grammar. By continuous exposure to the utterances of others, which are processed by the LAD, children learn the grammar, developing, in effect, grammatical competence. McNeill diagrams the LAD model simply as

Corpus   →   LAD   →   Grammatical competence

It should be remembered that *competence* (knowledge of the language) is not necessarily matched by *performance* (execution of that knowledge). For example, individuals who are born with or develop motor disabilities that affect speech production can have perfectly normal language competence despite limitations on their ability to produce spoken language.

This "black box" model of acquisition has been developed further to address how the language input (corpus) and the child's biological endowment (LAD) act to produce grammatical competence. Chomsky (1988) suggested that the language faculty includes invariant (universal) and variant features (parameters). Universal features account for properties that are standard across all languages; parameters must be set for those features that vary across languages. The parameters are set by exposure to language input, after which the settings become part of the child's language faculty. Pinker (1989) concentrated on how the language faculty organizes language input to let the child obtain grammatical proficiency. These two theories emphasize the unique role of the language faculty in processing language input. The language faculty is presumed to be innate, predetermined, and self-contained (i.e., "modular"). These three assumptions contrast markedly with other theories that emphasize the role of external forces (e.g., the behavioral approach) and general cognitive and maturational development (e.g., the cognitive approach) in language acquisition.

The Cognitive Approach

Cognitive development is a prerequisite to language development in the cognitive approach. Since the early 1920s, Piaget (1963) has been identified as one of the leading proponents of this approach. Piaget suggested that children's developing ability with language is a reflection of their progression through hierarchical stages of cognitive development. Language skills represent an application of general cognitive skills for the purpose of communication. Reflecting this assumption, cognitivists have attended to aspects of general, nonverbal development that are precursors to language development (e.g., Kelly & Dale, 1989).

In addition to cognitive maturation, experience is key in cognitive approaches. A child's first words code the people, objects, and actions that are experienced on a day-to-day basis. The acquisition of first words may represent a combination of the child's experiences and the increasing ability to represent those experiences with an abstract (linguistic) form. This account implicitly assumes that the child is forming cognitive notions about the world prior to coding them with language. Furthermore, the child's background knowledge (about people, settings, and events) provides additional support for effective communication. The close link among cognition, experience, and communication emphasizes the message of language rather than its form.

The cognitive approach assumes that the child's language skills, and the capacity for language development, pass through maturational stages. This theory stands in contrast to the nativist approach, which assumes that the child's language faculty is complete at birth and stable over time. Similar to the nativist approach, cognitive approaches may include innate predisposing factors. These factors are not language-specific but are general to many cognitive and linguistic skills. Language skills are assumed to rely on and develop in concert with emerging cognitive skills.

A recent evolution in the cognitivist tradition has been the application of computer models to the problem of language acquisition (e.g., Cartwright & Brent, 1997; Huiskens, Coppen, & Jagtman, 1991; McClelland & Rumelhart, 1986). In some ways, these computer models are a reaction to nativist claims that specialized, language-specific mechanisms underlie language competence and that language input to the child is insufficient to teach all the permutations that children quickly begin to produce. Few researchers would claim that a successful computer model proves how children acquire language. Instead, these models serve to broaden thinking about the possibilities that could account for acquisition. Simply put, the fact that a computer can mimic aspects of acquisition indicates that it is possible that those skills could be acquired without a language-specific mechanism.

These models start with the assumption that acquisition can be influenced by patterns available in the input. For example, let us suppose a child hears words associated with actions, like *jump* and *jumped*, *cry* and *cried*. He or she might learn the association between *–ed* and the ends of verbs. This child may even overextend this association to verbs that do not take the *–ed* ending (e.g., *runned, sitted*) for a while (as some children do). However, after he or she hears enough examples of the irregular forms (e.g., *ran, sat*), the child will use these forms correctly as well. If these irregular words occur quite frequently in the speech he or she hears, the child might learn these "exceptions to the rule" quite quickly. And in fact, irregular verbs are quite common in conversational speech.

This line of thinking led to the development of the cue-competition theory of language acquisition (Bates & McWhinney, 1987). This theory is based on the premise that all native languages provide the child with cues as to its underlying structure. The effectiveness, or strength, of these cues is related to how frequently they occur in the language and how reliably they lead the child to the correct conclusion about communication. For example, English speaking children hear "subject-verb-object" sentences quite frequently. Therefore, interpreting the initial noun of a sentence as the subject is quite reliable for understanding the sentence. This makes the "first-noun-as-subject" cue strong for English-speaking children. However, this same rule would not have high cue strength in other languages. This language-to-language variation in cues accounts for many of the differences in the age at which speakers of different languages acquire the specific components of their language.

The cue-competition theory accounts for the lack of a "universal" sequence for acquisition of linguistic structures among the languages of the world. It states that children are, in fact, learning their language through a process of associating language form with its meaning and communicative functions. Unlike the nativist theories, however, no language-specific mechanism is required for this learning. In fact, acquisition may occur simply by strengthening basic associations between form and function that prove productive over time. In contrast to the behaviorist approach, however, no reinforcement or "reward" is necessary to shape language acquisition.

The Biological Approach

Over the years, there has been increasing interest in the biological correlates of language and language acquisition. Evidence from the study of aphasia in both adults and children (see Chapters 7 and 8) indicates that the left hemisphere controls many aspects of the comprehension and production of language form. The right hemisphere seems to have much to do with rhythm, tonality, and the expression of emotions. Both hemispheres work in concert to facilitate communication (see Chapter 2).

Given this hemispheric processing bias for different aspects of communication, many investigators have directed their efforts toward describing biological features that may underlie these skills. Geschwind and Levitsky (1968) were the first to establish an asymmetry of one brain area associated with language processing. Later studies confirmed that this asymmetry occurs as early as the third prenatal trimester (Chi, Dooling, & Gilles, 1977). Researchers have suggested that this structural pattern may reflect a biological predisposition toward left-hemisphere control of language in the brain. How this lateralization of language is realized remains under investigation. We know that the proliferation of cell processes and connections in the language-associated areas of the brain occurs as babies are acquiring early communicative skills and their first words. These neurological events are correlates of language acquisition because neuroanatomical changes precede and accompany gains in language skills.

Some investigators have concentrated on the functional, or physiological, correlates of language acquisition. We now have several techniques for monitoring ongoing brain activity in adults and children. These methods are being applied to questions concerning language acquisition. For example,

Molfese (1990) demonstrated differences in toddlers' brain electrical response to words they had learned and words they did not yet know. This measured electrical activity is a reflection of brain physiology in response to the words these toddlers heard. Such methods provide a window on the brain's functional development as it relates to language acquisition. Others (e.g., Kutas & Hillyard, 1982; Neville, Nicol, Barss, Forster, & Garrett, 1991; Van Petten, Weckerly, McIsaac, & Kutas, 1997) have examined the electrical activity of adults' brains in response to the grammatical and semantic components of language.

The investigation of the biological bases of language is providing insights into possible mechanisms of language acquisition. Biological investigations can be guided by the assumptions drawn from any of the other theoretical approaches to language. Ultimately, the biological approach may provide evidence to support or refute the assumptions of other approaches to language acquisition.

A Summary of the Approaches to the Study of Language Acquisition

In many ways, the approaches described differ more in their focus than in their substantive claims. Indeed, writers frequently combine aspects of various positions or switch between them over time. Cognitive approaches tend to emphasize the importance of the communicative function of language. Nativist approaches are frequently designed to account for language form. Cognitive and behavioral approaches often address language content as it is mapped to the child's experiences. Biological approaches concentrate on anatomical and physiologic correlates of language. The differences in focus reflect, in part, the different disciplines that have contributed to the field of language. As the study of language becomes increasingly interdisciplinary, we can look forward to a greater integration of such approaches.

Several of these perspectives on language acquisition reflect a nature versus nurture argument. For example, nativist theories have historically emphasized the child's innate endowment (nature) for language. In contrast, behavioral theories have emphasized the role of the environment (nurture). Recent advances in the neurosciences demonstrate that strict nature-nurture dichotomies are unrealistic. We now know that experience shapes the structure and function of the brain at very basic levels. The pattern of neuron activation is shaped and changed by sensory input and experiences. Activation, in turn, promotes neuronal survival and outgrowth. These changes in the brain's basic organization make the brain a ready and increasingly efficient processor of experience, including experience with language.

This type of dynamic interaction between children's biological nature and their experiences forces a redefinition of innate versus experience-based skills. The word *innate* typically means "present from birth," although this definition no longer means that experience has had no effect. Many brain systems rely heavily on sensory input to develop normally, and such input may begin prenatally. For example, the auditory system becomes functional during the third prenatal trimester. Some aspects of spoken language, such as its prosodic patterns and certain sound contrasts, are audible in the womb. As we saw in Chapter 3, infants hear and respond differentially to sounds they were exposed to while in the womb (e.g., DeCasper & Spence, 1986). Thus, infants are born with some knowledge of acoustic characteristics of their language community, and this knowledge appears to be experience-based. These types of discoveries force a re-evaluation of the assumptions that underlie traditional approaches to language acquisition. As Locke (1990) suggested, language may be both innate and learned as certain biological characteristics may predispose a child to attend to language-relevant information, prompting the child to learn more about it. From this perspective, it is more productive to explore the interactions between the child and his or her experiences than to divide them artificially.

Language Development from Sounds to Sentences

In Chapter 3, we followed the development of a young boy named Abraham. We saw his communicative development progress from his first exposures to the sounds of language to the point where he was able to produce sounds recognizable as single words. This is a truly remarkable accomplishment. It signals coordination of the range of biological systems (respiratory, vocal, articulatory, hearing, and cognition) to support spoken language. Once the first words appear, others soon follow. A child learns words that characterize his environment. The family dog's name is learned and the word *dog* itself will follow. If there is no neighborhood cat, however, that word will take longer to appear. Sometimes these first words are highly context specific. For example, Abraham could name animals from his Noah's ark book that he did not name at the zoo. Nonetheless, with each day and every new experience, there were opportunities to learn new words and refine his understanding of words recently acquired. Let us continue to look at Abraham's communication from the perspective of his emerging language skills.

Twenty-One Months

Abraham visited us at the language clinic at twenty-one months of age. When he entered the large playroom, he was immediately attracted to the crayons and paper that we had set out on a child-sized picnic table. He loved to color, which at this point consisted of light marks scribbled mostly on the page, and occasionally on the table. Of course, at this age, Abraham's attention span for any one activity was fairly short, as we will see. When he began to color, his mother conducted the following conversation with him:

Mother: You like to color, huh?

Abraham: Gah!

Mother: Yeah, you like to color, huh?

Abraham: Ah deh. Out.

Mother: Want to get out? (She lifts him out from between the table and bench.) You want to go look in that bag? Bring your bag. Bring the bag over here. (Abraham brings the bag.) All right! (Laughs.) What's in there?

(Abraham and Mother look into the bag.)

Abraham: Bribee (baby).

Mother: Yeah.

Abraham: Beebee (baby).

Mother: That's your baby. (Takes it out.)

Abraham: Night night. Deh coo.

Mother: Blanket for the baby.

Abraham: Deh yi gah.

Mother: Yeah, that's your grrrr bear. (Takes it out.)

(Abraham wanders off…)

Mother: Where are you going, hun?

Abraham: Ow meh.

Mother: You're coming here?

Abraham: Eeehhh. (yes).

Mother: What else is in the bag?

Abraham: Ehhh off. (Abraham pulls at the vest he is wearing.)

Mother: Oh, we're gonna leave it on. Look how nice you look.

Abraham: Ah hah.

Mother: Very handsome.

This short conversation illustrates many aspects of Abraham's current stage of language acquisition. The first thing we notice is that, although he is now using words, we don't always understand what he is saying. Even his parents do not always understand everything he says. However, when the context gives clues to the meaning of the words (e.g., pulling objects out of a bag), his mother can translate his attempts into actual words. In fact, parents provide indirect feedback about the form of their children's language by repeating and expanding on their children's utterances (Demetras, Post, & Snow, 1986).

At this age, most of Abraham's language consists of single words. He is just beginning to use two-word combinations and an occasional three-word utterance as well. Clinicians often describe the stage of a child's early language development with reference to the average, or mean, length of utterance. In fact, this metric is so commonly used, it is typically referred to by the initials MLU. MLU is calculated by counting the number of morphemes in the child's utterances and calculating the average or mean number of morphemes used per utterance within the speech sample. At this age, Abraham's production of single words, with few multi-word combinations, is reflected by an overall MLU of 1.49. These utterances consist almost exclusively of content rich words (e.g., nouns, verbs). Completely absent are any of the grammatical morphemes (e.g., articles, plurals, verb tense markers). In contrast, Abraham can comprehend much longer utterances than he is able to produce. For example, his mother's request ("Bring your bag.") and her direction to him ("Oh, we're gonna leave it on.") are longer than what he produced.

Abraham has between 50 and 100 different words in his language repertoire. However, his understanding of the meanings of words may be different than those of an adult. This is the age when toddlers point to strange men in grocery stores and exclaim "Daddy!" For them, the word *Daddy* may be broadly defined as including all adult males. The narrower meaning of "my male parent" will develop later. Conversely, other words may have too narrow a definition. *Doggie* may be used only with the household pet, and not for other dogs. Other words are actually social routines (e.g., *Night night.*) or parts of songs, which may not be used outside of that specific context. As children grow in both experience and cognitive maturation, their understanding of the meaning of words will become more refined and adult-like.

Despite the fact that most of his language consists of single words, Abraham gets a lot of "mileage" out of those single words. He is actually able to convey a range of meanings with similar utterances, depending on the situational context and his intonation. When we look at his utterances from the perspective of language content and use, we can see this flexibility of expression.

Mother: We got a bunch of different books here.

Abraham: Elmo book! Elmo book!   (Content: Item name)

                                          (Use: Requests an action [reading])

Mother: You want to read the Elmo book?

Abraham: Elmo book.   (Content: Item name)

                                          (Use: Confirmation)

.

.

.

Mother: Who's that?

Abraham: Gower.   (Content: Character name)

                                          (Use: Labeling; reply to mother)

Mother: Grover.

Abraham: Gower coffee.   (Content: Possession)

                                          (Use: Comment)

Twenty-Eight Months

At two years of age, Abraham is quite the conversationalist. At this point, Abraham can be understood well by both family members and those who hear him speak less frequently. We can see an example when Abraham talks about his toddler gymnastics class.

Mother: What did you get to do at class?

Abraham: Jump!

Mother: You get to jump. On what?

Abraham: Trampoline.

Author: Did Mommy get to jump on the trampoline?

Abraham: Yeah.

Mother: Did I jump on that trampoline?

Abraham: No.

Mother: No.

Author: No? Why not?

Abraham: She want to get off.

Mother: Who else got to jump on it?

Abraham: Other boy turn.

Mother: Yeah. You guys shared, didn't you?

Abraham: Yeah. (Abraham crouches and makes a funny face.) Went nnnnnggggggggg.

Mother: Is that what he said?

Abraham: Yeah. I say that.

As this conversation illustrates, Abraham is talking in single words and short sentences. We hear the major content words (e.g., nouns, main verbs). We also hear the earliest acquired grammatical morphemes (e.g., "coming our house!" "Flowers."). However, most other grammatical units tend to be missing. In this early stage of language development, it is common to hear such "telegraphic speech" (Brown, 1976). Abraham's MLU on the day this conversation took place was 2.03, which is about average for children at this age.

We sometimes have difficulty understanding what Abraham says, not because the words themselves are mispronounced, but because he does not always provide enough information or background to convey the general context. For example, the word "jump" does not necessarily bring to mind bouncing on a trampoline when it is first said. In this case, Abraham's mother was filling in the background information and structure of the conversation by cueing him as to what information should be given next. In addition, children at this stage are likely to agree with what adults say, regardless of its actual truth, as we see here. Pragmatically, they understand that a positive response will continue the conversation, without appreciating that the listener's understanding has diverged from their own. Although Abraham's mother gets the conversation back on track, we can see that this tendency in young children can also lead to miscommunications.

Despite these limitations in form and content, Abraham is exhibiting a range of language use. During a play visit to the author at the clinic, we observed various pragmatic functions. The following is a small sample of these:

What that?   (request for information)
Mommy do it!   (request for action)

A doll.   (labeling)
Now him sad.   (commenting)
No! No!   (negating)

Thirty-Nine Months

Children's speech changes rapidly between the ages of two and four. In twelve months, we can already see changes in the form of Abraham's language. We recorded this interaction between Abraham and his mother when Abraham was thirty-nine months.

Mother: Oh, you know what? I should have brought your pictures of you and Christopher to show. They were so pretty. Remember?

Abraham: You forgot?

Mother: I forgot to bring them. They were really neat.

Abraham: The pictures that I made and colored?

Mother: Yep.

Author: You colored them by yourself?

Abraham: Mmmhmm. I made 'em mixed with for the sky.

Mother: Yep, you mixed the color of the sky.

Abraham: And I made the clouds inside.

Mother: You sure did.

Abraham: But the 'nuther one was messed up.

Mother: Well, yeah. You did make one that you didn't like much.

Abraham: It was messed up.

Mother: It was. But you really liked it because you put legs and feet and arms and hands.

Abraham: There wasn't enough room for the legs.

Although we still see a few form errors (e.g., *'the 'nuther one'* for *'another one'*) we see noteworthy gains as well. Abraham increased the length of his utterances. His MLU on this day was 5.28. This is actually above average for his age. MLUs for children at this age typically range between 2.71 to 4.23 (Miller, 1981). Abraham's MLU fluctuates from day to day as well. In a sample collected one month later, his MLU was 4.03. Other aspects of language form are entirely appropriate for Abraham's age. Most of his utterances now are complete sentences with nouns and verbs serving as subjects and predicates. Notice that Abraham now uses both content words and a number of grammatical morphemes (e.g., past tense *-ed*; plural *s*, articles *the* and *a*). Occasionally, we see complex sentences (e.g., "The pictures that I made and colored?").

Compared with the conversation we saw at age twenty-eight months, Abraham's contributions carry much more content. Instead of just providing input when prompted, he is now contributing new information spontaneously. There are still instances in which his meaning is not entirely clear (e.g., "And I made the clouds inside."), but most of the time others can follow his conversations with little effort.

We can clearly see how form, content, and use have developed and interact by revisiting some of the pragmatic functions we saw at twenty-eight months and looking at the form and content now being used to code those functions at thirty-nine months.

What does mine do?	(request for information)
Buy some at the store.	(request for action)
It is a tool.	(labeling)
That looks like a robot.	(commenting)
Mickey doesn't have shoes.	(negating)

At this age, Abraham is not just using language for communication with others, but for imaginative uses as well. He talks about what he is doing even when there is no one to hear or respond to him. The following excerpt was recorded while Abraham played alone with a large doll house and a family of dolls. What we hear is a verbal monologue of his ongoing thoughts as he plays. In this case, he is using language as a tool to organize and encode his thoughts and experiences in a pretend situation.

> Oh, wow, oh man, I need all these guys. There's a bunch of people. I don't want the bunch of people, just a little bit. A little bit means, this is a little bit. Yeah, this is a little bit. (Looks at one figure.) Gross. I don't want you. Well, get your mom and dad. I'll get the mom. I'll get the dad. (Talks for the boy doll.) Mom, could we go to the park? Dad, could we go to the park? This is the park already. Okay, I want to sit right. Let's go over . . . let's take . . . take a nap. Our bed. Oh wow. Your bed is . . . my bed is right down . . . your bed is right down there. That's right. These are not the big people's. No, these are ours. The baby's is right there where his is. Mommy and Daddy are busy down there. You guys, you can't wait to go to the nap like that. You need someone to help you get into bed. You guys already got back into bed and get the baby.

Forty-Four Months

At age four, children's language is adult-like in many respects. We rarely hear violations of language form, although we do hear false-starts and revisions (even adults produce these periodically). At forty-four months, Abraham's MLU is now 5.35, which was no increase in utterance length compared to five months before. In fact, Abraham has now passed the age where MLU is sensitive to gains in language acquisition. This is because his sentences are becoming more complex rather than becoming simply longer. We hear complex verb phrases ("He *wants to get* in there.") and conjoined sentences ("But not the boy, *'cause* he's hiding in a hiding place up there.").

The content of language continues to be dictated by experience. Children must hear new words to learn them (later, reading will contribute significantly to vocabulary growth). When children read a new book, play with others, go new places, or watch television programs, they are exposed to new words. Therefore, the words that children know depend, in large part, on their range of experience, which provides a context for new words to be learned. Once words are acquired, they are available to the child to help frame his or her future experiences and to support further learning. We can see this role of experience in building vocabulary when Abraham's preschool class made a trip to a local fire station. Although he had never been to one before, it was clear that he already had some very specific concepts about what a fire station is like and vocabulary to go along with the experience. In his case, a likely source of this vocabulary was a book that had been read to him many times. A home video captured the following conversation:

(The children enter the fire station.)

Abraham: What is . . . What's that? A fire truck. An old fire truck.

(The children go through the living areas.)

Abraham: We don't have one right here? We don't have a pole here?

Firefighter: We don't have a pole. There's only one or two left in the country that still has a pole and we don't . . .

Abraham: Whoa! Look at this. This is where the firefighter sleeps.

(The children look at the ambulance.)

Abraham: I have a question.

Firefighter: I have an answer. What can I do for you?

Abraham: These are the people that drive the ambulance?

Firefighter: That's right. Do you know I can drive this ambulance? That's my job.

In this conversation, we can see that Abraham is quite confident talking to others, although other children at this age may be shy. He is also beginning to show some of the subtleties of language use. For example, he uses the indirect "I have a question" before asking the actual question. We also see that his use of conversational conventions is still not perfect. Earlier, he asked a question and interrupted the adult before receiving the full answer. He will continue to refine skills within the domain of language use as he grows.

At 4 years of age, Abraham is developing skills in a second language modality—written language. His parents have been looking at books with him and reading to him since his first weeks. Through these activities, he has gained various preliteracy skills. These include awareness of print and the fact that information is carried by it. He also knows a set of social routines associated with reading: looking at a page and listening to the words, turning pages when the reading pauses, and even helping to fill in sentences for books he has heard over and over again. He enjoys both the books themselves and the attention he gets when he sits in his parent's lap to hear a book read. Abraham can identify the individual letters of the alphabet, although he makes some mistakes. He can print his name; typically with a giant A, a backwards b, and a letter or two that wanders above or below the horizontal plane on occasion. By this time next year, he will also recognize a handful of written words as well. All these skills are precursors to successful reading as he enters school. Within a few years of learning to read, this form of language will become an important tool for learning, exchange of ideas, and vocabulary growth.

In four short years, Abraham has gone from an infant, whose only means of expression was crying, to a preschooler whose language contains many of the features one would see in an adult speaker. In this chapter, we have seen the development of language *form* as he progressed from word attempts that were only approximations of the adult phonological form to fully intelligible speech. We saw single words progress to multiword phrases to sentences that contained clauses and complex verbs. We saw increased use of morphology as phrases and sentences emerged. We saw language *content* grow from the restricted meanings of the first few words to the multitude of words whose meanings approximate adult versions. Finally, we saw improvement in the *use* of language for a variety of communication functions. Although certain aspects of language form, content, and use will continue to expand as he grows, his language is, by age four, already a remarkable tool for communication.

Clinical Problem Solving

Here are two language samples obtained from Abraham at two different ages.

Twenty-eight months:

Mother: Is that a taco that you're making?

Abraham: Yeah.

Mother: Where do you eat tacos?

Abraham: With a mat.

Mother: On a placemat?

Abraham: (Pours beans into a bowl.) Put all in.

(They start to fall on the floor.)

Mother: Hey, honey, honey…

Abraham: Oh no, mommy!

Mother: Do you want help with the beans?

Abraham: It's a cooking beans!

Forty-four months:

Abraham: I ate eggs for breakfast.

Author: Did mommy make it?

Abraham: I got a gargoyle and I got a Casper today.

Author: What was the gargoyle on?

Abraham: They're just on my underwear.

Author: Oh, you have gargoyle underwear on.

Abraham: I have them *not* on today!

Author: You have Caspers on today?

Abraham: Yeah.

Look at the transcripts above and consider them from the perspective of language form, content, and use:

1. How has Abraham's language changed from twenty-eight to forty-four months?
2. Do you think that his content is typical of other children at each age? Why or why not?
3. What evidence can you find that Abraham has not yet reached adult-like competence in form, content, and use at each age?

References

Bandura, A. (1969). *Principles of Behavioral Modification*. New York: Holt, Rinehart & Winston.

Bates, E. (1976). Pragmatics and sociolinguistics in child language. In D. Morehead & A. Morehead (Eds.), *Normal and Deficient Child Language*. Baltimore: University Park Press.

Bates, E., Benigni, L., Bretherton, I., Camaioni, L., & Volterra, V. (1977). From gesture to the first word: On cognitive and social prerequisites. In M. Lewis & L. Rosenblum (Eds.), *Interaction, Conversation, and the Development of Language*. New York: Wiley.

Bates, E., & MacWhinney, B. (1987). Competition, variation, and language learning. In B. MacWhinney (Ed.), *Mechanisms of Language Acquisition* (pp. 157–193). Hillsdale, NJ: Lawrence Erlbaum Associates.

Bloom, L. (1988). What is language? In M. Lahey, *Language Disorders and Language Development*, New York: Macmillan.

Brown, R. (1973). *A First Language: The Early Stages*. Cambridge, MA: Harvard University Press.

Brown, R. (1976). *A First Language*. New York: Penguin.

Bruner, J. S. (1975). The ontogenesis of speech acts. *Journal of Child Language*, 2:1–19.

Cartwright, T.A., & Brent, M.R. (1997). Syntactic categorization in early language acquisition: Formalizing the role of distributional analysis. *Cognition, 63*, 121–170.

Chi, J.C., Dooling, F.C., & Gilles, F.H. (1977). Gyral development of the human brain. *Annals of Neurology, 1*:86–93.

Chomsky, N. (1965). *Aspects of the Theory of Syntax*. Cambridge, MA: MIT Press

Chomsky, N. (1988). *Language and Problems of Knowledge: The Managua Lectures*. Cambridge, MA: MIT Press

Clark, E. (1979) What's in a word? On the child's acquisition of semantics in his first language. In V. Lee (Ed.), *Language Development*. New York: Wiley.

Crommer, R. (1988). Differentiating language and cognition. In R.L. Schiefelbusch & L.L. Lloyd (Eds.), *Language Perspectives: Acquisition, Retardation, and Intervention* (2nd ed.). Austin, TX: Pro Ed.

Cruttenden, A. (1979). *Language in Infancy and Childhood*. New York: St. Martin's.

DeCasper, A. B., & Spence, M. B. (1986). Prenatal maternal speech influences newborns' perception of speech sounds. *Infant Behavior and Development, 9*:133–150.

Demetras, M.J., Post, K.N., & Snow, C.E. (1986). Feedback to first language learners: The role of repetitions and clarification questions. *Journal of Child Language, 13*, 275–292.

Geschwind, N. (1977). Specializations of the human brain. *Scientific American, 241*:180-201

Geschwind, N., & Levitsky, W. (1968). Human brain: Asymmetries in temporal speech region. *Science, 7*:5097–5100.

Halliday, M. (1975). *Learning How to Mean: Explorations in the Development of Language*. London: Edward Arnold.

Hubbell, R. (1985). Language and linguistics. In P. Skinner & R. Shelton (Eds.), *Speech, Language, and Hearing* (2nd ed.). New York: Wiley.

Huiskens, L., Coppen, P.A., & Jagtaman, M. (1991). Developing a tool for the description of language acquisition. *Linguistics, 29*, 451–479.

Ingram, D. (1981). Transitivity in child language. *Language, 47*:888–910.

Johnson, W. (1946). *People in Quandaries*. New York: Harper & Row.

Kelly, C.A., & Dale, P.S. (1989). Cognitive skills associated with the onset of multiword utterances. *Journal of Speech and Hearing Research, 32*:645–656.

Kutas, M., & Hillyard, S. A. (1983). Event related brain potentials to grammatical errors and semantic anomalies. *Memory and Cognition, 11*:539–550.

Lahey, M. (1988). *Language Disorders and Language Development*. New York: Macmillan.

Lenneberg, F. (1967). *Biological Foundations of Language*. New York: Wiley.

Locke, J. (1990). Structure and stimulation in the ontogeny of spoken language. *Developmental Psychobiology, 23*:621–643.

McClelland, J., & Rumelhart, D. (1986). A PDP model of the acquisition of morphology. In B. MacWhinney (Ed.), *Mechanisms of Language Acquisition*. Hillsdale, NJ: Lawrence Erlbaum.

McNeill, D. (1970). *The Acquisition of Language*. New York: Harper & Row.

Miller, J. (1981). *Experimental Procedures. Assessing Language Production in Children*. Baltimore, MD: University Park Press.

Molfese, D.L. (1990). Auditory evoked responses recorded from 16 month old infants to words they did and did not know. *Brain and Language, 38*:345–363.

Neville, H., Nicol, B. L., Barss, A., Forster,I., & Garrett, M. (1991). Syntactically based sentence processing classes: Evidence from event related potentials. *Journal of Cognitive Neuroscience, 3*:151–165.

Oller, D. (1980). The emergence of speech sounds in infancy. In G. Yeni-Komshian, J. Kavanaugh, & C. Ferguson (Eds.), *Child Phonology*. Vol. 1. *Production*. New York: Academic Press.

Piaget, J. (1963). *The Origins of Intelligence in Children*. New York: Norton.

Pinker, S. (1984). *Language Learnability and Language Development*. Cambridge, MA: Harvard University Press.

Pinker, S. (1989). Resolving a learnability paradox in the acquisition of the verb lexicon. In M.L. & R.L. Schiefelbusch (Eds.), *The Teachability of Language*. Baltimore: Paul A. Brooks.

Prutting, C., Bagshaw, N., Goldstein, H., Juskowitz, S., & Umen, I. (1978). Clinician-child discourse: Some preliminary questions. *Journal of Speech and Hearing Disorders, 43*:123–129.

Searle, B. (1969). *Speech Acts*. London: Cambridge University Press.

Sinclair-De Zwart, H. (1979). Language acquisition and cognitive development. In V. Lee (Ed.), *Language Development*. New York: Wiley.

Skinner, B. F. (1957). *Verbal Behavior*. New York: Appleton-Century-Crofts.

Staats, A. (1968). *Learning, Language, and Cognition*. New York: Holt, Rinehart & Winston.

Van Petten, C., Weckerly, J., McIsaac, H.K., & Kutas, M. (1997). Working memory dissociates lexical and sentential context effects. *Psychological Science, 8*, 238–242.

Watson, B.B. (1970). *Behaviorism*. New York: Norton.

Chapter 5

Disorders of Hearing
in Children

Anne Marie Tharpe

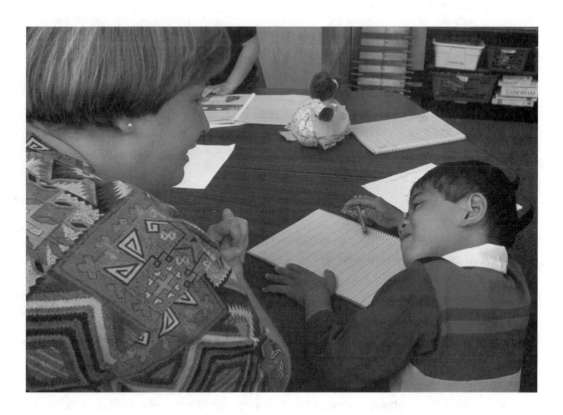

Preview

For the vast majority of children, listening and learning through the auditory modality is a passive and natural process. However, some children experience a hearing loss that impairs their ability to communicate and may require some level of habilitation. Audiologists are uniquely trained professionals with the skills to evaluate the hearing of children of any age, even newborns. Audiologists are also prepared to initiate intervention, provide support and counseling to families, and work with educators and other professionals to design habilitation and educational programs for children with hearing loss. This chapter will begin with a discussion of the various causes, types, and degrees of hearing loss in children. We will investigate the identification and impact of hearing loss on the receptive and expressive communication of children.

Between 1 and 6 per 1000 children experience a hearing loss that impairs their ability to communicate and may require some level of habilitation (Parving, 1993; Watkin, Baldwin, & McEnery, 1991). The presence of a hearing loss can create challenges for the developing child related to communication, education, and socialization. To understand the potential impact for the child, the following questions must be addressed: How severe is the hearing loss? Is it permanent or temporary? Which frequencies are affected by the hearing loss? A hearing test will begin to answer these, and other, questions. The graph that is used by audiologists to plot hearing test results is the audiogram (see Chapter 3). Recall that the audiogram displays frequency (in Hertz) across the top and intensity (in decibels) along the side. Air and bone conduction responses are plotted on the audiogram.

Air conduction audiometry refers to the presentation of speech or pure-tone stimuli transmitted through earphones to the patient. The test signal travels through the ear canal, across the eardrum and middle ear space, to the inner ear, and is ultimately transmitted to the auditory centers in the brain. You can follow the path of an air conducted signal by viewing Figure 5-1A. As you can see, if someone has difficulty hearing a signal by air conduction, the problem could be in any of the areas through which the signal travels.

Bone conduction audiometry refers to the transmission of sounds presented to the patient by a bone vibrator that is usually placed behind the ear on the mastoid bone. The vibrator causes the bones of the skull to vibrate, which in turn stimulate the inner ear or **cochlea**. The cochlea is a labyrinth carved into the skull that is lined with a membranous surface and filled with fluid. When a signal causes the skull to vibrate, the cochlea is stimulated directly and hearing does not depend on the outer and middle ears. You can follow the path of a bone conducted signal by viewing Figure 5-1B. If someone has difficulty hearing by bone conduction, the damage must be in the inner ear or auditory nerve. Such hearing losses result in fairly equal air and bone conduction thresholds, and the condition is known as a sensorineural hearing loss (Figure 5-2A).

When someone demonstrates normal hearing by bone conduction, but has difficulty hearing signals presented by air conduction, the problem must be in the outer or middle ears. This condition is known as a conductive hearing loss (Figure 5-2B). The difference between the air and bone conduction responses is referred to as an air-bone gap. When an individual has both a sensorineural and a conductive hearing loss it is referred to as a **mixed hearing loss** (Figure 5-2C).

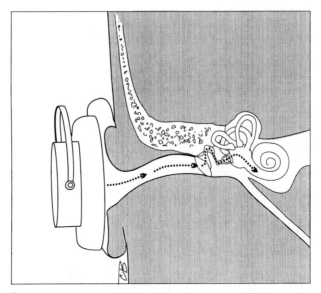

A

B

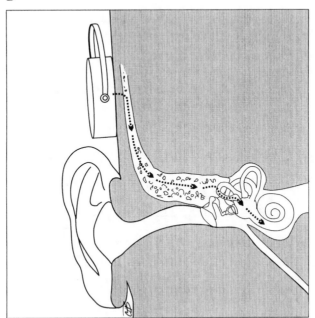

FIGURE 5-1   The two pathways of sound in the ear.
Broken arrows demonstrate the route of (A) air conduction hearing and (B) bone conduction hearing.

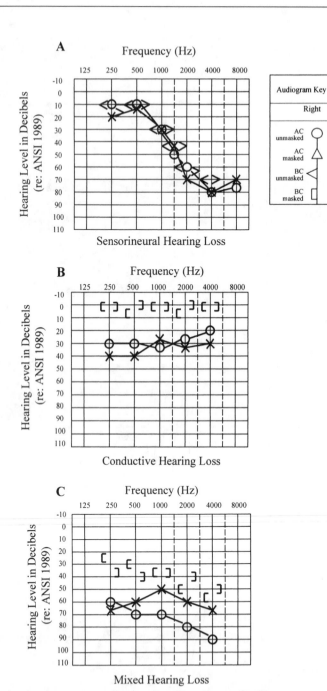

FIGURE 5-2   Pure tone air and bone conduction audiograms. (A) Severe high-frequency sensorineural hearing loss. (B) Mild conductive hearing loss. (C) Moderate to severe mixed hearing loss.

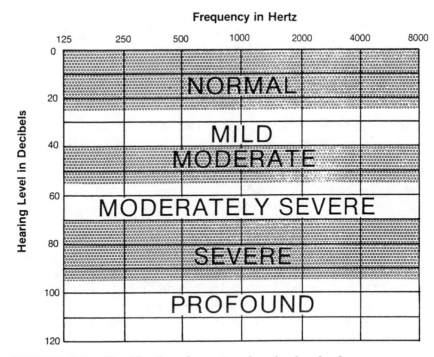

FIGURE 5-3   Classification of pure tone hearing loss by degree.

In addition to classifying the type of hearing loss, the audiogram is also used to classify the degree of hearing loss. Figure 5-3 illustrates a widely accepted classification of the degree of hearing loss.

As valuable as the audiogram is for describing the type and degree of hearing loss, it is important to note that we cannot predict academic, social, or communicative success or limitations from the audiogram alone. It simply defines the line between hearing and not hearing at various frequencies. It does not describe the quality of what is heard or the difficulties that the hearing loss may impose on an individual. Those issues will be addressed later in this chapter.

Auditory Pathologies

Disorders associated with hearing loss in children can be genetic, **congenital** (present at birth), or acquired at any point in development. It is important to note that these categories can overlap. For example, not all genetic disorders are congenital and not all congenital disorders are genetic. For example, mucopolysaccharidoses syndrome (MPS) is a genetically inherited metabolic disorder but children with MPS are normal at birth. Over time, the genetic effect of this disorder results in a progressive hearing loss with age. On the other hand, children whose mothers abuse alcohol during pregnancy may incur damage to the auditory mechanism in utero as one of several symptoms of fetal alcohol syndrome. The resulting hearing loss is congenital, acquired during prenatal development, but not genetic. The estimated percentage of acquired versus genetic hearing loss is illustrated in Figure 5-4. We will review a variety of disorders using the following categories: *genetic without associated abnormalities, genetic with associated abnormalities, acquired prenatally, acquired perinatally,* and *acquired postnatally.*

Genetically Inherited Hearing Loss

As illustrated in Figure 5-4, it is estimated that 50% of all hearing loss is genetically transmitted (or **endogenous**). Approximately two-thirds of genetic hearing losses occur as the only abnormality, and one third occurs in association with additional abnormalities or as part of a syndrome. Pediatric audiologists frequently must draw on knowledge of genetics to counsel families. We see this in the following case:

> Caesar's parents were taken totally by surprise when they were told that he had a moderate sensorineural hearing loss in both ears. After a couple of weeks of thinking and talking with each other about the hearing loss, they returned to Caesar's audiologist and asked him whether their future children were at risk for hearing loss. Although not a geneticist, their audiologist knew that because Caesar had no other risk factors for hearing loss, there was a high likelihood that the hearing loss was the result of a recessive mode of genetic inheritance. After explaining the possible causes of hearing loss to Caesar's parents, they were referred for further genetic counseling.

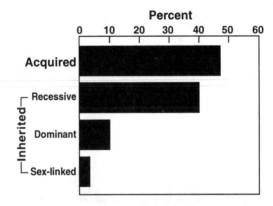

FIGURE 5-4   Percentage of individuals who exhibit acquired and inherited types of hearing loss. (Reprinted with permission from F.H. Bess & L.E. Humes: *Audiology: The Fundamentals* **(2nd ed.), Williams & Wilkins, 1995.)**

Genes occur in pairs and are located on 23 pairs of **chromosomes**. One member of each gene pair is inherited from each parent. Each egg and sperm carries one-half of the chromosomes from each parent so that when the egg is fertilized by the sperm, a child inherits half of the genes from the father and half from the mother. There are three primary patterns of inheritance: *autosomal dominant*, *autosomal recessive*, and *x-linked*.

Autosomal Dominant

Approximately 20% of genetic hearing loss is the result of dominant inheritance (Rose, Conneally, & Nance, 1977). With this type of inheritance, only one copy of the gene is required to transfer the trait to the next generation. As illustrated in Figure 5-5, one parent typically exhibits the trait and each offspring has a 50% chance of inheriting the gene for hearing loss.

This does not mean that half of the children of a parent with an autosomal dominant gene will be affected. It does mean, rather, that each child has a 50% chance of being affected. Furthermore, a dominant type of hearing loss may present a different clinical picture from one child to the next. If different children exibit different features of the same genetic disorder, the disorder is said to have a *variable expression*. In other cases, some children who inherit the gene may not exhibit any features of the syndrome, or the disorder may be very mild. This is known as *reduced penetrance*. Some of the most common types of dominantly inherited syndromes associated with hearing loss can be found in Table 5-1.

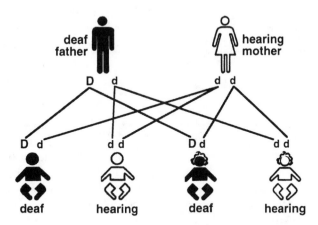

FIGURE 5-5   Persons with dominant deafness have one dominant gene (D) and a corresponding normal gene (d). Each child has a 50/50 chance to inherit the deafness gene (D) from the parent who has this trait. (From Shaver, 1988. Reprinted with permission.)

TABLE 5-1   Genetic Disorders Associated with Hearing Loss

Disorder	Clinical Signs
Autosomal Dominant Disorders	
Waardenburg's syndrome	Pigment abnormalities including a white forelock and different colored irides; unilateral or bilateral sensorineural hearing loss.
Alport's syndrome	Nephritis; ocular lesions; progressive hearing loss.
Stickler syndrome	Ocular anomalies; cleft palate, progressive hearing loss.
Treacher Collins syndrome	Facial malformations including depressed cheek bones, deformed pinna, receding chin; conductive or mixed hearing loss.
Branchio-oto-renal syndrome	Ear malformation; renal anomalies, mixed hearing loss.
Neurofibromatosis	Tumor disorder; variable audiological findings.
Autosomal Recessive Disorders	
Usher syndromes	Retinitis pigmentosa; congenital sensorineural hearing loss.
Friedrich's ataxia	Nervous system disorder; ocular abnormalities; abnormal movement; progressive sensorineural hearing loss.
Hurler's syndrome	Growth failure; mental retardation; progressive hearing loss.
X-linked Disorders	
Hunter's syndrome	Growth failure; mental retardation; mixed or conductive hearing loss.
Norrie's syndrome	Progressive visual impairment; mental retardation, progressive sensorineural hearing loss.
Alport's syndrome	Renal disorder; ocular abnormalities; progressive sensorineural hearing loss.

Autosomal Recessive

Recessive inheritance accounts for the vast majority of genetic hearing loss or approximately 80% (Shaver, 1988). A child must receive two copies of the gene for **hearing impairment** in order for the trait to be expressed. This means the parents of a child with recessive hearing loss each carry one normal and one abnormal gene in the pair so both have normal hearing. However, if their child receives both copies of the abnormal gene, a hearing loss will occur. As shown in Figure 5-6, when both parents are carriers of the recessive gene for hearing loss, each child of that union has a 25% chance of being affected. If only one abnormal gene is inherited, the child will be a carrier for that trait but will not be affected. Some of the more common examples of recessively inherited syndromes that include hearing loss are provided in Table 5-1

Although approximately one in eight individuals carries a gene for hearing loss, there are so many different types of recessive genes for hearing loss that it is extremely rare for two individuals carrying the same gene for hearing loss to mate. When blood relatives mate, referred to as a **consanguineous** union, however, it is more common for recessive hearing loss to appear because of the increased likelihood that parents have inherited the abnormal gene from a common ancestor.

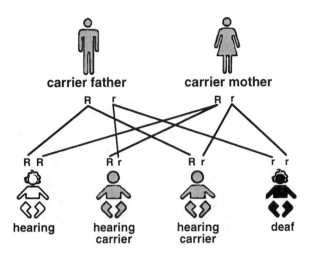

FIGURE 5-6   **Persons with recessive deafness have a double dose of the deafness gene (r), one inherited from each of the parents. The parents are hearing carriers and have a 25% chance to produce a deaf child with each pregnancy. (From Shaver, 1988. Reprinted with permission.)**

X-Linked (also known as sex-linked)

In the x-linked mode of inheritance, traits are determined by genes located on the one pair of 23 chromosomes referred to as the sex chromosomes. Genes for hearing loss can be located on the X chromosome. Females inherit two X chromosomes (one from each parent) and males inherit one X chromosome from their mother and one Y chromosome from their father. As exhibited in Figure 5-7, a female with a recessive gene for hearing loss on one of her X chromosomes will not exhibit hearing loss but each son has a 50% chance of having the trait, and each daughter has a 50% chance of being a carrier. If an affected male's wife is not a carrier, all of their daughters will be carriers and all of their sons will have normal hearing because they inherit the Y chromosome from their father. Approximately 2 to 3% of hearing loss is the result of x-linked transmission.

Acquired Hearing Loss

Acquired hearing losses are those that are caused by factors that are **exogenous** (outside the genes), such as disease, toxicity, or accident. These factors can occur during pregnancy (**prenatally**), shortly before, during, or shortly after delivery (**perinatally**), or after birth (**postnatally**). In the case of prenatal damage, gestational age of the fetus is an important factor in the effect on hearing. For example, if the infection occurs during the development of the organs (**organogenesis**), or during the first trimester, the fetus is more likely to incur damage than when the fetus is exposed later in the gestational period. It is important for pediatric audiologists to be familiar with the **sequelae** (consequences of conditions or events) of these infections in order to appropriately counsel families

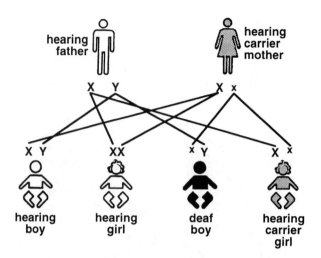

FIGURE 5-7   X-linked recessive deafness is caused by a gene on the X chromosome and occurs only in males. The sons of a woman who is a carrier of x-linked deafness have a 50% chance to be deaf and the daughters have a 50% chance to be carriers. (From Shaver, 1988. Reprinted with permission.)

regarding expectations for their children. For example, some infections result in hearing losses that are progressive and audiologists should prepare families for that eventuality. Other prenatal infections result in hearing losses that are not present at birth but appear later in childhood. Again, the pediatric audiologist is alert to these possibilities and can arrange for periodic audiological monitoring of these children.

STORCH Infections

Many of the pre- and perinatal diseases have come to be known as part of the STORCH complex of infections. STORCH is an acronym for (S)yphilis, (T)oxoplasmosis, (O)ther, (R)ubella, (C)yto-megalovirus, and (H)erpes simplex. All of these diseases put infants at high risk for hearing loss, and each will be discussed here briefly.

Syphilis.   Syphilis is a sexually transmitted disease that can affect the developing fetus. Hearing loss secondary to syphilis may not be present at birth. Onset in infancy is usually associated with bilateral sensorineural hearing loss of sudden onset and rapid progression. When the onset is later in life it is generally a bilateral sensorineural hearing loss with sudden onset and slow progression (Dennis & Neely, 1991; Schuknecht, 1974).

Toxoplasmosis.   Toxoplasmosis is a condition caused by a parasitic infection acquired by adults from accidental ingestion of the parasite. The parasite is found in material contaminated by the feces of cats or by the ingestion of another form of the parasite found principally in raw or undercooked meat (Robillard & Gersdorff, 1986). When the infection is transmitted from mother to fetus, a congenital infection may result that ranges in severity and can be fatal in some cases. Premature birth, mental retardation, blindness, and, less often, deafness have all been linked to toxoplasmosis (Vaughan, McKay, & Behrman, 1979).

Rubella (also known as German Measles).   Hearing loss occurs in 50% of surviving infants exposed to rubella during the first trimester of gestation and is the most common of the rubella defects (Davis & Johnson, 1983). Fetal exposure to the rubella virus after 4 months rarely results in any damage. The sensorineural loss may appear at birth or with delayed onset and may progress or fluctuate over the life of the affected individual (Bergstrom, 1988; Newton & Rowson, 1988). The rubella epidemic of 1964–1965 resulted in more than 20,000 neonates born with congenital rubella syndrome. Although immunization is available, congenital rubella remains a cause of severe to profound sensorineural hearing loss in severely involved children and congenital conductive loss in less severe cases.

Cytomegalovirus.   A member of the herpes group of viruses, cytomegalovirus (CMV) is the leading cause of congenital viral infection and the most common viral agent causing sensorineural hearing loss among neonates. Individuals at greatest risk for serious problems due to CMV are immuno-compromised patients (e.g., those receiving chemotherapy or with HIV) and pregnant women. Transmission occurs through intimate contact and exposure to saliva, urine, feces, or tears. The most likely source of maternal infection is from children because women of childbearing age are frequently care-providers for young children, thus making them highly susceptible to CMV. Ten to 15% of children with congenital CMV demonstrate mental retardation or hearing loss. The hearing loss associated with congenital or prenatally acquired CMV is sensorineural with variable configuration; it can be unilateral or bilateral, mild to profound, and frequently is progressive (Dahle, McCollister, Stagno, Reynolds, & Hoffman, 1979). Onset may occur as late as 7 years of age (Stagno, Reynolds, Amos, Dahle, McCollister, Hohindra, Ermocilla, & Alford, 1977).

Herpes Simplex.   A common sexually transmitted disease, herpes simplex is generally transmitted to the fetus when passing through the birth canal if the mother has an active infection. Ninety-six percent of infected newborns have sequelae including central nervous system involvement, visual impairments, and hearing loss (Gershon, 1981).

Prematurity

Approximately 11% of all births are less than 37 weeks gestation and are considered preterm. Low birthweight due to preterm birth is a strong predictor of developmental problems and mortality. Imagine the concerns of a new mother who has delivered her infant two months early.

Maya weighed only 1450 grams (approximately 3.2 lbs.) at birth and could be held in the palm of one hand. Maya's mother knew from her prenatal classes that premature babies are about 30 times less likely to survive than are full-term infants, and those who survive are at high risk for health and developmental problems. Immediately after birth, Maya had her first test—the APGAR. Fortunately, she scored within normal limits on this measure.

The **APGAR** scoring system was devised in 1953 to quickly identify infants who are severely stressed and in need of resuscitation (Apgar, 1953). The five signs used to score the baby's condition can be remembered easily using the mnemonic (A)ppearance, (P)ulse, (G)rimace, (A)ctivity, and (R)espiration. Immediately prior to birth and during the delivery process, an infant may receive insufficient oxygen across the placenta from her mother. This results in reduced oxygen and increased carbon dioxide in the blood and tissues, or *asphyxia*. Because asphyxia commonly occurs in premature infants who have other medical conditions, it is difficult to pinpoint asphyxia as a cause of hearing loss. Simmons (1980), however, identified asphyxia as the most common high risk factor in the medical histories of babies with hearing loss.

> Maya's mother noticed her daughter's skin was a yellowish color. She was told by her nurse that this was caused by jaundice or hyperbilirubinemia, the result of excessive *bilirubin* (a bile pigment in the blood). Maya seemed to enjoy lying naked under warm lights for her phototherapy (treatment by exposure to light) and in a few days, the yellow tinge to her skin was gone.

If Maya had had a more serious case of jaundice, she would have required a blood transfusion and may have been at risk for hearing loss. Although some researchers have reported that up to 80% of infants surviving hyperbilirubinemia demonstrate some degree of sensorineural hearing loss, others have reported no such relationship (Bergman, Hirsch, Fria, Shapiro, Holzman, & Painter, 1985; de Vries, Lary, & Dubowitz, 1985; Sabo, Brown, & Watchko, 1992; Salamy, Eldredge, & Tooley, 1989).

In addition to these medical concerns, preterm infants are susceptible to bleeding within the skull or *intracranial hemorrhage*. Mental retardation and hearing loss are common sequelae of intracranial hemorrhage (Krishnamoorthy, Shannon, DeLong, Todres, & Davis, 1979).

> In Maya's case, a brain scan showed no evidence of intracranial hemorrhage. Other than being very small, Maya was in good health overall. Once it was clear that Maya's health was not in any danger, her physician recommended that she receive a hearing evaluation by the audiologist. The results of her evaluation were normal. (Later in this chapter, information on hearing testing techniques for infants will be described.) It was required that Maya stay in the hospital until her weight was increased, and then she went home with her mother to begin her new life.

Other premature infants are not as lucky as Maya. Some infants, because they are born before their immune systems are fully developed, are susceptible to a variety of infections. Because of this, they are given medications to help them fight off the bacteria. Some antibiotics (e.g., streptomycin, kanamycin) are known to cause sensorineural hearing loss by damaging structures of the inner ear. In addition, diuretics, commonly used with neonates with chronic lung disease, have been shown to have a negative effect on hearing (Sabo et al., 1992), and when used with other ototoxic drugs, the effects may be multiplied (Salamy et al., 1989). The typical hearing loss associated with ototoxicity is bilateral, sensorineural, and high frequency.

The precise risk of hearing loss associated with each of the factors we have discussed is difficult to establish since premature infants generally have multiple risk factors simultaneously. Consequently, researchers have had heated debates regarding the contributions of each of these risk factors to subsequent hearing loss. As a general rule, however, all premature infants requiring a stay in the neonatal intensive care unit are considered at risk for hearing loss and should have their hearing screened prior to discharge (Davis, Wood, Healy, Webb, & Rowe, 1995).

Postnatal Infections

In contrast to Maya, Cole had an uneventful pre- and postnatal course.

> Cole was the product of a full-term gestation and normal delivery. After 24 hours in the hospital, he and his mother went home. Cole continued to develop normally, babbling and sitting up around 6 months of age, walking and producing his first words around 1 year of age. By the time Cole was in kindergarten, he was quite a precocious child. He seemed to be into everything and was always full of stories about his latest adventures to tell his mother. One day during his first year of kindergarten, Cole had flu-like symptoms. He ran a fever and slept a great deal. After several days with no break in his fever, Cole's mother took him to the doctor. Following a brief examination, his pediatrician instructed Cole's mother to take him to the emergency room at the hospital. A test at the hospital confirmed that Cole had *bacterial meningitis*.

The age at which children are most likely to contract meningitis is 6 to 12 months, however, it is possible for older children to contract the disease as well. Approximately 15% of meningitis survivors have neurologic sequelae that may include seizures, paresis, learning or developmental disabilities, and hearing loss (Kallio, Kilpi, Anttila, & Peltola, 1994). The hearing loss is usually bilateral, sensorineural, mild to profound in degree, and permanent.

> With this knowledge in mind, when Cole was feeling better his physician ordered a hearing test. A pediatric audiologist found that Cole demonstrated a profound hearing loss in both ears.

Audiologists should be seeing fewer cases like Cole in the future. The recent release of a preventive vaccine should result in a marked decline in hearing loss secondary to meningitis (Klein, 1994; Stein & Boyer, 1994).

Viral infections can also lead to hearing loss. A common viral cause of unilateral sensorineural hearing loss in children is mumps. The associated hearing loss occurs suddenly and can range in severity from mild to profound. Approximately 5% of mumps patients acquire hearing loss (Vuori, Lahikainen, & Peltonen, 1962). *Measles* is another viral cause of sensorineural hearing loss in children. Approximately 10% of those with measles have resulting hearing loss. The pattern is typically a bilateral severe-to-profound, high frequency hearing loss (Bergstrom, 1984).

Other Hearing High Risk Factors

Fetal Alcohol Syndrome (FAS)

One of the most common birth defects today, FAS has been estimated to occur in one of every 750 live births (Streissguth, Landesman-Dwyer, Martin, & Smith, 1980). FAS, and the milder version called fetal alcohol effects (FAE), result from drinking during pregnancy because alcohol affects the developing fetus. FAS is characterized by mental retardation, low birthweight, and abnormal facial features (Clarren & Smith, 1978). Only a few investigations of hearing status in this population have been conducted, however, they suggest a high incidence of recurrent otitis media and bilateral sensorineural hearing loss (Church & Gerkin, 1988; Streissguth, Clarren, & Jones, 1985).

Persistent Pulmonary Hypertension of the Newborn (PPHN)

Also known as persistent fetal circulation, PPHN is a cardiac abnormality exhibiting persistence of the fetal vessel joining the pulmonary artery to the aorta, which results in deficient oxygenation of the blood, or severe hypoxemia. Twenty to 40% of infants diagnosed with PPHN have sensorineural hearing loss (Leavitt, Watchko, Bennett, & Folsom, 1987; Sell, Gaines, Gluckman, & Williams, 1985; Walton & Hendricks-Munoz, 1991). The onset of hearing loss is thought to be related to the combined effects of the very medical procedures (e.g., drug therapy, ventilation) used to keep these babies alive (Hendricks-Munoz & Walton, 1988; Walton & Hendricks-Munoz, 1991). Hearing loss associated with PPHN has been described as bilateral, progressive, and sensorineural, with variability in degree and the possibility of delayed onset (Hendricks-Menoz & Walton, 1988; Naulty, Weiss, & Herer, 1986).

Otitis Media

Inflammation of the middle ear space, or **otitis media**, is the most frequent cause of hearing loss in young children. Approximately one-third of children in the United States have recurrent and severe middle ear disease by age 3; the peak age for acute otitis media is 7 to 12 months (Klein, 1992). Hearing loss associated with otitis media when fluid is present in the middle ear (called otitis media with **effusion** [OME]) is conductive, unilateral or bilateral, and fluctuates. The average hearing loss caused by otitis media is between approximately 25 and 30 dB (Brookhouser, Worthington, & Kelly, 1993; Fria, Cantekin, & Eichler, 1985). Several factors contribute to the likelihood of the occurrence of otitis media (Table 5-2). These include placement in day care centers (Alho, Koivu, Sorri, & Rantakallio, 1990; Pukander, 1982; Sipila, Karma, Pukander, Timonen, & Kataja, 1988), parental smoking (Sipila et al., 1988; Stahlberg, Ruuskanen, & Virolainen, 1986), and the autumn season (Alho, Oja, Koivu, & Sorri, 1995). Antibiotic therapy is the most common form of treatment for OME. The insertion of tubes into the eardrum for treatment of OME usually eliminates the conductive hearing loss by allowing drainage of middle ear fluid and is the most common operation for children in the United States and usually completely eliminates conductive hearing loss by allowing drainage of middle ear fluid (Kleinman, Kosecoff, DuBois, & Brook, 1994).

TABLE 5-2   High Risk Factors for Middle Ear Disease in Children

1. First episode of acute otitis media prior to 6 months of age
2. Infants who have been bottle-fed
3. Children with craniofacial anomalies, stigmata, or other findings associated with syndromes known to affect the outer and middle ear
4. Ethnic populations with documented increased incidence of outer and middle ear disease (e.g., Native American and Eskimo populations)
5. Family history of chronic or recurrent OME
6. Children in group day care settings or crowded living conditions
7. Children exposed to excessive cigarette smoke
8. Children diagnosed with sensorineural hearing loss, learning disabilities, behavior disorders, or developmental delays and disorders

From Bluestone and Klein (1996).

Degree of Hearing Loss and Its Effect on Communication

The identification of hearing loss is usually a bit different for children than for adults. Hearing loss in adults has been defined as an average of greater than 25 dB of the thresholds at the frequencies 500, 1000, 2000, and 3000 Hz (American Academy of Otolaryngology and American Council of Oto-laryngology, 1979). In children, however, hearing loss is frequently regarded as an average threshold of greater than 20 or even 15 dB over the same range of frequencies (Northern & Downs, 1991). After all, young children are in the process of learning speech and language and cannot always "fill in the gaps" of conversation the way that adults can. If some words or sounds are missed in conversation, an adult can often determine what was said by the context. For example, if an adult hears "*The ole of my shoe needs repairing,*" he or she will figure out that the misunderstood word must be "sole" based on the other key words in the sentence. Children, on the other hand, do not have the extensive vocabularies, linguistic experiences, or strategies to assist them in interpreting misunderstood words. Even a slight hearing loss can result in speech perception that is missing critical vowel or consonant sounds. In reviewing Figure 5-8, note that the unvoiced consonants /th/, /f/, /k/, /t/ fall at or below normal hearing thresholds for soft conversational speech.

An audiogram will provide a good starting place for understanding the impact of a hearing loss, because greater degrees of loss are typically associated with more severe consequences to the individual. We can see this relationship in Table 5-3. However, it is impossible to characterize the type or severity of communication problems an individual child with hearing impairment will have from

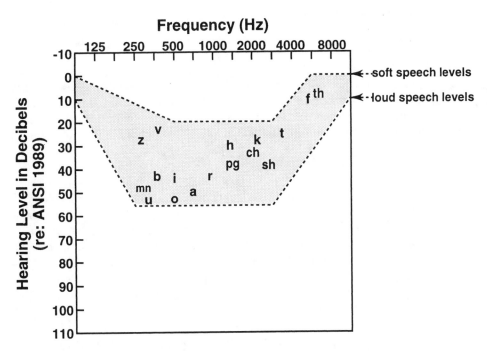

FIGURE 5-8 **Distribution of various speech sounds at conversational levels. (Adapted with permission from F.H. Bess & L.E. Humes: *Audiology: The Fundamentals,* 2nd ed., Williams & Wilkins, 1995.)**

TABLE 5-3   Impact of Hearing Loss

Minimal Hearing Loss (16 to 25 dB HL)	At 15 dB a student can miss up to 10% of the speech signal when a teacher is at a distance greater than 3 feet and when the classroom is noisy.
Mild Hearing Loss (26 to 40 dB HL)	With a 30 dB loss, a student can miss 25–40% of a speech signal. Without amplification, the child with 35–40 dB loss may miss at least 50% of class discussion.
Moderate Hearing Loss (41 to 55 dB HL)	Child understands conversational speech at a distance of 3–5 feet (face-to-face) only if structure and vocabulary controlled. Without amplification, the amount of speech signal missed can be 50–75% with a 40 dB loss, and 80–100% with a 50 dB loss.
Moderate to Severe Hearing Loss (56 to 70 dB HL)	Without amplification, conversation must be very loud to be understood. A 55 dB loss can cause a child to miss up to 100% of speech information.
Severe Hearing Loss (71 to 90 dB HL)	Without amplification, may hear loud voices about 1 foot from ear. When amplified optimally, children with hearing ability of 90 dB or better should be able to identify environmental sounds and detect all the sounds of speech.
Profound Hearing Loss ($\geq$ 91 dB HL)	Aware of vibrations more than tonal patterns. May rely on vision rather than hearing as primary avenue for communication and learning.
Unilateral Hearing Loss (Normal hearing in one ear with the other ear exhibiting at least a mild permanent loss.)	May have difficulty hearing faint or distant speech. Usually has difficulty localizing sounds and has greater difficulty understanding speech in background noise.

the audiogram alone. Many factors contribute to communication ability such as severity, configuration, and age of onset of hearing loss. Additional factors such as intelligence, extent and quality of intervention, and family support also influence a child's communication development. With those factors in mind, we will attempt to describe general effects of hearing loss on communication in the following scenarios.

Julia, age 7, has a mild conductive hearing loss (15–30 dB) bilaterally. Julia's hearing loss is the result of otitis media with effusion (OME). This temporary loss should disappear as the middle ear fluid resolves. As can be seen in Figure 5-9, Julia has a mild hearing loss that is "flat" in that all frequencies are affected to a similar degree. She can hear vowels clearly but has some difficulty hearing voiceless consonants. As shown in the figure, Julia cannot hear the fricatives (/f/, /th/, /v/, /z/) because they are below her threshold. This type of hearing loss would be similar to trying to listen with cotton balls in your ears. Her teachers noticed that Julia seemed to have difficulty paying attention in class and frequently appeared to daydream.

Numerous studies suggest that some children with recurrent bouts of otitis media are at risk for language delays or disorders. However, the research has not been clear regarding the long-term effects of otitis media on speech and language, that is, the impact after the otitis media has cleared up.

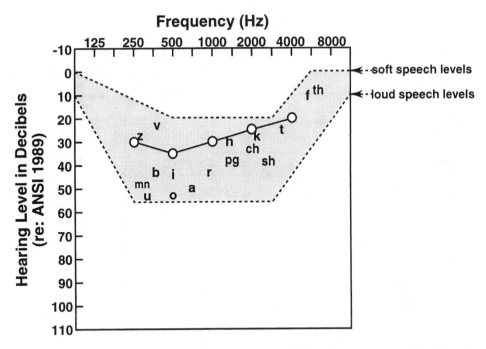

FIGURE 5-9 **Effects of a mild hearing loss on ability to hear conversational levels of speech.**

Suzanne, age 10, has a mild to moderate hearing loss (30–50 dB) bilaterally. As illustrated in Figure 5-10, without her hearing aids, Suzanne missed almost all of the speech sounds at normal conversational loudness levels. She can hear vowels better than consonants and has difficulty discriminating between consonants. Therefore, she misunderstands similar-sounding words such as *sue, shoe, two, coo*. In addition, her speech is sometimes difficult to understand because she frequently distorts or omits consonants. Suzanne is considered at risk for academic problems even though her hearing loss is relatively mild (Tharpe & Bess, 1991).

Catherine, age 2 years, has a severe to profound sensorineural hearing loss (80 sloping to 100 dB) bilaterally. Catherine's parents initially requested a hearing test because they were concerned about her lack of speech and language development. As illustrated in Figure 5-11, she cannot hear conversational level speech or many environmental sounds. Catherine can hear loud environmental sounds and loud speech if the speaker is close by. Without the use of hearing aids, Catherine will not develop speech. Even though she now uses hearing aids, she still exhibits severe speech and language deficits. Her speech is characterized by excessive nasality, substitutions, omissions, intrusive voicing, restricted range of voice pitch, and extended duration of phonation.

Roy, age 9 years, has a profound hearing loss (90 dB or greater) in his right ear with normal hearing in his left ear. Roy's parents never noticed that he had difficulty hearing until age 4 when they observed that he would always switch the telephone to his left ear

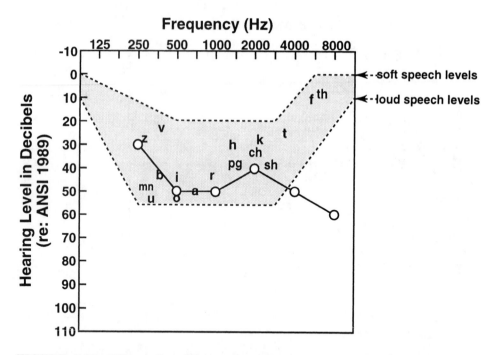

FIGURE 5-10   Effects of a mild to moderate hearing loss on ability to hear conversational levels of speech.

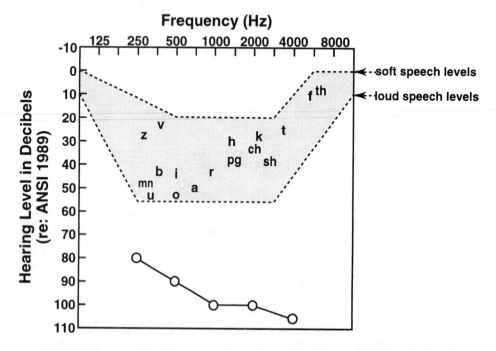

FIGURE 5-11   Effects of a severe to profound hearing loss on ability to hear conversational levels of speech.

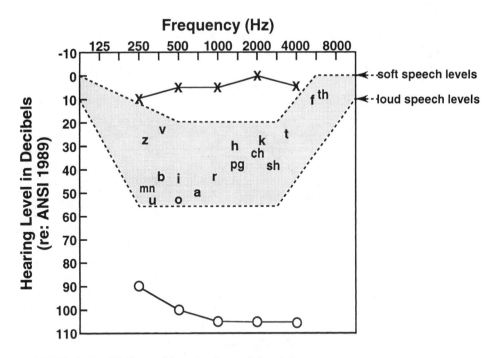

FIGURE 5-12   Unilateral hearing loss of the right ear.

when his grandparents called him. When he started school at age 5, Roy's teacher reported problems of inattention and daydreaming. Figure 5-12 demonstrates Roy's unilateral hearing loss. It was once believed that such losses would result in little if any problems as long as a child was seated preferentially in the classroom, with the normal hearing ear toward the teacher. Unilateral hearing losses, however, have been found to put children at risk for communication and academic problems (Bess & Tharpe, 1986). In fact, approximately 30% of children with unilateral hearing loss have been found to need grade repetition or resource assistance in school (Bess & Tharpe, 1986; Oyler, Oyler & Matkin, 1988).

Audiological Testing

In the last decade, several organizations and lawmakers have called for earlier identification and intervention of infants with hearing impairment (Healthy People 2000, 1990; Joint Committee on Infant Hearing, 1994; NIH, 1993). As a result, audiologists are identifying and evaluating younger children than ever before. This evaluation of infants and children requires the use of behavioral and electrophysiological test procedures.

Behavioral Testing

Even with the widespread use of advanced technological evaluation tools, behavioral testing remains a valuable part of hearing assessment for children. The behavioral technique employed depends largely on the age and developmental level of the child. Some general principles hold across all behavioral tests. Testing is conducted in sound-treated rooms that meet the requirements for accurate measurements set forth by the American National Standards Institute (1991). Test signals are increased and decreased systematically until the softest level at which the infant or child responds (usually 50% of the time) is reached. This level is called the *threshold* or *minimum response level* (*MRL*) in the case of young infants because they may actually hear a sound at a lower level to which they are able or willing to respond. Thresholds or MRLs can be determined via earphones for air conduction testing, via a bone vibrator for bone conduction testing, or via loud speakers for soundfield testing.

When testing is conducted via earphones or a bone vibrator, one problem that must be addressed is *cross-over*. This refers to the fact that the two ears are not totally isolated, and sometimes a sound going to one ear can cause the skull to vibrate and actually stimulate the other, or nontest, ear. The audiologist must eliminate participation of the nontest ear during testing. To do so, noise is delivered to the nontest ear with a frequency spectrum similar to the test signal, but at a higher intensity, so that any sound crossing over from the test ear will not be heard. This is called masking noise, and responses obtained in this manner are referred to as *masked thresholds*.

Behavioral testing usually begins with the use of speech stimuli. A *speech reception threshold* is determined by asking the child to repeat two-syllable words that have equal stress on each syllable, called **spondaic words**. These are words such as *baseball*, *hotdog*, or *airplane*. For children whose speech is difficult to understand, or if they are shy, they may point to the picture of the word that they heard rather than say the word. If a child is unable to repeat words or identify pictures, a *speech awareness threshold* is obtained that simply identifies the softest intensity level at which a child responds. Pure tone air conduction testing is typically done next. Several techniques for obtaining pure tone thresholds from children of different ages are discussed below.

Behavioral Observation Audiometry

For infants from birth to approximately 5 months of age, *Behavioral Observation Audiometry* (*BOA*) is typically employed. With this technique, the audiologist looks for gross body movements such as eye-widening, startles, breathing changes, facial grimaces, or cessation of movements that are time-locked with sound presented through speakers. Although POA is a useful clinical procedure for infants, responses are highly variable and subjective (Moore & Wilson, 1978). One reason that BOA is so subjective is that the infant's responses to sound are variable and open to the observer's interpretation. Thus, BOA allows only a limited number of responses before the infant gradually adapts, or **habituates**, to the sound. With maturation, the child responds to lower and lower signal intensity levels until approximately 2 years of age (Thompson & Weber, 1974). These factors contribute to a wide range of results in normally developing infants, so it is impossible to define hearing loss as a change or deviation from this "norm" (Thompson & Weber, 1974). Rather than measuring the softest sound that infants can hear, audiologists measure the lowest level at which they respond to sound (the *minimum response level*). Therefore, BOA is probably best viewed as a hearing screening assessment procedure that allows one to conclude that an infant's hearing is grossly within or outside the range of normal hearing.

Visual Reinforcement Audiometry (VRA)

Visual Reinforcement Audiometry is a procedure that addresses many of the problems inherent in BOA. Used for infants and young children from approximately 6 months to 2 years of age, VRA depends on the child's natural inclination to turn toward a sound source. The schematic in Figure 5-13

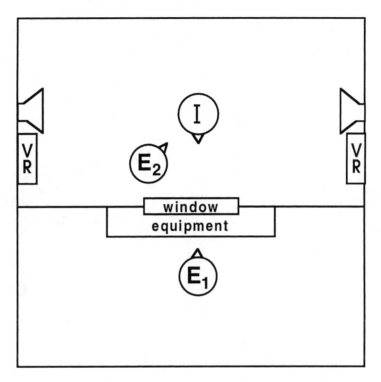

**FIGURE 5-13   Typical two-room test suite arrangement for
conducting VRA. E1 = Examiner 1, E2 = Examiner 2, I =
Infant, VR = Visual Reinforcer.**

illustrates the VRA procedure. An infant (I) is seated in a high chair or parent's lap facing forward toward an observation window. Examiner 1 (E_1) is in a darkened room and cannot be seen by the infant. When E_1 determines that the infant is in a quiet state, an auditory signal is delivered through earphones or speakers. When the infant turns in response to the signal, a toy in a Plexiglas box, the visual reinforcer (VR), is animated and lights up on the side where the sound emanated. Examiner 2 (E_2) (perhaps the infant's parent) serves as an assistant who is needed to keep the infant content and sitting quietly during the test.

Figure 5-14 illustrates several aspects of the VRA procedure. In the first panel of Figure 5-14, note that the assistant who is in the booth with the baby is wearing earphones. Because the infant is being tested through speakers, the assistant is wearing earphones with masking music or noise to keep from accidentally cuing the infant when a sound occurs. The middle panel demonstrates the use of earphones in the VRA procedure in order to obtain individual ear information from the infant. The bottom panel illustrates the infant head-turn to the sound being reinforced by the mechanical toy.

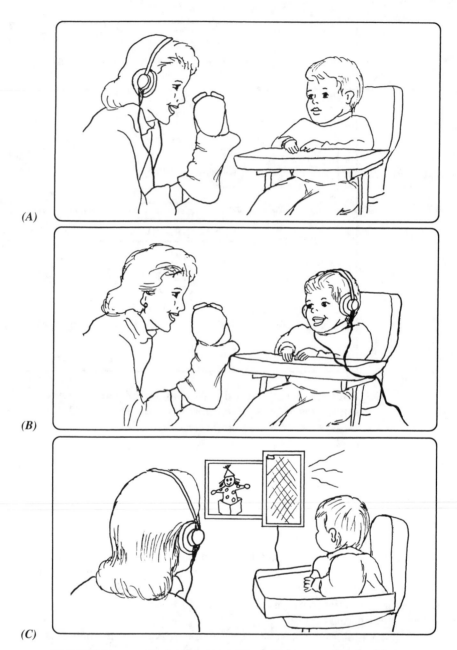

(A)

(B)

(C)

FIGURE 5-14   Illustrations of various aspects of visual reinforcement audiometry (VRA). Panel A illustrates the assistant with masking earphones on while the child is being tested through speakers. Panel B illustrates the VRA procedure with the infant wearing earphones. Panel C illustrates the infant head-turn in response to sound and the subsequent animation of the mechanical toy as reinforcement.

Tangible Reinforcement Operant Conditioning Audiometry (TROCA)

At approximately 2 to 2 1/2 years of age, play audiometry becomes the behavioral technique of choice. *Tangible Reinforcement Operant Conditioning Audiometry (TROCA)* is one form of play audiometry developed by Lloyd and colleagues (Lloyd, Spradlin, & Reid, 1968). For this technique, the child is conditioned to push a button when a sound is heard. The button push is followed by the delivery of an edible reinforcement controlled by the examiner. The reinforcement is small, preferably sugarless, and quick to eat. The treat may be varied to keep a restless or experienced child's interest. More traditional play audiometric techniques include placement of a peg in a pegboard or a block in a box when the child hears the sound. The audiologist chooses tasks that are fun and interesting to the child.

Speech Discrimination Testing

As discussed earlier in this chapter, the pure tone audiogram does not tell precisely how well a person understands the most important sound stimulus, speech. *Speech discrimination* testing is usually conducted after pure tone testing for children who are approximately 3 years of age or older. Unlike threshold tests, speech discrimination testing is conducted at a comfortable loudness level in an attempt to determine the child's ability to understand conversational speech. Typical materials for discrimination testing consist of monosyllabic words that can be repeated or pointed to on picture cards.

Auditory Brainstem Response Testing

Sometimes valid behavioral tests cannot be obtained from children. This may be because the child is too young (under 4 or 5 months of age) or uncooperative due to behavioral or developmental disabilities. For those children, alternative testing procedures that do not require voluntary responses are quite useful. You will recall from Chapter 2 that information about sounds must be transmitted from the inner ear to the brain via the brainstem pathways. The **auditory brainstem response** (ABR) reflects the electrical activity along the auditory pathway rather than testing hearing directly. A waveform can be recorded in response to acoustic stimuli with electrodes placed on the scalp and on the earlobes or mastoids of the patient. The normal waveform consists of five waves that occur at specific time intervals or latencies. At high intensity levels (approximately 80 dB), all five waves should be observable. One of these waves (V) is observable even with very soft intensity levels, within approximately 10 dB of true auditory threshold. It is this feature of the ABR that is useful for estimating hearing threshold. Since a child does not have to provide a voluntary response and can even be asleep for this test, the ABR makes a valuable contribution to the pediatric test battery, particularly for children who are unable or unwilling to cooperate for behavioral testing.

Immittance Audiometry

A standard component of the pediatric test battery is immittance audiometry, which includes *tympanometry* and *acoustic reflex thresholds*. Tympanometry is a measurement of the mobility of the middle ear system as air pressure is varied in the external auditory canal. It is a valuable tool for identifying the presence of middle ear fluid associated with otitis media and other middle ear pathologies commonly seen in children. The procedure is quick and painless, making it ideal for children. A rubber tipped probe is inserted gently into the child's ear canal, and air pressure is pumped into the cavity formed between the end of the probe and the eardrum (tympanic membrane). As the air pressure in the cavity is varied above and below ambient air pressure, the middle ear mobility is measured and plotted on a graph called a *tympanogram*. In a normally functioning ear, maximum middle ear mobility should occur at or near ambient air pressure. This is an important measurement because pathology, such as otitis media, will influence the movement of the eardrum.

The acoustic reflex threshold is the lowest intensity required to elicit a contraction of the middle ear muscle. This contraction can be evoked by introducing a loud sound (usually a pure tone) to the ear canal either through the probe or through an earphone placed on the opposite ear from the probe. This test provides information about the functioning of the middle and inner ear as well as the auditory nerve. In a normal functioning ear, a reflex is elicited when the sound is between about 65 and 95 dB. A hearing loss may result in an elevation of the sound needed to evoke the acoustic reflex or an absence of it altogether. If middle ear fluid is present or the acoustic nerve is damaged, it may also affect the acoustic reflex. The acoustic reflex thresholds, viewed in conjunction with the tympanogram and audiogram, can assist the pediatric audiologist in determining the type and degree of hearing loss.

Otoacoustic Emissions

Evoked otoacoustic emissions (OAEs) were discovered in 1978 (see Chapter 2) and have quickly been incorporated into the audiologist's clinical armamentarium. Although there are several types of evoked OAEs, they are all produced by presenting sound to the ear and then examining the sound recorded by a miniature microphone in the ear canal. The presence of OAEs suggests a normal functioning cochlea; absent or reduced OAEs are the result of conductive or cochlear hearing loss. Like immittance audiometry, this tool is particularly useful for children because it is quick, painless, and requires no voluntary response.

It is important to note that no one test should be depended upon when testing infants or young children. Rather, a battery of tests is used by pediatric audiologists. Let us look at a typical evaluation.

Juan's mother brought him in for a hearing evaluation at age 2 years because of concern about his lack of speech and language development. Juan had several aunts and uncles on his mother's side of the family with hearing loss so she was particularly concerned that his hearing might be a factor in his communication problems. His medical history included a normal gestation and delivery, a few colds and upper respiratory infections, and several episodes of otitis media that had been treated with antibiotics. When testing began, Juan refused to wear earphones by crying and yanking them off. As an alternative to the earphones, Juan was tested in soundfield through speakers utilizing visual reinforcement audiometry. Responses were consistent with a mild (35–45 dB) hearing loss for all of the test frequencies and speech. In an effort to determine if the hearing loss was conductive or sensorineural, the audiologist attempted to put a bone vibrator on Juan. Again, he resisted the placement of anything on his head so the audiologist had to abandon that tactic. By having an assistant blow bubbles to distract him while he sat on his mother's lap, the audiologist was able to place the probe for tympanometry in his ear canal and obtain a tympanogram. The results were consistent with the presence of middle ear fluid in both ears. Even though the audiologist was not able to obtain all of the test results that she would like, the overall pattern of the test results (i.e., the mild hearing loss and abnormal tympanograms) suggested that the hearing loss was conductive. She then recommended that Juan be seen by his pediatrician for treatment of the middle ear fluid, and then return for another hearing test to determine if his hearing loss resolved following medical treatment.

Hearing Screening

One of the many responsibilities of the pediatric audiologist is to organize and oversee the **screening** of neonates, infants, preschoolers, and school-age children for hearing loss and middle ear disease (otitis media). The process of screening involves identifying those at risk for hearing loss or ear disease so they can be referred for further evaluation. Screening tests provide a quick, simple, safe, valid, reliable, and cost-effective means of identification of risk status; they are not intended to diagnose hearing loss.

Guidelines for screening procedures are available for children at various ages. For infants, both brainstem response testing and evoked otoacoustic emissions are used for screening purposes. The Joint Committee on Infant Hearing (1994) and the American Speech-Hearing-Language Association (ASHA) (1997) recommend screening infants with identified indicators associated with sensorineural or conductive hearing loss if screening for all newborns is not available. As recently as 1995, eighteen states had mandated newborn hearing screening statutes or regulations (Tharpe & Clayton, 1997).

ASHA (1997) recommended screening preschoolers who have any indicators associated with late-onset or progressive hearing loss or parental or health care provider concerns regarding hearing, speech, language, or developmental delay. Play audiometric techniques are recommended although visual reinforcement audiometry may be used if necessary. ASHA (1997) recommended screening school-age children upon initial entry to school, and annually in kindergarten through third grade, and in seventh and eleventh grades. Further, all children entering special education, those repeating a grade, or entering the school system without evidence of having passed a previous hearing screening are typically screened. In addition, school-age children reporting exposure to high levels of noise should receive a hearing screening. The recommended screening procedure is play or conventional audiometry with earphones.

There has been considerable debate on the issue of *who* should be screened for middle ear disease. Some professionals feel that *all* children should be screened while others believe only those considered at greatest risk for middle ear disease should be screened. Currently, ASHA has left that decision to each individual screening program (1997). ASHA recommended a middle ear screening protocol that includes a case history from the parent or guardian; visual inspection of the ears to identify risk factors for outer and middle ear disease, and any contraindications for performing tympanometry; examination of the external ear canal and tympanic membrane; and tympanometry with a screening or diagnostic tympanometer (1997).

Management of Children with Hearing Impairment

Once hearing loss has been identified and described in terms of type and degree, a decision regarding the most appropriate intervention, medical or audiological, or both, must be made. Consideration is given to possible medications, surgical interventions, or the fitting of hearing aids. As a general rule, conductive types of hearing loss are most likely to benefit from surgical approaches or amplification whereas the options for sensorineural hearing losses are usually limited to amplification.

Amplification

The early identification of hearing loss in children has little value if intervention is not initiated in a timely manner. The first, and perhaps the most important, step in intervention is the fitting of appropriate sound amplification. It is the role of the pediatric audiologist to ensure that children receive a consistent and audible speech signal at intensity levels that are safe and comfortable. The Pediatric Working Group (1996) developed recommendations for fitting amplification on infants and children. Although no hard and fast rules exist regarding the specific degree of hearing loss at which amplification should be fit, the group concurred that any child with thresholds exceeding 25 dB HL should be considered a candidate for amplification. This includes children with unilateral or bilateral hearing loss.

There are several different types of hearing aids available today. These include (1) *the body aid*, (2) *behind-the-ear aid* (*BTE*), (3) *in-the-ear aid* (*ITE*), and (4) *in-the-canal aid* (*ITC*). These are worn by both adults and children (see Chapter 6 for a photograph of these types of aids). By far, the most common hearing aid type for children is the BTE (see Figure 5-15). All of these hearing aid types contain similar internal components and function similarly. The hearing aid microphone picks up the acoustic signal and converts it to an electrical signal that is amplified (made louder), filtered, and converted back to an acoustic signal by a receiver. In BTEs, the amplified sound is routed to the child's ear by tubing that leads to an earmold. The earmold is made specifically for an individual child's ear, allows the sound to be directed to the ear canal, and keeps the hearing aid in place.

It is particularly important when fitting children to know exactly how much the sound is being amplified since it is difficult or impossible for an infant or young child to tell you when the amplified sound is too loud or not loud enough. Although initial hearing aid settings can be made with computerized prescriptive formulae, amplified sound levels are typically verified by an audiologist using *probe microphone measures*. A probe microphone is one that is small enough to be inserted into the ear canal of a child while the hearing aid is worn (see Figure 5-16). A sound signal is presented from

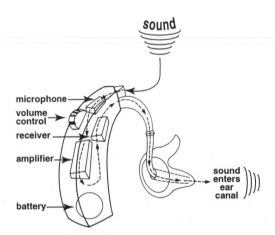

FIGURE 5-15   Schematic of a behind-the-ear hearing aid.

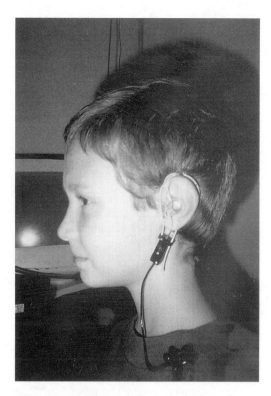

FIGURE 5-16   Probe microphone measurements with a cooperative child.

a small speaker and the probe microphone system records the intensity level of the test signal amplified through the hearing aid from within the child's ear canal. Several techniques are available for making needed measurements quickly from a child.

Sometimes, traditional hearing aids are not sufficient to overcome the hearing deficits of those with profound hearing losses. An alternative to traditional hearing aids for those children is the **cochlear implant**. The cochlear implant is a surgically implanted device with electrodes that are coiled into the cochlea to stimulate the auditory nerve with electrical current (see Figure 5-17). A microphone is worn on the child's ear, in a casing that looks like a hearing aid, and converts the acoustic signal to an electrical signal. The electrical signal is modified by a processor and is then sent to a receiver worn behind the child's ear. The signal is then transmitted through the skin to an internal receiver implanted in the mastoid bone where it is transmitted to electrodes implanted in the cochlea. Although cochlear implants do not restore normal hearing, and children vary markedly in terms of the benefits received from the implant, most children experience at least an awareness of sound and benefit from the prosodic aspects of speech. The pediatric audiologist assists in determining whether a child is an appropriate candidate for the cochlear implant, counsels families on the benefits and limitations of the implant, sets the stimulus levels of the speech processor after implantation, and works with the child to develop or improve listening skills.

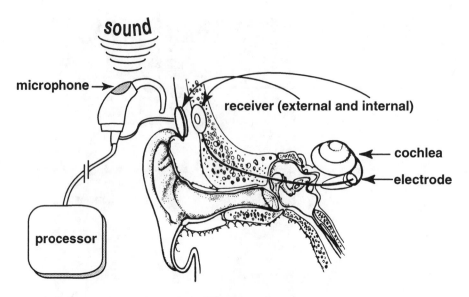

FIGURE 5-17   Schematic of a cochlear implant.

Communication and Education Approaches

One of the most difficult decisions facing parents of a child newly identified with hearing loss is how to communicate most effectively with their child. The most common communication options are *auditory-oral*, *total communication*, and *manual* modes. Auditory-oral communication emphasizes listening and oral communication. A total communication approach includes listening, speech reading, signing, finger spelling, and oral expression. A manual mode of communication uses one of the signed languages, typically without oral speech. The decision regarding which communication mode to adopt usually is highly influenced by the degree of the child's hearing loss. Children with mild or moderate hearing losses generally use an auditory-oral approach because they have a considerable amount of residual hearing. Children with severe to profound hearing loss, however, may have a more difficult time acquiring spoken language and may require the additional visual input afforded by a total or manual communication approach. It is not uncommon, however, for children or their parents to adopt communication modes for cultural reasons. For example, when a child with moderate hearing loss is born to parents who are deaf and who use a manual communication approach, the child is most likely to use a manual approach also. Many factors, audiological, educational, and cultural, are considered when choosing the communication mode that is best for an individual family. After all, the best communication mode is the one that will be most comfortable for the entire family to use.

Federal law has strongly influenced the education of children with hearing loss. Public Law 99-457, or Individuals with Disabilities Education Act (IDEA), was intended to fulfill four primary purposes: (1) to ensure that all children with handicaps have available to them a *free, appropriate public education* that emphasizes special education and related services designed to meet their unique needs; (2) to ensure that the rights of handicapped children and their parents or guardians are protected; (3) to help states pay for education of all children with handicaps; and (4) to ensure and assess the effectiveness of educational programs. Children who are deaf or hard-of-hearing are covered by this legislation. Under PL 99-457, *deaf* means a hearing impairment that is so severe that the child is impaired in processing linguistic information through hearing, with or without amplification, which adversely affects educational performance. *Hard-of-hearing* means a hearing loss, permanent or fluctuating, that adversely affects a child's educational performance. Children with handicaps from birth to age 3 years and their families are provided with early intervention programs under Part H of PL 99-457. Part B provides free and appropriate public education and related services to children with disabilities 3 to 5 years of age.

Whereas in the past, children with hearing loss received their education in segregated schools and classrooms, most are now enrolled in general education programs in their local schools with their normal hearing peers. This trend is referred to as *inclusion* and may occur on a full-time or part-time basis. If additional services are needed for these children, they may attend resource classrooms by leaving their general education classroom for short periods during the day. Another alternative is to receive additional support from an itinerant teacher who travels from class to class. Special services are designed to meet the unique needs of children with hearing loss and maximize the benefit they receive from their educational program. These special services may include speech-language pathology, audiology, psychology, counseling, or physical therapy, among others.

The role of the audiologist in the schools is an important one. Duties include developing and supervising the school's hearing screening program, monitoring the hearing of children identified with hearing loss, participating in the educational planning for children with hearing loss, monitoring individual hearing aids or other assistive devices to ensure their proper function, and educating teachers and other school personnel regarding hearing loss, hearing aids, and communication with children having hearing loss.

Counseling

Counseling is an important component of the overall services that audiologists provide to children and their families and, more specifically, a critical part of the management process. Counseling can range from explaining test results, to making recommendations for habilitation services, to assisting families as they work through feelings of confusion and disappointment about their child's hearing loss. Although not trained as professional counselors, audiologists can provide educational and supportive counseling to assist families in making practical life changes to ease the unexpected disruptions that hearing loss can cause.

Parents often look to professionals for answers and direction. The audiologist's goal in counseling, however, is to provide the information and guidance that families need to make their own decisions and solve their own problems. For example, not every child or family is the same and there is not one approach to communication and education that is right for every child. Parents must ultimately find the answers they are seeking; audiologists simply provide the tools to help that happen.

Most counseling takes place informally while discussing test results or responding to a parent's phone call. Support groups can provide a more structured setting where families share their feelings of fear, confusion, and perhaps guilt, with other parents of hearing-impaired children. It is through communication with other families that parents learn that they are not alone. Support groups may include parents, siblings, and even extended family members such as grandparents, aunts, and uncles.

Clinical Problem Solving

The parents of 4-year-old Josh were shocked to learn that his articulation problems were the result of a moderate sensorineural hearing loss in both ears. After all, neither of them had a hearing loss nor did any of their parents or siblings. The pregnancy with Josh was normal as was his entire postnatal course.

1. What are some possible causes of Josh's hearing loss?
2. Is it more likely that Josh's hearing loss will be treated medically or with hearing aids?
3. What receptive communication difficulties might you expect with this degree of hearing loss?
4. What expressive communication difficulties might you expect with this degree of hearing loss?

References

Alho, O.P., Oja, J., Koivu, M., & Sorri, M. (1995). Risk factors for chronic otitis media with effusion in infancy. *Archives of Otolaryngology Head and Neck Surgery, 121*: 839–843.

Alho, O.P., Koivu, M., Sorri, M., & Rantakallio, P. (1990). Risk factors for recurrent acute otitis media and respiratory infection in infancy. *International Journal of Pediatric Otorhinolaryngology, 19*: 151–161.

American Academy of Otolaryngology and American Council of Otolaryngology (1979). Guide for the evaluation of hearing handicap. *Journal of the American Medical Association, 241*: 2055–2059.

American National Standards Institute (1991). Maximum permissible ambient noise levels for audiometric test rooms (ANSI S3.1-1991). New York: Acoustical Society of America.

American Speech-Hearing-Language Association Panel on Audiologic Assessment (1997). *Guidelines for Audiologic Screening*. Rockville, MD: ASHA.

Apgar, V. (1953). A proposal for a new method of evaluation of the newborn infant. *Anesthesia and Analgesia, 32*: 260.

Bergman, I., Hirsch, R.P., Fria, T.J., Shapiro, S.M., Holzman, I., & Painter, M.J.U. (1985). Cause of hearing loss in the high-risk-premature infant. *Journal of Pediatrics, 106*: 95–101.

Bergstrom, L. (1984). Congenital hearing loss. In J.L. Northern (Ed.), *Hearing Disorders* (2nd ed.). Boston: Little, Brown.

Bergstrom, L. (1988). Infectious agents that deafen. In F.H. Bess (Ed.), *Hearing Impairment in Children*. Parkton, MD: York Press.

Bess, F.H., & Humes, L.E. (1995). *Audiology: The Fundamentals* (2nd ed.). Baltimore, MD: Williams & Wilkins.

Bess, F.H., & Tharpe, A.M. (1986). Case history data on unilaterally hearing-impaired children. In F.H. Bess et al., Children with unilateral hearing loss. *Ear and Hearing Monograph*, Jan-Feb.

Bluestone, C.D., & Klein, J.O. (1996). Otitis media, atelectasis, and eustachian tube disfunction. In C.D. Bluestone, S.E. Stool, & M.A. Kenna (Eds.), *Pediatric Otolaryngology* (3rd ed., vol. I, pp. 388–582). Philadelphia: Saunders.

Brookhouser, P.E., Worthington, D.W., & Kelly, W.J. (1993). Middle ear disease in young children with sensorineural hearing loss. *Laryngoscope, 103*(4): 371–378.

Church, M.W., & Gerkin, K.P. (1988). Hearing disorders in children with fetal alcohol syndrome: Findings from case reports. *Pediatrics, 82*(2): 147–154.

Clarren, S.K., & Smith, D.W. (1978). The fetal alcohol syndrome. *New England Journal of Medicine, 198*: 1063–1067.

Dahle, A.J., McCollister, F.P., Stagno, S., Reynolds, D.W., & Hoffman, H.E. (1979). Progressive hearing impairment in children with congenital cytomegalovirus infection. *Journal of Speech and Hearing Disorders, 44*: 220–229.

Davis, A., Wood, S. Healy, R., Webb, H., & Rowe, S. (1995). Risk factors for hearing disorders: Epidemiologic evidence of change over time in the United Kingdom. *Journal of the American Academy of Audiology, 6*(5): 365–370.

Davis, L.E., & Johnson, L.G. (1983). Viral infections of the inner ear. Clinical virologic and pathologic studies in humans and animals. *American Journal of Otolaryngology, 4:* 347–362.

Dehner, L.P., & Gersell, D.J. (1994). Congenital syphilis: A reminder about the return of an old scourge. *Missouri Medicine, 91*(10): 630—635.

Dennis, J.M., & Neely, J.G. (1991). Otoneurologic diseases and associated audiologic profiles. In J.T. Jacobson & J.L. Northern (Eds.), *Diagnostic Audiology.* Austin, TX: Pro-Ed.

deVries, L.S., Lary, S., & Dubowitz, L.M.S. (1985). Relationship of serum bilirubin level to ototoxicity and deafness in high-risk low-birth-weight infants. *Pediatrics, 76:* 351–354.

Fria, T.J., Cantekin, E.I., & Eichler, J.A. (1985). Hearing acuity of children with otitis media with effusion. *Archives of Otolaryngology, 111:* 10–16.

Gershon, A. (1981). Infections of fetus and newborn infants. *Journal of Perinatal Medicine, 9:* 204–206.

Healthy People 2000. (1990). U.S. Department of Health and Human Services, Public Health Service, DHHS Publication No. (PHS) 91-50213. Washington, DC: U.S. Government Printing Office.

Hendricks-Munoz, K.D., & Walton, J.P. (1988). Hearing loss in infants with persistent fetal circulation. *Pediatrics, 81:* 650–656.

Joint Committee on Infant Hearing (1994). Joint Committee on Infant Hearing 1994 Position Statement. *Pediatrics, 95*(1): 152–156.

Kallio, M.J.T., Kilpi, T., Anttila, M., & Peltola, H. (1994). The effect of a recent previous visit to a physician on outcome after childhood bacterial meningitis. *Journal of the American Medical Association, 272*(10): 787–791.

Kemp, D.T. (1978). Stimulated acoustic emissions from the human auditory system. *Journal of the Acoustical Society of America, 64:* 1386–1391.

Klein, J.O. (1992). Epidemiology and natural history of otitis media. In F.H. Bess & J.W. Hall, III (Eds.), *Screening Children for Auditory Function.* Nashville, TN: Bill Wilkerson Center Press.

Klein, J.O. (1994). Antimicrobial therapy and prevention of meningitis. *Pediatric Annals, 23*(2): 76–81.

Kleinman, L.C., Kosecoff, J., DuBois, R.W., & Brook, R.H. (1994). The medical appropriateness of tympanostomy tubes proposed for children younger than 16 years in the United States. *Journal of the American Medical Association, 271*(16): 1250–1255.

Krishnamoorthy, K.S., Shannon, D.C., DeLong, G.R., Todres, I.D., & Davis, K.R. (1979). Neurologic sequelae in the survivors of neonatal intraventricular hemorrhage. *Pediatrics, 64*(2): 233–237.

Leavitt, A.M., Watchko, J.F., Bennett, F.C., & Folsom, R.C. (1987). Neurodevelopmental outcome following persistent pulmonary hypertension of the neonate. *Journal of Perinatology, 7*(4): 288–291.

Lieberman, J.M., Greenberg, D.P., & Ward, J.I. (1990). Prevention of bacterial meningitis: Vaccines and chemoprophylaxis. *Infectious Disease Clinics of North America, 4*(4): 703–729.

Lloyd, L.L., Spradlin, J.E., & Reid, M.J. (1968). An operant audiometric procedure for difficult-to-test patients. *Journal of Speech and Hearing Disorders, 33:* 236–245.

Moore & Wilson (1978). Visual reinforcement audiometry (VRA) with infants. In S.E. Gerber & G.T. Mencher (Eds.), *Early Diagnosis of Hearing Loss.* New York: Grune & Stratton.

Naulty, C.M., Weiss, I.P., & Herer, G. (1986). Progressive sensorineural hearing loss in survivors of persistent fetal circulation. *Ear and Hearing, 7:* 74–77.

Newton, V.E., & Rowson, V.J. (1988). Progressive hearing loss in childhood. *British Journal of Audiology, 22*(4): 287–295.

NIH Consensus Statement (1993). *Early Identification of Hearing Impairment in Infants and Young Children.* March 1–3, *11:* 1–24.

Northern, J.L., & Downs, M.P. (1991). *Hearing in Children* (p. 7), Baltimore: Williams & Wilkins.

Oyler, R.F., Oyler, A.L., & Matkin, N.D. (1988). Unilateral hearing loss: Demographics and educational impact. *Language, Speech, and Hearing Services in Schools, 19:* 201–210.

Parving, A. (1993). Congenital hearing disability: Epidemiology and identification; A comparison between two health authority districts. *International Journal of Pediatric Otolaryngology, 27*: 29–46.

Pediatric Working Group. (1996). Amplification for infants and children with hearing loss. *American Journal of Audiology, 5*(1): 53–68.

Pukander, J. (1982). Acute otitis media among rural children in Finland. *International Journal of Pediatric Otorhinolaryngology, 4*: 325–332.

Robillard, T.A.J., & Gersdorff, M.C.H. (1986). Prevention of pre- and perinatal acquired hearing defects: Part I—study of causes. *Journal of Auditory Research, 26*: 207–237.

Rose, S.P., Conneally, P.M., & Nance, W.E. (1977). Genetic analysis of childhood deafness. In F.H. Bess (Ed.), *Childhood Deafness* (pp. 19–35). New York: Grune and Stratton.

Sabo, D.L., Brown, D.R., & Watchko, J.F. (1992). Sensorineural hearing loss in high-risk infants. In F.H. Bess & J.W. Hall (Eds.), *Screening Children for Auditory Function*. Nashville, TN: Bill Wilkerson Center Press.

Salamy, A., Eldredge, L., & Tooley, W.J. (1989). Neonatal status and hearing loss in high-risk infants. *Journal of Pediatrics, 114*: 847–852.

Schuknecht, H.F. (1974). *Pathology of the Ear*. Cambridge, MA: Harvard University Press.

Sell, E., Gaines, J., Gluckman, C., & Williams, E. (1985). Persistent fetal circulation. *Archives of the Journal of Disorders of Children, 139*: 25–28.

Shaver, K. (1988). Genetics and deafness. In F.H. Bess (Ed.), *Hearing Impairment in Children* (pp. 15–32). Parkton, MD: York Press.

Simmons, F.B. (1980). Patterns of deafness in newborns. *Laryngoscope, 90*:448.

Sipila, M., Karma, P., Pukander, J., Timonen, M., & Kataja, M. (1988). The Bayesian approach to the evaluation of risk factors in acute and recurrent acute otitis media. *Acta Otolaryngology, 106*:94–101.

Stagno, S., Reynolds, D.W., Amos, C.S., Dahle, A.J., McCollister, F.P., Hohindra, I., Ermocilla, R., & Alford, C.A. (1977). Auditory and visual defects resulting from symptomatic and subclinical congenital cytomegaloviral and toxoplasma infections. *Pediatrics, 59*: 669–678.

Stahlberg, M.R., Ruuskanen, O., & Virolainen, E. (1986). Risk factors for recurrent otitis media. *Pediatric Infectious Disease Journal, 5*:30–32.

Starling, S.P. (1994). Syphilis in infants and young children. *Pediatric Annals, 23*(7): 334–340.

Stein, L.K., & Boyer, K.M. (1994). Progress in the prevention of hearing loss in infants. *Ear and Hearing, 15*(2): 116–125.

Streissguth, A.P., Clarren, S.K., & Jones, K.L. (1985). Natural history of the fetal alcohol syndrome: A 10-year follow-up of eleven patients. *Lancet, 2*:85–91.

Streissguth, A.P., Landesman-Dwyer, S., Martin, J.C., & Smith, D.W. (1980). Teratogenic effects of alcohol in humans and laboratory animals. *Science, 209*:353–361.

Tharpe, A.M., & Bess, F.H. (1991). Identification and management of children with minimal hearing loss. *International Journal of Pediatric Otolaryngology, 21*.

Tharpe, A.M., & Clayton, E.W. (1997). Newborn hearing screening: Issues in legal liability and quality assurance. *American Journal of Audiology, 6*(2):5–12.

Thompson, G., & Weber, B.A. (1974). Responses of infants and young children to behavior observation audiometry (BOA). *Journal of Speech and Hearing Disorders, 2*:140–147.

Vaughan, V., McKay, R.J., & Behrman, R. (1979). *Nelson Textbook of Pediatrics*. (11th ed.). Philadelphia: Saunders.

Vuori, M., Lahikainen, E.A., & Peltonen, T. (1962). Perceptive deafness in connection with mumps. *Acta Otolaryngol, 55*:231–236.

Walton, J.P., & Hendricks-Munoz, K. (1991). Profile and stability of sensorineural hearing loss in persistent pulmonary hypertension of the newborn, *Journal of Speech and Hearing Research, 34*: 1362–1370.

Watkin, P., Baldwin, M., & McEnery, G. (1991). Neonatal at risk screening and the identification of deafness. *Archives of Diseases in Children, 66*:1130–1135.

Zizz, C.A., & Glattke, T.J. (1988). Reliability of spontaneous otoacoustic emission suppression tuning curve measures. *Journal of Speech and Hearing Research, 31*: 616–619.

Disorders of Hearing in Adults

Linda Norrix, Ph.D.

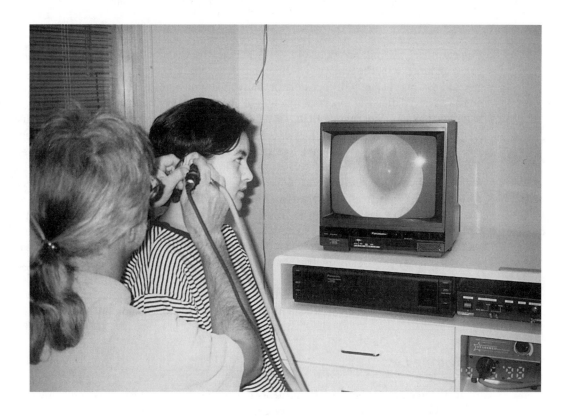

Preview

According to a 1991 survey by the National Center for Health Statistics, about 21 million Americans report difficulties with their hearing. This was an increase from the 1971 estimate of 13 million, a number much greater than that expected from population growth. The increase can partly be explained by the aging of the population as well as higher levels of environmental noise that are present today compared with the past (Sandor, 1994). Of the 21 million Americans, the majority developed hearing impairment in adulthood. Hearing impairment in adulthood can have devastating effects on one's ability to communicate and may significantly impact family relationships, social interactions, vocation, self-identity, and economic well-being. Because communication is such a vital part of human existence, hearing difficulties can decrease one's quality of life (Mulrow, Aguilar, Endicott, Tuley, Velez, Charlip, Rhodes, Hill, & DeNino, 1990). The audiologist plays a critical role in the assessment and rehabilitation of adults with acquired hearing impairment. This chapter focuses on causes, effects, and treatments of adult-onset hearing impairments.

Approximately 21 million adults (45% of whom are 65 years of age or older) have difficulty hearing (Sandor, 1994). The majority of these individuals developed their hearing impairment after the age of 18. This chapter will focus on the individual with adult-onset hearing impairment. Hearing impairment is defined as abnormal function of the auditory system that can be measured using laboratory techniques (Stephens & Hetu, 1991). Hearing-impaired individuals may have reduced sensitivity, or poor hearing, for tones, may exhibit poor understanding of words, or both. As recommended by Giolas (1994), the term **hearing loss** will be used to quantify the degree of the impairment (e.g., Frank has a 50 dB hearing loss). A hearing impairment, if left untreated, may result in disability or handicap. **Hearing disability** refers to the auditory problems that the person experiences and therefore is influenced by one's social environment (Stephens & Hetu, 1991). For example, an individual who is socially active and who has a high frequency hearing impairment is likely to report difficulties understanding speech in noisy environments. In contrast, the same impairment in a person who has few social contacts may not report difficulties hearing in noise. The **handicap**, or nonauditory effects that develop, might include social isolation, reduced economic resources, and difficulty maintaining independence. Audiologists working with the adult population need to understand not only the hearing impairment but also the disability and handicap that are associated with the impairment. Only then can the best rehabilitation plan be developed and implemented.

Conductive Hearing Loss

A small percentage of hearing impairments in adulthood are conductive. A conductive hearing impairment occurs when the sound cannot efficiently get to the inner ear to stimulate the sensory receptors for hearing (see Chapters 2 and 5). The audiogram for a conductive impairment will exhibit elevated thresholds by air conduction and normal thresholds by bone conduction, so that an air-bone gap will be present. The hearing-impaired person typically has good word recognition provided that speech is loud enough to be heard. Causes of conductive impairments include *cerumen*, or ear wax, blocking the ear canal, fluid behind the eardrum within the middle ear space (see Chapter 5 for a discussion of middle ear fluid in children), a perforated eardrum, or damage to the ossicles that lie in the middle ear. **Otosclerosis** is an example of a disorder that occurs in adulthood and causes a progressive, conductive hearing impairment. In otosclerosis, bony tissue is replaced by spongy or fibrous bone growth. The most common place for this abnormal bone growth to occur is in the area of the oval window resulting in reduced motion of the stapes and a conductive hearing impairment. Otosclerosis is more commonly found in both ears than in one, in women than in men, and in Caucasians rather than Asian or African Americans. Genetics seem to play a role because a family history is often reported.

Mrs. Garrett, age 35, reported that within the last several years she has had difficulties understanding speech when there was background noise, localizing sounds, hearing people talk when they were positioned to her left, and she could not use the left ear on the telephone. Figure 6-1 illustrates Mrs. Garrett's audiogram and word recognition ability. She has otosclerosis in the left ear. Notice that when tested in the left ear at a normal conversational intensity level (45 dB) she only repeated 44% of the single syllable words correctly. This was because the entire speech signal was not audible to her.

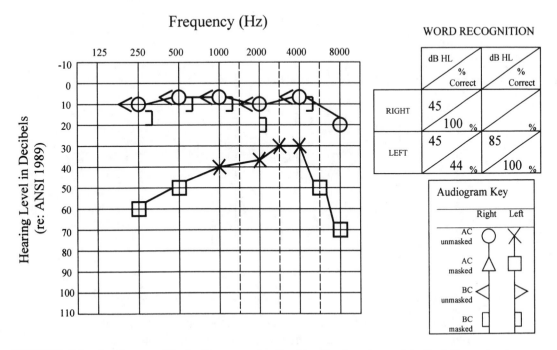

FIGURE 6-1 **Audiogram illustrating a conductive hearing impairment in the left ear due to otosclerosis.**

In order to appreciate the effect of hearing loss on the ability to understand speech, it is helpful to examine the relative contribution of the different frequency and intensity combinations for speech audibility as shown in Figure 6-2. One hundred dots are displayed on the graph. The denser the dots, the greater the amount of speech energy that falls within that frequency band. An **articulation index** is calculated by assigning 0.01 (one percent) to each dot that is audible. Mrs. Garrett's left ear air conduction thresholds are superimposed on the graph.

Mrs. Garrett has approximately 36 audible dots that fall below her audiometric curve. This suggests that at a normal conversational intensity level approximately 36% of the speech signal is audible to her in the left ear, thus reducing the likelihood of understanding speech. When words were presented at a higher intensity level (85 dB), Mrs. Garrett's word recognition ability was excellent (100% correct).

Mrs. Garrett's profile indicates that she is an excellent candidate for wearing a hearing aid because her hearing impairment is primarily conductive so there is little or no sound distortion. When provided with appropriate amplification, the individual with a conductive hearing impairment will have little if any disability or handicap. Depending on the cause of the conductive impairment,

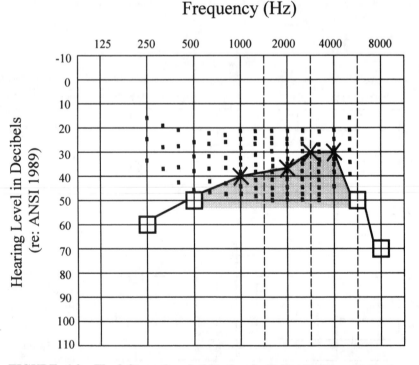

FIGURE 6-2   The left ear thresholds of an individual with unilateral otosclerosis superimposed on the Count-the-Dot audiogram for calculation of the articulation index. (Adapted from Mueller & Killion, 1990.) The shaded portion of the graph indicates the dots that are audible.

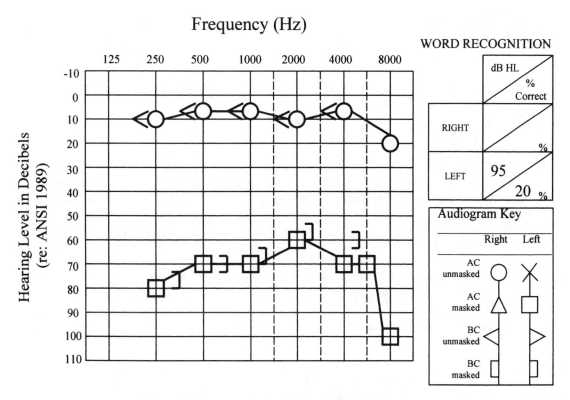

FIGURE 6-3 **Audiometric results after an unsuccessful stapedectomy that resulted in a moderate to severe sensorineural hearing impairment in the left ear. Word recognition was also very poor.**

surgery or medical treatment may improve or restore an individual's hearing. Surgeries, however, are not risk-free, as we see as we continue to follow Mrs. Garrett's history.

Mrs. Garrett had surgery in an attempt to eliminate the conductive hearing impairment due to otosclerosis. The surgery, performed by an ear, nose, and throat (ENT) specialist, is known as a **stapedectomy** and often reduces or nearly eliminates the conductive component of a hearing impairment. During her surgery, the footplate of the stapes was removed and replaced with a wire prosthesis. Although initial results indicated almost complete elimination of the conductive hearing impairment, one month after the surgery she returned to the clinic because she was hearing loud noise in the left ear. Figure 6-3 illustrates the audiogram obtained from this visit. Her thresholds deteriorated and her audiogram revealed a sensorineural hearing impairment with very poor word recognition ability (20% correct) when words were presented well above her thresholds for tones (95 dB). Because of the poor word recognition ability, she was no longer a candidate for amplification in this ear.[1] Amplification would make sounds audible but not very clear, possibly interfering with speech understanding in the good ear.

---

[1]Only 1 to 3% of stapedectomies result in sensorineural hearing impairment.

Sensorineural Hearing Loss

The majority of hearing impairments in adulthood are sensorineural. A sensorineural hearing impairment occurs when there is damage to the inner ear or the VIIIth nerve (see Chapter 2). The three most common conditions associated with hearing impairments in adulthood are the aging process, noise exposure, and Ménière's disease.

Aging Process

A slowly progressive decrease in hearing associated with the aging process is known as **presbycusis**. A lifetime of environmental noise exposure, disease processes, drug effects, and genetic predisposition to hearing impairment contribute to presbycusis. Although changes in the cochlea probably begin early in life, it is not until middle age that people most commonly begin to have difficulties understanding speech. Initial changes occur in the high frequency range, which reflect the basal end of the cochlea. Because low frequency hearing is relatively normal, individuals with early presbycusis typically report that they can hear people talk but they can't understand what is being said. This is because the low frequency, high intensity vowels are audible, but the high frequency, low intensity consonants, which are most important for intelligibility, are inaudible. Figure 6-4 depicts the frequency and intensity characteristics of four classes of speech sounds: nasals, vowels, stops, and fricatives (Olsen, Hawkings, & Van Tasell, 1987). Notice that the cues for stops and fricatives are high in fre-

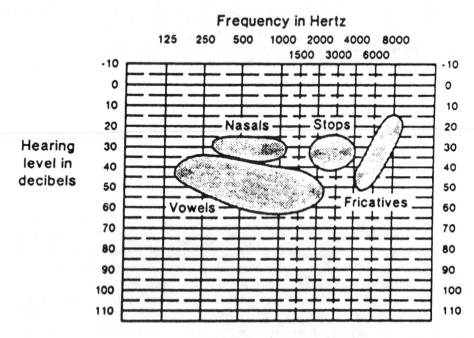

FIGURE 6-4   The frequency and intensity characteristics of several classes of speech sounds. (From Olsen, W., Hawkins, D., & Van Tasell, D. [1987]. Representations of the long-term spectra of speech. *Ear and Hearing, 8*(5), 1003–1085.)

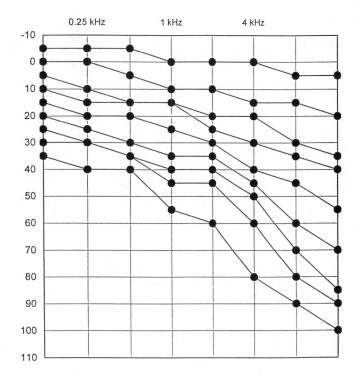

FIGURE 6-5 Audiogram illustrating the patterns of normal aging. (From Goodhill, V., *Presbycusis in Ear Diseases, Deafness and Dizziness*. Hagerstown, MD: Harper and Row, p. 719 [1979]. Reprinted by permission of St. Mary's Ear, Nose and Throat Specialists.) Each curve represents the following age group (from top to bottom):

0-20 years	**60-70 years**
20-30 years	**70-80 years**
30-40 years	**80-90 years**
40-50 years	**90-100 years**
50-60 years	

quency compared to the cues for nasals and vowels.[2] Therefore, stops and fricatives are easily missed by the person with a high frequency hearing impairment. Place of articulation cues (e.g., distinguishing /b/ from /d/ from /g/) are also high frequency and easily misinterpreted. It is not uncommon for a person with a high frequency hearing impairment to report hearing "van" for "than," "gay" for "day," and "pin" for "kin." Another common complaint of individuals with high frequency hearing impairment is the inability to understand speech in the presence of background noise that masks the weaker components of the speech signal (e.g., the high frequency consonants and place of articulation cues). Rooms with reverberation (echoes) are also difficult listening environments for those with hearing impairment.

Typical thresholds for individuals of various ages are illustrated in Figure 6-5. Notice that with increases in age, the low frequency sounds also become more difficult to detect. With advanced pres-

---

[2]In addition to frequency cues, temporal and intensity cues are important for understanding speech.

bycusis, a loss of central auditory neurons may accompany the changes within the cochlea resulting in central presbycusis or a **central auditory processing disorder** (CAPD). A sign of central presbycusis is **phonemic regression**. This refers to word recognition that is very poor and cannot be explained based on the amount of hearing loss for pure tones. A common report of individuals with central presbycusis is "I can hear fine but everyone mumbles."

Mr. Robinson, age 70, came to the clinic to have his hearing evaluated. He was accompanied by his two daughters who reported that their father was answering questions inappropriately and saying "huh" constantly. Although Mr. Robinson admitted that he had some difficulty hearing, he commented that his hearing "was not all that bad" and that he would be able to hear better if people "would speak more clearly." Figure 6-6 illustrates Mr. Robinson's audiogram. He has central presbycusis. His word recognition ability was 28% in his left ear and 32% in his right ear when presented at an intensity level well above his threshold levels.

In contrast to Mr. Robinson's test results, the same degree of hearing loss in a 44-year-old man tested at the same clinic was associated with 80% word recognition ability. Stach, Spretnjak, and Jerger (1990) estimated that by the age of 65 years, over 50% of the elderly will have CAPD. This

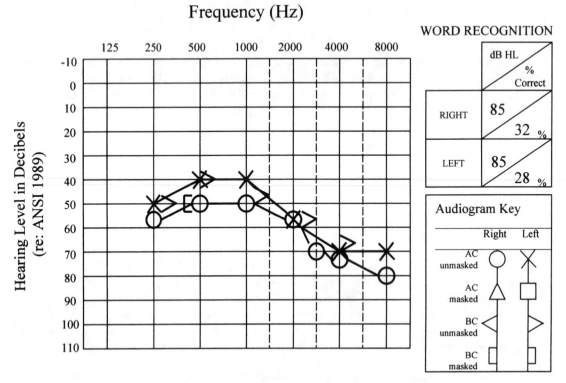

FIGURE 6-6   **Audiogram illustrating a sensorineural hearing impairment due to central presbycusis.**

population, compared to the non-CAPD hearing-impaired population, has greater difficulty extracting speech from noise, understanding speech when reverberation is present, and successfully using amplification devices.

Many factors contribute to hearing impairment in the aged population, therefore, the presbycusic individual's hearing capabilities are unique, and therapies must be tailored to each individual's needs. Rehabilitating the presbycusic individual presents an exciting challenge for the audiologist.

Noise Exposure

Many Americans are exposed to potentially hazardous noise levels in the workplace as well as during recreational activities. Noise exposure can cause a "threshold shift" initially observed around 4000 Hz. That is, hearing a tone in the 4000 Hz frequency region will be more difficult after noise exposure than before.

Mr. McGee, age 52, has been employed in a manufacturing plant for 25 years. He also enjoys carpentry work and snowmobiling as recreational activities. He reported that he hears

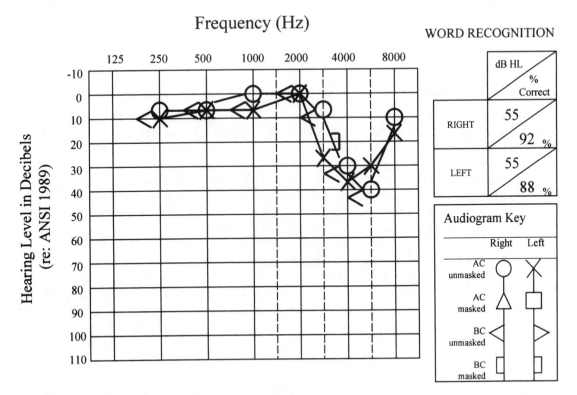

FIGURE 6-7 Audiogram illustrating a sensorineural hearing impairment centered around the 4000 Hz region as a result of excessive noise exposure.

ringing in his ears (**tinnitus**) and that speech sounds are muffled. The audiologist employed by his company evaluated his hearing (see Figure 6-7) and compared the results to previous evaluations. She noted a threshold shift, that is, his hearing for the frequencies 3000, 4000, and 6000 Hz has worsened since his previous tests.

Poor thresholds that are worst around 4000 Hz (4 kHz) and improve at 8000 Hz are known as the "**4k notch**." This threshold shift is due to damaged sensory cells in the inner ear resulting in sensorineural hearing impairment. Initially the threshold shift may be temporary. After removing oneself from the loud noise (or removing the noise from oneself, as in the case of portable tape player headphones) thresholds may return to normal. This is known as a *temporary threshold shift* or TTS. However, it is likely that some damage has been done. Furthermore, with repeated exposures, exposure for a longer period of time, or in an individual with susceptibility to noise damage, the recovery may not be complete, resulting in *permanent threshold shift* or PTS. Like those with presbycusis, individuals with noise-induced hearing impairment have difficulties understanding speech in noisy environments and in rooms with a lot of reverberation.

Mr. McGee received a complete audiometric evaluation and was counseled about the harm that noise exposure causes, as well as the effects of that hearing impairment on communication ability. He was shown how to wear earplugs appropriately, instructed to limit his exposure to noise, and to wear hearing protectors at work and during recreational activities when loud noise is present.

Ménière's Disease

Mrs. Hill, age 55, experiences episodic attacks of vertigo, nausea, tinnitus, and a sensorineural hearing impairment in the right ear that is more severe in the low frequencies than in the high frequencies. A feeling of pressure in her right ear often precedes the attacks. The most distressing symptom for her is the vertigo that comes on suddenly with little warning. Because of the unpredictability of these attacks and the embarrassment she feels, Mrs. Hill is no longer employed and has stopped socializing with friends. She has **Ménière's disease**. Figure 6-8 displays her audiogram. She has had Ménière's disease for ten years. The hearing impairment has become slightly worse over the last five years.

Although the exact cause of Ménière's disease is unknown, it is thought to be due to an excess buildup of inner ear fluid called *endolymph*. The organ of Corti and sensory cells are surrounded by this fluid. Ménière's disease is often unilateral, although one-third of those with the disease will develop it in both ears. It is common for the first episode to occur between 40 and 60 years of age. As the disease progresses, the low frequency hearing loss becomes more severe and permanent. The role of the audiologist with this population is to provide support and education to the individual about the disease and the available audiologic rehabilitation methods. Amplification may be necessary depending on whether a stable or deteriorating hearing impairment is present. Noise maskers may also be necessary to help the patient with Ménière's disease become less aware of the tinnitus.

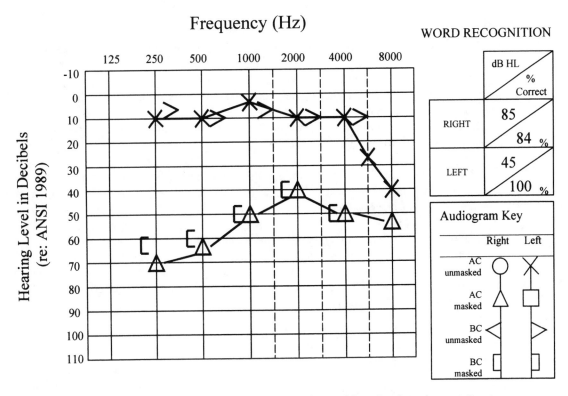

FIGURE 6-8   Audiogram illustrating a right sensorineural hearing impairment due to Ménière's disease.

Although sensorineural hearing impairments associated with the aging process, noise exposure, and Ménière's disease are the most prevalent causes of hearing impairments in the adult population, the audiologist will test and provide rehabilitation for adults with impairments due to other causes. The audiologist must know about toxins to and disorders of the auditory system such as ototoxicity, acoustic neuromas, and diseases of the central auditory system.

Ototoxicity

Ototoxicity results when certain drugs damage the inner ear resulting in sensorineural hearing impairment. The damage is usually in the high frequencies and can be reversible or permanent. Examples of ototoxic drugs are the aminoglycosides used for treatment of many and often life-threatening infectious diseases, diuretics used to reduce edema or excessive fluid from renal failure, high doses of acetylsalicylic acid (e.g., aspirin), and cisplatin, a drug used to treat cancer. The audiologist's role is to obtain periodic audiograms prior, during, and after drug therapy. For those individuals who develop hearing impairment, the audiologist provides rehabilitation services that may consist of providing amplification, support, and encouragement. Education about hearing conservation is also important because individuals on drug therapies may be more susceptible to noise damage.

Acoustic Neuroma

Ms. Parker, age 56, came to the ENT clinic because she was having pain on the left side of her face, tinnitus in the left ear, and dizziness. Her audiogram (Figure 6-9) revealed a sloping, mild to moderate sensorineural hearing loss in the left ear and mild high frequency sensorineural hearing loss in the right ear. Her word recognition was excellent in the right ear when words were presented at normal and loud conversational intensity levels (50 and 90dB, respectively). Left ear results revealed good word recognition at 70dB but poor recognition when words were presented at 90 dB.

This dramatic decrease in word recognition as the intensity of the words is increased is known as **rollover** and is often associated with pathology beyond the cochlea and along the central auditory pathway, that is, retrocochlear pathology.

The audiologist evaluated Ms. Parker using the auditory brainstem response (ABR) test. Four electrodes were placed on the surface of her skin and clicking sounds were presented to each ear. The electrodes detected the electrical activity that occurred on the surface of her scalp in response to the clicks. Samples of the electrical activity that occurred after each click were averaged with a computer.

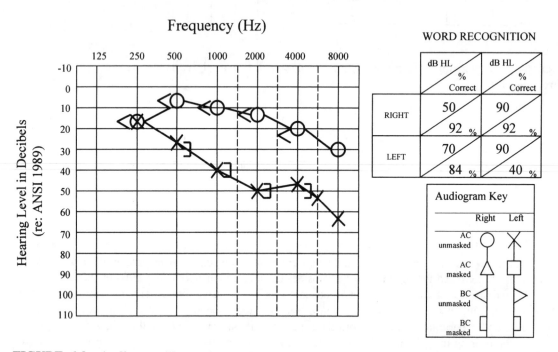

FIGURE 6-9   Audiogram illustrating a left sensorineural hearing impairment associated with an acoustic neuroma. Word recognition ability was decreased at a loud intensity level in the left ear compared to a softer intensity level (rollover).

In neurologically normal individuals, several positive peaks can be identified that occur within a certain number of milliseconds following the clicks. Delayed peaks or delayed intervals between peaks are a strong indication of *retrocochlear* pathology.

Figure 6-10 exhibits Ms. Parker's ABR results. The peaks for waves III and V for the left ear were 5.16 ms and 7.44 ms, respectively. These were much longer than the latencies for waves III and V for the right ear (4.64 ms and 6.72 ms, respectively). Ms. Parker subsequently had an MRI (magnetic resonance image) of the internal auditory canal (the bony canal that extends from each cochlear nucleus to its corresponding cochlea) and an **acoustic neuroma** (tumor) on the VIIIth nerve was confirmed. The tumor was surgically removed but the surgery, unfortunately, resulted in no measurable hearing in the left ear. Ms. Parker, being active in her vocation and community, found that the unilateral hearing loss was quite disabling. As is common with unilateral hearing impairment, she had difficulties localizing sounds, understanding a talker when positioned on the side of the poor ear, and understanding speech in noise. The audiologist fit her with a hearing aid that placed a microphone at the unusable right ear. The microphone picked up the signal reaching the impaired ear and sent it to a receiver placed on the good left ear.

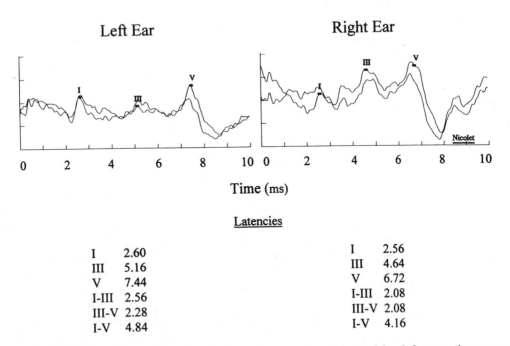

FIGURE 6-10 **The auditory brainstem response of a patient with a left acoustic neuroma. When clicks were presented to the left ear, waves III and V were abnormally delayed compared to the waves associated with right ear click stimulation.**

A hearing aid arrangement in which a microphone is placed behind an unaidable ear and sends the signal to the good ear is known as *contralateral routing of signals* or a CROS hearing aid. Wearing a CROS hearing aid makes it easier for the individual with a unilateral hearing impairment to hear sounds directed to the impaired ear. It also restores a sense of sound balance to sound perception and an improvement in the signal-to-noise ratio when the signal is on the side of the poorer ear. Although acoustic neuromas only affect 1 out of 100,000 people, if undetected they can result in death by exerting pressure on brainstem structures as they grow. If detected early and surgically removed, hearing may be preserved. Therefore, patients experiencing unilateral hearing impairment or unilateral tinnitus should be tested to determine if an acoustic neuroma is the cause of their symptoms.

Diseases of the Central Auditory System

Audiologists may also test and participate in the rehabilitation of patients who have lesions to the brain or brainstem that affect hearing. Such disorders include multiple sclerosis, strokes, and cortical and brainstem tumors. A central lesion can disturb the blood supply to the cochlea resulting in damage to the hair cells and resulting in a reduced ability to hear pure tones. However, most often a central auditory disorder will cause difficulties with speech processing without affecting pure tone hearing sensitivity. Individuals with central auditory lesions report difficulties listening when there is background noise or reverberation, when visual cues are not available, and when speech is spoken at a rapid rate. An elderly person with a central auditory lesion will likely have some difficulty hearing pure tones due to aging of the cochlea. As a result of the central lesion, difficulties processing speech in adverse listening situations will also be reported. As in central presbycusis, the difficulties in speech understanding will be greater than expected from the pure tone audiogram.

Mixed Hearing Impairment

Finally, a hearing impairment can have both conductive and sensorineural components and is known as a **mixed hearing impairment**.

> Mrs. Leon, age 84 years, reported a sudden decrease in her hearing. Her family, who accompanied her to the evaluation, reported that for many years she had some difficulties understanding speech and had to turn the television to higher-than-normal loudness in order to hear most programs. Recently, her neighbors complained about the loud noise coming from her apartment. Mrs. Leon reported a sudden hearing impairment coincident with a cold she developed approximately 2 months prior. She expressed much concern about her deteriorating hearing ability, as it was a sign of "getting old" and "one more thing going wrong."
>
> Mrs. Leon's audiometric results are displayed in Figure 6-11. The audiogram showed that she had a mixed hearing loss. Notice the 30 to 40 dB air-bone gap, which reflects the conductive component of the hearing loss, in addition to a mild to moderate 30 to 50 dB sensorineural hearing loss (thresholds for bone conduction range from 30 to 50 dB). The conductive component of her hearing impairment was due to bilateral middle ear infection (otitis media, see Chapter 5). The sensorineural component was diagnosed as presbycusis.

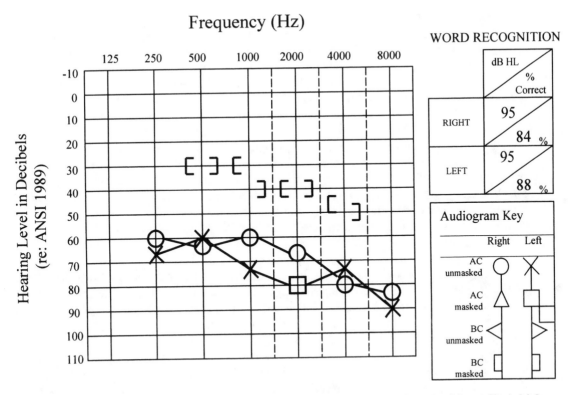

FIGURE 6-11 **Audiogram illustrating a mixed hearing impairment due to otitis media (which caused the conductive component) and presbycusis (which caused the sensorineural component).**

Pressure equalization (PE) tubes were placed in her ears by an ENT specialist.[3] After medical intervention, the audiologist prescribed a hearing aid and assisted her in the rehabilitation process. Mrs. Leon adapted quite well to her new hearing aids and showed a renewed interest in communicating with her family and friends. Comforted by the knowledge that she was not rapidly going deaf, and assisted with amplification, she was better able to participate in community functions and in her Sunday church service.

Psychosocial Impact of Hearing Loss

Both conductive and sensorineural hearing impairments can result in social, emotional, and communication difficulties for an individual. For example, hearing impairment can be associated with low self-esteem, a change in self-image, loss of independence, isolation, cognitive decline, and depression. Avoidance of social interactions and activities is often a result of hearing impairment if left untreated.

---

[3]Some audiologists work in an ENT clinic. Others work more autonomously as part of a rehabilitation unit in a hospital or in private practice. If the patient with a conductive hearing impairment has not been evaluated by an ENT, an ENT referral is made.

Mr. Cohen, a 42-year old salesman, experienced a sudden, severe, and bilateral sensorineural hearing loss. Mr. Cohen had provided the sole financial support for his family that included three children. Because of the severity of the loss and the communication demands that his job required, he quit his job. His wife became employed and Mr. Cohen became more responsible for daily activities in the home. He often declined social invitations because he tired easily when trying to participate in the conversation. He relied on his wife to interpret for him and often pretended to understand what people were saying.

Ramsdell (1960) distinguished three psychological levels of hearing: primitive level or the auditory background of daily living, signal/warning level, and symbolic or social level. Any or all of these levels can be affected by a hearing impairment. For example, an individual with a sudden and total hearing loss will have difficulties at all three levels. In contrast, a person with a mild hearing loss still feels connected to the world (still hears background noises) and is able to hear warning signals. However, the social level of hearing is affected by a mild hearing loss because communication difficulties arise.

The rehabilitation methods employed by an audiologist working with an individual with a sudden hearing loss versus a gradual hearing loss are quite different. The person with a sudden, total hearing loss will need immediate coping strategies such as the use of alerting devices, use of writing to communicate, trial period with amplification, and greater use of visual cues. Long-term goals and coping strategies might consist of learning sign language, obtaining a cochlear implant if appropriate, and the maintenance of established or development of new social networks. In contrast, the person with a mild, gradual hearing loss may have social needs met by wearing appropriate amplification and using good communication strategies. How an individual reacts to hearing impairment is not easily predicted. Factors that influence the adjustment include the severity and progression of the hearing impairment, age of onset, lifestyle and personality, and support of friends and family members.

A hearing impairment also impacts the family. Often a hearing-impaired individual is seen in the clinic at the urging of a spouse. Family members may become frustrated at continually repeating and interpreting for the hearing-impaired individual. The extra effort required to include the hearing-impaired individual in conversations and spectator activities such as plays, movies, and lectures can put stress on family relationships and result in exclusion of the hearing-impaired person. It is not uncommon to hear an elderly hearing-impaired man say "If I don't do something about my hearing, my wife will leave me." Although usually said in jest, the statement reflects the seriousness of communication breakdown and its impact on relationships. Likewise, hearing impairment can interfere with activities of daily living. Communicating on the telephone or asking a passerby for directions are just two examples of the many activities that may become more difficult with hearing impairment.

For the nursing home resident, hearing impairment may result in poor patient-staff relationships. Hearing-impaired residents are often labeled withdrawn, uncommunicative, or confused. Hearing impairment can also be associated with poor performance on cognitive tests, especially if administered verbally. For example, Weinstein and Amsel (1986) tested hearing-impaired patients using a test of mental function. Patients were tested with and without their hearing aids. Results indicated that 33% of the patients were reclassified as less severely demented when amplification was used compared to no amplification. Thus, the use of amplification with nursing home residents may have profound implications for their perceived versus actual mental status. The impact that a hearing impairment can have on the nursing home resident is particularly important given that Schow and Nerbonne (1980) estimated that 48% of residents have a hearing impairment that interferes with communication. Although some residents may own personal hearing aids, many are likely to be malfunctioning (Thibodeau & Schmitt, 1988). In addition, few health care providers have received formal training in the management of patients with communication disorders. Because of the high prevalence of hearing impairment in this population, an audiologist might be employed to provide audiological evaluations, fit hearing aids, and train staff members on how to use strategies to enhance communication and how to troubleshoot malfunctioning hearing aids. These services are important because isolation as a result of hearing impairment can dramatically decrease the quality of life for those living their last years in a nursing home facility.

Audiological Evaluation

Hearing Screenings

The audiologist working with adults has a variety of responsibilities. For one, the audiologist may screen for hearing impairment or handicap or oversee such a screening program. Hearing screenings serve to identify a hearing impairment that may warrant medical or audiological rehabilitation referrals. Common settings for screenings include industries, health fairs, medical centers, and nursing facilities. High-noise industries are particularly important sites for screening because noise damage to the cochlea can be avoided. Nursing homes are also important screening sites because of the high prevalence of hearing impairments that exist in the elderly population.

Hearing screenings consist of presenting pure tones at a predetermined loudness level for the individual to hear. Criteria are established to determine whether the individual passes or fails the screening. For example, does the person being screened hear a 1000, 2000, and 4000 Hz tone presented at 25 dB? In addition to pure tone screening, a hearing disability index (HDI) can be used to identify individuals who perceive themselves as having a disability or handicap related to their hearing impairment. One such index is the Hearing Handicap Inventory for the Elderly-Screening Version (HIEE-S) developed by Ventry and Weinstein (1982) and displayed in Table 6-1. The HIEE-S consists of 10 short questions that can be answered in 5 to 10 minutes. The test was designed to detect emotional and social problems associated with hearing impairment. Individuals who fail the pure tone screening or the HDI should be referred for further audiological testing. Use of an HDI in conjunction with pure tone screens can help to identify those individuals who believe they have a disability or handicap and thus will be most motivated to attempt rehabilitation.

Hearing Assessment

A second task of the audiologist is to accurately assess a client's hearing status. Complete audiometric testing (including case history, otoscopic examination, pure tone thresholds, speech testing, and impedance testing) will determine which individuals need medical referral. If a medical referral is made (or if the audiogram was obtained as part of the ENT evaluation), the audiometric test results will assist the ENT specialist in diagnosing and treating the patient. Complete audiometric testing also provides the basis for development of a rehabilitation plan.

The audiological evaluation begins with a case history. The audiologist obtains information about the hearing difficulties that the person is experiencing, family history of hearing loss, medical history, and whether hearing aids have been previously worn. The audiologist examines the patient's external ears using an **otoscope**. If excessive **cerumen** (wax) is observed in the ear canal, it must be

TABLE 6-1   Hearing Handicaps Inventory for the Elderly—Screening Version (HHIE-S)

	Yes (4)	Sometimes (2)	No (0)
E-1 Does a hearing problem cause you to feel embarassed when meeting new people?	_____	_____	_____
E-2 Does a hearing problem cause you to feel frustrated when talking to members of your family?	_____	_____	_____
S-1 Do you have difficulty hearing when someone speaks in a whisper?	_____	_____	_____
E-3 Do you feel handicapped by a hearing problem?	_____	_____	_____
S-2 Does a hearing problem cause you difficulty when visiting friends, relatives, or neighbors?	_____	_____	_____
S-3 Does a hearing problem cause you to attend religious services less often than you would like?	_____	_____	_____
E-4 Does a hearing problem cause you to have arguments with family members?	_____	_____	_____
S-4 Does a hearing problem cause you difficulty when listening to TV or radio?	_____	_____	_____
E-5 Do you feel that any difficulty with your hearing limits or hampers your personal or social life?	_____	_____	_____
S-5 Does a hearing problem cause you difficulty when in a restaurant with relatives or friends?	_____	_____	_____

From Ventry, I., & Weinstein, B. (1982). Identification of elderly people with hearing problems. *Ear and Hearing, 3*: 128–134. Reprinted with permission from Williams & Wilkins.

A "yes," "no," and "sometimes" response scores 4, 0, and 2 points, respectively. Possible scores range from 0 to 40. Ventry and Weinstein suggest that scores of 0-8 indicate no perceived handicap, scores of 10–22 indicate mild to moderate handicap, and scores of 24–40 indicate severe handicap. (E-emotional, S-social)

removed prior to testing. Cerumen removal can be performed by an audiologist with specialized training or by appropriate medical personnel. Audiological testing is performed to determine if a hearing impairment exists, the type of impairment (conductive, sensorineural, or mixed), and the severity of the impairment for various frequencies and for speech. We can examine the stages of audiological exam by following the case of Mr. Peterson.

Mr. Peterson came to the clinic because he was having difficulties hearing his coworkers. He reported having more difficulty hearing from his right ear than his left ear. After a case history was obtained and an otoscopic examination revealed the ear canals to be free of cerumen, impedance measures were obtained (see Chapter 5 for a discussion of impedance). Next, Mr. Peterson was seated inside a sound-treated booth with earphones. The audiologist tested the hearing of each ear individually using an audiometer. The test began with the audiologist saying two-syllable words (such as "cowboy" and "armchair") to Mr. Peterson, who was not allowed to see the audiologist's face to prevent speechreading. The lowest level at which Mr. Peterson was able to repeat the two-syllable words 50% of the time in each ear was written on the audiogram and is called the speech reception threshold (SRT). Next, the pure tone air-conduction audiogram was obtained. The lowest level at which Mr. Peterson detected pure tones 50% of the time was plotted on the audiogram for both ears and is known as his hearing thresholds. The frequencies that were tested ranged from 250 to 8000 Hz. The air conduction thresholds were judged to be valid because of the close agreement between the SRT and the average of the pure-tone thresholds for 500, 1000, and 2000 Hz. Word recognition ability was then assessed. Single-syllable words were presented to Mr. Peterson in quiet at normal and loud conversational intensity levels. He reported what he heard using an oral response and the audiologist recorded the percent of words he repeated correctly. Finally, bone conduction audiometry was performed. A bone vibrator was placed on Mr. Peterson's mastoid bone, located behind the ear, causing the skull to vibrate. The fluids within both cochleae, being housed in the skull, moved producing a perception of sound. Because both cochleae can respond to bone conduction (regardless of the mastoid on which the vibrator is placed), masking of Mr. Peterson's better ear (with noise) was used to determine bone conduction thresholds for his poorer ear.

Audiologists also test some adults who are not able to respond orally to the test stimuli, such as adults with developmental disabilities, severe head injury, or stroke. Written or picture-pointing responses can be used during word recognition testing. *Otoacoustic emissions* (OAEs; see Chapter 2) can be used to screen for hearing loss in difficult-to-test adults because they do not require a volitional response. If a person fails the screening, an ABR threshold search can be performed to estimate hearing sensitivity for the high frequency (2–4 kHz) region of the cochlea. As the intensity of test sounds sounds (clicks) approach an individual's thresholds, all waves of the ABR response disappear (see section on acoustic neuroma, this chapter).

Assessing Hearing Handicap

For those hearing impairments that are not medically correctable or treatable, the audiologist has a third task of developing and implementing a rehabilitation plan in conjunction with the patient. Results from the audiological evaluation are useful in determining the appropriate rehabilitation plan. However, the same degree of hearing loss in two individuals can result in significantly different handicaps. Furthermore, word recognition ability for single words in quiet may not be predictive of communicative performance in noisier environments. Word recognition does not assess how the individual is able to use syntactic and semantic context, visual cues, or previous knowledge of the topic during communicative interactions. These abilities can have a dramatic affect on the degree of handicap that an individual experiences as a result of hearing impairment. The communication demands may be quite variable between individuals. Some elderly individuals may be housebound with few visitors; other elderly individuals are actively involved in their vocation and other social activities. Because of the range of communicative needs and the lack of good correspondence between audiological results and degree of perceived handicap (Matthews, Lee, Mills, & Schum, 1990; Weinstein & Ventry, 1983), self-assessment tools have been used to assess functional communication. Some of the more popular tools include:

- Communication Profile for the Hearing Impaired, or CPHI (Demorest & Erdman, 1987).
- Hearing Performance Inventory, or HPI (Giolas, Owens, Lamb, & Schubert, 1979).

- Self-Assessment of Communication, or SAC, and the Significant Other Assessment of Communication, or SOAC (Schow & Nerbonne, 1982).
- Hearing Handicap Scale, or HHS (High, Fairbanks, & Glorig, 1964).
- Performance Inventory for Profound and Severe Loss, or PIPSL (Owens & Raggio, 1988).

The audiologist must understand the individual's hearing abilities as they relate to their communication demands. An understanding of the needs of the patient will assist the audiologist in jointly developing rehabilitation goals with the patient and the patient's family.

Management Strategies

The goal of rehabilitation is to reduce the disability and to reduce or avoid the handicap associated with hearing impairment. The audiologist is knowledgeable in several types of rehabilitation tools: counseling techniques, hearing aids, speechreading, auditory training, cochlear implants, and assistive listening devices. The most important components of rehabilitation are the selection, fitting, and evaluation of appropriate hearing aids, education of the client and significant other(s) in the use and care of the hearing aids, and follow-up with the client. Appropriate use and care of amplification are critical because when a greater percentage of the speech signal is audible, a greater the number of acoustic cues are available, resulting in a greater chance for accurate speech understanding.

Hearing Aids

Hearing aids come in various styles. Eyeglass hearing aids attach to the stem of glasses and are infrequently sold these days. Body-worn hearing aids also represent a small percentage of the hearing aids sold. This hearing aid, with its microphone, is worn on the chest with hardwire connections to the earmold that fits in the ear canal. Ear level hearing aids include *behind-the-ear* (*BTE*), *in-the-ear* (*ITE*), *in-the-canal* (*ITC*), and *completely-in-the-canal* (*CIC*). The largest is the *body hearing aid* and the smallest is the CIC (Figure 6-12). The CIC hearing aid is removed by a small wire and is almost unnoticeable unless one looks directly into the canal.

The audiologist must consider the degree of impairment when recommending a particular style of hearing aid. In general, the larger the device the greater amount of amplification possible. It is also important to consider what type the patient is willing to wear and able to handle. The audiologist must determine the type of amplification and circuitry that is best for the individual's hearing loss and listening needs. For example, those with hearing impairment may have a narrow dynamic range or a reduced range of useable hearing in the impaired frequency region(s). The range between the softest sound heard and the dB level at which sounds become too loud is reduced compared to normal-hearing individuals. Those with a narrow dynamic range; that is, when a small increase above threshold results in the perception of an intolerably loud sound, are said to have **recruitment**. Special circuitry can adjust the speech signal so that soft sounds are amplified more than loud sounds and all sounds fit within an individual's comfortable loudness range. Binaural amplification is almost always recommended for the individual with a bilateral hearing impairment. Binaural hearing is important for localizing sounds, improving the signal relative to the noise, and producing greater ease of listening.

The quality of hearing aids has improved dramatically in recent years. Digital and programmable hearing aids offer more efficient and precise settings of the frequency and gain characteristics of

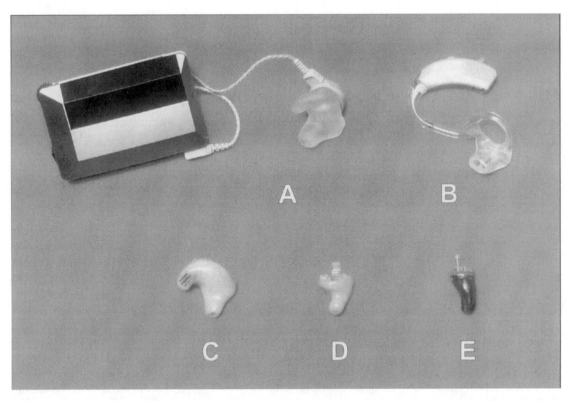

FIGURE 6-12   Types of hearing aids. From top to bottom, left to right: (A) body aid; (B) behind-the-ear aid; (C) in-the-ear aid; (D) in-the-canal aid; and (E) completely-in-the-canal aid.

the hearing aid. The frequency response (frequency and sound pressure level characteristics) of these hearing aids can be set in the audiologist's office and changed if the patient's listening demands or hearing thresholds change. Some programmable hearing aids come with a remote control that allow the patient to change the frequency response and loudness of the hearing aid(s) to best match the listening environment. These technologies are available in the behind-the-ear (BTE) hearing aid and in any hearing aid that sits in the ear or in the ear canal.

Digital hearing aids use a computer chip and special mathematical formulas to enhance the speech signal while reducing the amplification in frequency regions where background noise is thought to exist. The incoming signal is analyzed and manipulated depending on its characteristics, and therefore no loudness control is needed. With continued research, complex signal processing strategies will be developed and applied to digital hearing aids to further improve the quality of the speech signal.

After fitting the hearing aid, the audiologist must verify the fitting by one of several methods. One method is to compare the aided with the unaided thresholds for particular frequencies. Tones are presented through speakers in the sound booth, and the levels at which the hearing-impaired person detects the signal 50% of the time are recorded. The difference between the aided and unaided thresholds is known as **functional gain**. Another method is to obtain the **real ear insertion response (REIR)** using probe-microphone measurements. Frequencies are presented through a loudspeaker while a probe-microphone, placed close to the eardrum, measures the SPL with the hearing aid in the ear and turned on (aided condition) and without the hearing aid in the ear (unaided condition). The difference in SPL between the aided and unaided conditions as a function of frequency is the REIR. Because probe-microphone measurements require no response from the patient, they are reliable and can be used to verify hearing aid fittings even with the difficult-to-test patient.

The patient is instructed in the use and care of hearing aids. Let us examine this aspect of the rehabilitation process by following Mrs. Leon, the woman who received PE tubes to correct the conductive component of a mixed hearing impairment (see Figure 6-11).

> Written and oral instructions were provided to Mrs. Leon and her family regarding her hearing aids. A gradual listening program was recommended. Mrs. Leon was instructed to initially wear the hearing aids in quiet environments such as when watching television or having a conversation with one or two people. After she became comfortable using the hearing aids in quiet, she was instructed to wear them in noisier environments. Listening activities were also recommended. Mrs. Leon was instructed to make a list of common, everyday background sounds in her environment (e.g., water running, the refrigerator humming) and to listen to these sounds while wearing the hearing aids. She was informed that these exercises would assist her in relearning how to tune out or ignore the background noises that she may not have heard for quite some time due to her hearing impairment.

Although hearing aids are the most common form of treatment for sensorineural hearing impairment, less than 20% of the people with hearing impairment wear them (Gallup, 1980; Ries, 1982). This low percentage is likely due to denial, embarrassment, or a belief that a hearing aid will not help. Technological advances as well as skillful counseling are likely to increase the number of adults who become successful hearing aid users. One of the greatest predictors of hearing aid success is a patient's motivation and perception of handicap. An individual who purchases a hearing aid because he or she is missing out on conversations during social interactions is much more likely to make a successful adjustment than a person who has stopped socializing and purchases a hearing aid because of family pressure. Presbycusic listeners with severe CAPD are also less likely to successfully wear hearing aids. For these individuals, assistive listening devices may be more appropriate.

Assistive Listening Devices (ALDs)

An **assistive listening device** or **ALD** is any device, excluding hearing aids, designed to improve a hearing-impaired individual's ability to communicate and therefore function more independently than without the device. The ALD can transmit amplified sound more directly from its source to the listener or can transform the signal into a tactile or visual signal (Wayner, 1997). With some ALDs, the signal to noise ratio is improved by placing the microphone close to the sound source. This technology is beneficial for those who have difficulty hearing in noise and reverberation and who must listen to talkers from a distance. (There is a loss of 6 dB every time the distance from the source is doubled.) A frequency-modulated, or **FM system**, is an example of an ALD used for one-on-one communication. It consists of a microphone, amplifier, and receiver. The signal is transmitted by radio waves from the microphone (placed near the sound source) to the receiver and hearing instrument (worn by the hearing-impaired individual). Radio waves are not affected by reverberation or noise, therefore the signal at the source is transmitted with high fidelity. Because an FM system is wireless, that is, there are no wires between the source and the listener, the hearing-impaired individual and the talker are able to move around freely within the listening environment. This type of system is ideal for tours, lectures, religious services, and other group functions. Another ALD used for one-on-one communication is the PockeTalker® (Williams Sound). The PockeTalker consists of a microphone, amplifier and earphones. Like the FM system, the microphone can be placed near the person speaking. However, a wire extends between the microphone and amplifier and also between the amplifier and earphones that are worn by the hearing-impaired individual. The PockeTalker is ideal for one-on-one communication. For example, individuals with CAPD and decreased mobility are excellent candidates for this device. The PockeTalker is often used in hospital or nursing home settings for rehabilitation evaluations and treatments if a personal hearing aid is not available or not functioning.

Various types of telephone amplifiers are available. A simple amplified handset is often sufficient to allow the hearing-impaired individual to communicate over the telephone. For more profound hearing impairments, the telephone message can be typed by a relay operator and transmitted to a special **telecommunication device for the deaf** (**TDD**) for the hearing-impaired individual to read.

Understanding television or music is often difficult for hearing-impaired individuals. Direct audio input that is sent directly to the hearing aid via a cord can be used to improve the signal quality. Because the signal is carried through a wire there is no interference from room reverberation or background noise. Those who have difficulty understanding the spoken message on television can use a **closed caption decoder** that displays the television dialogue in written form at the bottom of the television screen.

In addition to ALDs, assistive sensory devices are also available for the hearing-impaired individual. These include visual alerting devices to monitor the doorbell, a knock on the door, a baby's cry, a smoke alarm, or an alarm clock. Auditory alerting devices such as a loud ringer or buzzer might be used to indicate that the phone is ringing or that there is smoke in the house. Finally, tactile devices such as a pillow, wrist, or bed vibrator or blowing fan might be used to indicate danger situations and alert the hearing-impaired person to sounds that a normal hearing individual takes for granted (e.g., hearing the morning alarm clock). Hearing-ear dogs are also trained to help alert their owners to auditory signals. The audiologist is familiar with methods that will assist the hearing-impaired individual to function independently at home, at work, and at recreational activities.

Not all hearing-impaired persons come to the audiologist's office with the intent to purchase hearing aids or to inquire about ALDs or assistive sensory devices. Mrs. Lough is an example of a woman who continued to deny that she had a hearing problem and had no intention of trying amplification.

Mrs. Lough came in for testing urged by her husband who was having difficulty communicating with her. He reported that when she does not hear him (which was most of the time) he raises his voice and then Mrs. Lough gets angry because she feels like he is yelling at her. Mrs. Lough's first comment to the audiologist was "I hope you're not going to fit me with hearing aids because I don't want them." She had tried hearing aids twice previously at another clinic and was very dissatisfied with them. The hearing evaluation was performed, and as Figure 6-13 indicates, Mrs. Lough had a moderate sensorineural hearing loss in both ears. Her word recognition ability was fair at a high intensity level. Once the testing was completed the audiologist used a Pocketalker to describe the hearing impairment and its implications for speech. Oral and written information was provided to Mrs. Lough and her husband about hearing aids (what hearing aids could and could not do) and strate-

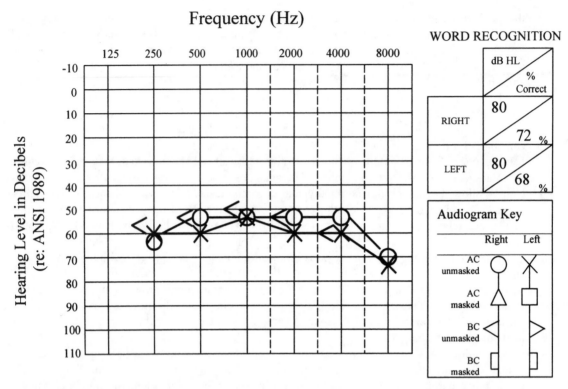

FIGURE 6-13   Audiogram of a moderate sensorineural hearing impairment with fair word recognition ability. Although amplification would make more speech sounds audible to this client, she refused to try any type of amplification.

gies that could facilitate the communication process. Assistive listening devices (ALDs) were also discussed as an alternative to hearing aids. Mrs. Lough was resistant to purchasing any type of amplification including ALDs.

Unfortunately, sometimes counseling cannot undo the negative impact of bad experiences with prior amplification or poor motivation to communicate more effectively. A patient must accept the hearing loss and be ready to work with the audiologist to improve his or her communication abilities.

Cochlear Implants

For those with profound hearing loss who do not benefit substantially from amplification, cochlear implants might be recommended. The implant consists of either single or multiple electrodes surgically placed within the cochlea that convert sound into electrical current and directly stimulate auditory nerve fibers to produce hearing sensations. The external components, worn outside of the head, include a microphone, transmitter, and signal processor (see Chapter 5 for a discussion of cochlear implants). To date the cochlear implant has been most successful in adults with acquired deafness. It codes pitch by rate of stimulation (pulses per second), place (which electrode is stimulated), or both.

Place coding for pitch requires that more than one channel or electrode be implanted. Low frequency sounds are associated with electrical stimulation near the apex of the cochlea while high frequency sounds are associated with stimulation at the base. Loudness is coded by the amount of electrical stimulation. In general, the greater the amount of current, the louder the sound is perceived. Although only a small minority of audiologists are employed in cochlear implant centers, they play an important role in education and counseling of potential candidates for cochlear implants.

Speechreading

Speechreading refers to perceiving speech by observing visual articulation and facial gestures. In everyday speech perception, speechreading is combined with whatever auditory information is available to determine the speaker's message. Sumby and Pollack (1954) found that listeners who watched a speaker's mouth could improve speech intelligibility. The improvement was comparable to the level expected if the signal-to-noise ratio was increased by 5 to 22 dB. This improvement is due to the complementary nature of visual and acoustic cues to speech perception. Acoustic cues that indicate place of articulation are most severely affected by background noise and high frequency hearing impairment. Fortunately, it is the place cues that are most readily available from watching a speaker's mouth.[4] Although the ability to speechread varies widely across subjects, there are some factors that can increase the likelihood of successful speechreading (see also Montgomery, 1993, for suggestions to maximize lipreading in combination with amplification).

- Position yourself so that there is good lighting behind you (the listener) and the speaker's face is well lit.
- Have reasonably good visual acuity; use eyeglasses if necessary.
- Let the talker know you are hearing-impaired. Ask speakers to articulate clearly with unexaggerated movements of the facial structures.
- Try to understand phrases and ideas rather than identify individual words.
- Watch for ideas rather than isolated words. It is also helpful to keep up with current events and the topic of discussion so as to guess the content or ask for clarification if necessary.

Although a minority of audiologists provide speechreading training (White, Dancer, & Burl, 1996), the strategies listed above may assist the hearing-impaired individual to "fill-in" missing auditory information.[5] These strategies will be particularly beneficial for the individual who typically does not attend to the talker's face during communication. The audiologist will need to give special attention to the client who is both visually and hearing-impaired. ALDs to maximize the signal-to-noise ratio may be of great benefit to this population especially if communication typically occurs in noisy environments.

---

[4]Forty percent or more of the speech sounds are considered homophenous. That is, they look alike on the lips (Nitchie, 1930).

[5]The lack of enthusiasm for speechreading training is probably a result of unreliable assessment tools. Training methods that allow the individual to generalize to everyday communication settings also need to be developed.

Auditory Training

Historically, speechreading and **auditory training** were the most common techniques used to teach children who were deafened before or shortly after birth to understand speech. Although speechreading and auditory training are large components of the rehabilitation process for cochlear implant patients, neither is typically part of rehabilitation for adults who are fitted with hearing aids. These techniques, however, may be useful for individuals who use amplification but still have difficulty understanding speech. Auditory training involves teaching the individual to optimally use the available sound cues. There certainly is evidence from the second language learning literature that training can facilitate the discrimination of certain phonemes (Logan, Lively, & Pisoni, 1991). However, the short- and long-term effects of auditory training on speech perception in those with acquired hearing impairment are not known.

Several approaches to auditory training exist. The hearing-impaired individual can be trained in the discrimination and identification of nonsense syllables such as /ba/ and /da/. Simple words might also be used as training stimuli. Feedback and repetition reinforce correct responses. Alternatively, a more holistic approach can be used in which listening exercises and conversational strategies are employed to understand the meaning of sentences, paragraphs, and stories. Examples of such strategies are: prepare for the listening situation by staying informed of events, guess when uncertain, listen carefully, and stay relaxed. Beiter and Brimacombe (1993) recommended a multisensory approach to auditory training. Auditory visual speech materials, with the most cues available, are used initially during training. Once the patient reached a high level of performance, auditory only material (fewer cues available) are presented.

Counseling

The audiologist provides information to the patient and family. Individuals and their families must understand the nature of the hearing impairment; its implications for understanding speech, and the limitations of amplification, cochlear implants, or other rehabilitative methods employed. For example, it is important for the hearing-impaired individual and family to understand that hearing aids will not enable the impaired individual to have normal hearing. Rather, hearing aids are amplifiers that do not "fix" distortion within the cochlea or central auditory system. Hearing aids, if properly fit, will increase the audibility of speech sounds and thus increase the probability that understanding will occur. The audiologist counsels the hearing-impaired person on how to use and care for the amplification device(s). Other strategies to improve the communication process are also discussed with the patient and significant other(s). Kaplan (1988) listed several strategies for the person talking with the hearing-impaired individual. Strategies such as these should also be used by health care professionals who work with or care for hearing-impaired individuals. Examples include:

- Allow and encourage the hearing-impaired person to be involved in the communication process.
- Rather than shout, speak in a normal audible voice facing the hearing-impaired person.
- Use clear and distinct articulation.
- Inform the hearing-impaired person about the topic of conversation.
- Speak to, not about, the hearing-impaired person.
- Help the hearing-impaired person manipulate the environment (e.g., reduce background noise, if possible).
- Restate what you've said when you detect that the hearing-impaired person has misunderstood.

Examples of strategies that the hearing-impaired person can use (Kaplan, 1988) include:

- Ask a speaker to repeat or rephrase a statement that you did not understand.
- Before going to a movie or theater, read the reviews in advance to familiarize yourself with the plot.
- Try to avoid rooms with poor acoustics. If noise is present, move yourself and the speaker away from the noise source if possible.
- Ask speakers to face you so that speechreading can be used.
- If you cannot hear a speaker at a meeting, request that he or she use a microphone.

In addition to informational counseling, the audiologist must be sensitive to how an individual reacts to his or her hearing impairment and to any adjustment problems related to the impairment. Tanner (1980) provided an excellent article about loss related to communication disorders and Kubler-Ross's (1969) five stages of the grieving process (i.e., denial, anger, bargaining, depression, acceptance). It is important to keep in mind that an individual may not only be grieving the loss of hearing but also the loss of independence, vocation, and group or self-identity. Hard-of-hearing support groups offer an excellent opportunity for those with hearing handicaps to share their experiences and feelings with others experiencing similar handicaps.

Support Groups

Members of national and local support groups work together to improve communication and teach self-management skills. Information about hearing impairment is often provided at support group meetings as are discussions about communication problems and solutions. The meetings provide an opportunity for the hearing-impaired individual to practice assertive communication strategies in a nonthreatening environment. The groups also offer an opportunity for members to be proactive in political issues related to the civil rights of those with hearing-impairment. For example, members of Self-Help for the Hard of Hearing (SHHH) were actively involved in developing regulations for section 255 of the Telecommunications Act of 1996. This section requires telecommunication products and services to be accessible to people with disabilities. The group was also instrumental in developing regulations for the Americans with Disabilities Act (ADA) of 1990. The ADA was designed to ensure that those with disabilities were not discriminated against in employment, public accommodations, transportation, state and local government services, and telecommunications.

Clinical Problem Solving

Mr. Westrich, age 76, reported he has difficulty understanding his wife and grandchildren when they talk. He also has difficulty understanding speakers on television. He suggested that "all newscasters must go to the same school of mumbling." At family gatherings he relies on his wife to repeat what people have said and often gets left out of conversations. He was a pilot in the military for 30 years and enjoyed hunting before he retired. Figure 6-14 displays his audiogram and word recognition ability.

1. What type of hearing impairment does Mr. Westrich have?
2. What factors are likely to have contributed to Mr. Westrich's hearing impairment?

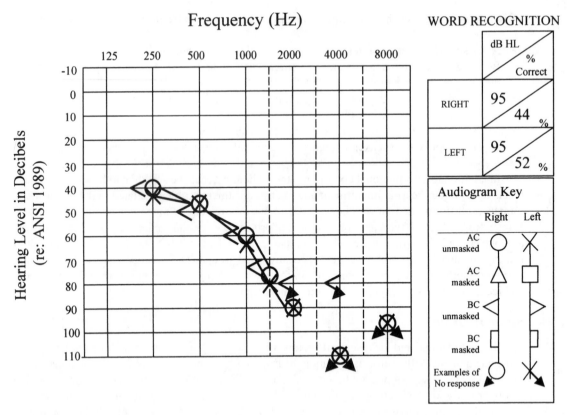

FIGURE 6-14   Audiogram of a client who came to the clinic because of difficulties communicating with his family.

3. What class(es) of speech sounds will Mr. Westrich have most difficulty hearing?
4. Is Mr. Westrich a candidate for amplification? Why or why not?
5. What types of communication strategies might Mr. Westrich use when communicating? What might the speaker do to facilitate Mr. Westrich's speech understanding?

References

Beiter, A.L., & Brimacombe, J.A. (1993). Cochlear implants, In J. Alpiner & P. McCarthy (Eds.), *Rehabilitative Audiology: Children and Adults* (pp. 417–437). Baltimore: Williams & Wilkins.

Demorest, M.E., & Erdman, S.A. (1987). Development of the communication profile for the hearing impaired. *Journal of Speech and Hearing Disorders, 52:* 129–142.

Gallup, F. (1980). *A Survey Concerning Hearing Problems and Hearing Aids in the United States.* Washington, DC: Hearing Industries Association.

Giolas, T.G. (1994). Aural rehabilitation of adults with hearing impairment. In J. Katz (ed.), *Handbook of Clinical Audiology* (pp. 776–789). Baltimore: Williams & Wilkins.

Giolas, T.G., Owens, E., Lamb, S.H., & Schubert, E.D.

(1979). Hearing performance inventory. *Journal of Speech and Hearing Disorders*, *44*: 169–195.

Goodhill, V. (1979). *Presbycusis in Ear Diseases, Deafness and Dizziness* (p. 719). Hagerstown, MD: Harper and Row.

High, W.S., Fairbanks, G., & Glorig, A. (1964). Scale of self-assessment of hearing handicap. *Journal of Speech and Hearing Disorders*, *29*: 215–230.

Kaplan, H. (1988). Communication problems of the hearing-impaired elderly: What can be done? *Pride Institute Journal of Long Term Home Health Care*, *7*: 10–22.

Kubler-Ross, E. (1969). *On Death and Dying*. New York: Macmillan.

Logan, J.S., Lively, S.E., & Pisoni, D.B. (1991). Training Japanese listeners to identify /r/ and /l/: A first report. *Journal of the Acoustical Society of America*, *89*: 874–886.

Matthews, L. J., Lee, F., Mills, J. H., & Schum, D. J. (1990). Audiometric and subjective assessment of hearing handicap. *Archives of Otolaryngology—Head and Neck Surgery*, *116*: 1325–1330.

Montgomery, A.A. (1993). Management of the hearing-impaired adult, In J. Alpiner & P. McCarthy (Eds.), *Rehabilitative Audiology*: *Children and Adults* (pp. 311–330). Baltimore: Williams & Wilkins.

Mueller, H., & Killion, M. (1990). An easy method for calculating the articulation index. *Hearing Journal*, *3*: 14–17.

Mulrow, C.D., Aguilar, C., Endicott, J.E., Tuley, M.R., Velez, R., Charlip, W.S., Rhodes, M.C., Hill, J.A., & DeNino, L.A. (1990). Quality-of-life changes and hearing impairment. *Annals of Internal Medicine*, *113*: 188–194.

Nitchie, E. B. (1930). *Lip-reading Principles and Practice*. New York: F. Stokes & Co.

Olsen, W., Hawkins, D., & Van Tasell, D. (1987). Representations of the long-term spectra of speech. *Ear and Hearing*, *8* (5): 1003–1085.

Owens, E., & Raggio, M. (1988). Performance inventory for profound and severe loss (PIPSL). *Journal of Speech and Hearing Disorders*, *53*: 42–56.

Ramsdell, D. (1960). The psychology of the hard of hearing and deafened adult. In H. Davis & S. Silverman (Eds.), *Hearing and Deafness*. New York: Holt, Rinehart & Silverman.

Ries, P.W. (1982). Hearing ability of persons by sociodemographic and health characteristics: United States (Vital and Health Statistics, Series 10, No. 140, DHHS Publication No. [PHS] 82-1568). Washington, DC: U.S. Government Printing Office.

Sandor, G. (1994). Hearing a new market. *American Demographics*, November, 48-55.

Schow, R., & Nerbonne, M. (1980). Hearing level in nursing home residents. *Journal of Speech and Hearing Disorders*, *45*: 124–132.

Schow, R., & Nerbonne, M. (1982). Communication screening profile; use with elderly clients. *Ear and Hearing*, *3*: 135–147.

Stach, B.A., Spretnjak, M.L., & Jerger, J. (1990). The prevalence of central presbycusis in a clinical population. *Journal of the American Academy of Audiology*, *1*: 109–115.

Stephens, D., & Hetu, R. (1991). Impairment, disability and handicap in audiology: Towards a consensus. *Audiology*, *30*: 185–200.

Sumby, W.G., & Pollack, I. (1954). Visual contributions to speech intelligibility in noise. *Journal of the Acoustical Society of America*, *26*: 212–215.

Tanner, D. (1980). Loss and grief: Implications for the speech-language pathologist and audiologist. *ASHA*, *22*: 916–928.

Thibodeau, L.M., & Schmitt, J. (1988). A report on condition of hearing aids in nursing homes and retirement centers. *Journal of the American Academy of Audiology*, *21*: 99–112.

Ventry, I., & Weinstein, B. (1982). Identification of elderly people with hearing problems. *Ear and Hearing*, *3*: 128–134.

Wayner, D.S. (1997). ALDs: Building a practice in communication accessibility. *The Hearing Review*, *4*(6): 18–22.

Weinstein, B.E., & Amsel, L. (1986). Hearing loss and senile dementia in the institutionalized elderly. *Clinical Gerontology*, *4*: 3–15.

Weinstein, B. E., & Ventry, I. M. (1983). Audiometric correlates of hearing handicapped inventory for the elderly. *Journal of Speech and Hearing Disorders*, *48*: 379–384.

White, S., Dancer, J., & Burl, N. (1996). Speechreading and speechreading tests: A survey of rehabilitative audiologists. *American Annals of the Deaf*, *141* (3): 236–239.

Chapter 7

Disorders of Language in Children

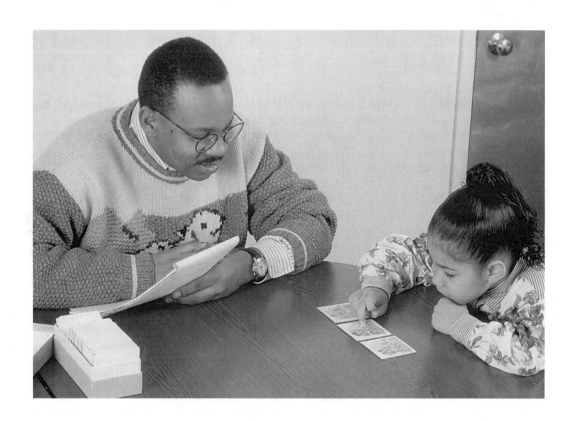

Preview

Normal development is critical for the development of normal language skills. When normal development is impeded because of congenital disability or childhood illness, a language disorder may occur. In this chapter, we will describe selected conditions that are associated with impaired language in children. The early language difficulties of these children evolve as they pass through the preschool and school years. In later childhood, solid language skills are important for not only listening and speaking, but also for reading and writing. Language in its various modalities is assessed through a variety of methods, including case histories, observation, and standardized assessment tools. Information from the assessment may be used to identify and describe a language disorder and, possibly, to determine preliminary goals for intervention. We will describe some of the approaches available for addressing children's language needs at various ages.

As we discussed in Chapters 3 and 4, the development of language follows a fairly predictable sequence. Infants begin with an awareness of sound and quickly develop a preference for the sounds and patterns of their native language(s). Sounds, first produced reflexively, are soon produced intentionally and take on the characteristics of speech. Across cultures and languages, the child's first words appear around the child's first birthday. By age 2, most children know many words and are combining them into short phrases. By age 4, children sound remarkably adult-like in their spoken language.

Not all children are so fortunate as to experience normal language acquisition. Language disorders may affect up to 13% of children (Tomblin, Records, & Zhang, 1996). A variety of conditions can lead to a language disorder. Genetic conditions may disturb the development of the brain and alter its capacity for normal language development. We learned in Chapter 5 that the presence of a hearing impairment can have a profound effect on language development. Injury or illness can arrest language development after a period of normal development. Finally, there are a wide variety of developmental syndromes that include impaired language as part of the presenting signs.

Although many conditions can lead to a language disorder, the types of skills affected may vary considerably. For this reason, a good working definition of a language disorder will be necessarily broad. One such definition would be that a language disorder includes impaired ability to understand or use language—spoken, signed, or written—as well as same-age peers of the same community. Several components of this definition deserve further comment. The definition does not specify severity; indeed severity can vary widely among types of language disorders and even among children who are identified as having the same type of language disorder. The definition specifies that language disorders can affect language in either spoken, signed, or written modalities. In fact, it is often the case (although there are exceptions) that all modalities are affected to some extent when language is impaired. We included the comparison to the child's age-mates for two reasons. First, language disorders are often first suspected because the child's language development lags behind the expected norms for children of the same age. Second, the nature of the language disorder may change as age-expected language skills expand as the child grows. For example, language skills will not affect reading until the child has reached an age at which reading skills would be expected. Finally, we include a reference to the child's community. This comparison is critical as language form, content, and use all vary from region to region and culture to culture.

Language Differences

There are children from particular cultural and social groups whose speech may demonstrate phonological, morphosyntactic, semantic, and pragmatic differences from that of standard English. However, these differences do not, in themselves, constitute a language disorder. Such children have learned the language code of their community, which simply differs in some aspect from that used by the majority of speakers in the country. So, these children may be quite competent in their use of the native language.

Some linguistic variation reflects regional differences in language, known as dialects. We recognize dialectal differences in how certain sounds are produced in the Northeast, or the Deep South, or the Midwest. Other differences may affect the choice of words that are used within a region. Carbonated drinks may be "soda" in one region and "pop" in another. Large-scale sandwiches on long rolls are "submarines," "hoagies," or "po' boys" depending on the region. Dialects can vary with social or cultural groups within a particular region. Communities with strong Hispanic roots may use a variant of English that includes influences from Spanish. Residents of both inner cities and rural districts may speak one or more versions of a dialect known as Black English (sometimes called Ebonics). Although these dialects are culturally influenced, speakers do not necessarily have to be a member of the particular minority group to speak the dialect. Furthermore, any given speaker of a dialect may not use it at all times. Social rules may dictate when a dialect, or even which variant of a dialect, is appropriate to the situation. So, an individual who uses one version of Black English among friends may use another with parents and switch to standard English when addressing a teacher. This situational shifting of speech and language patterns is referred to as **code switching**.

The variations in language *form* observed in dialects are rule governed, meaning that there are strict conventions that dictate correct use of these forms. However, for the listener who is unfamiliar with the conventions of a dialect, it may seem as if the speaker is making linguistic errors. For example, residents of Maryland may "go down the shore for the weekend," omitting the preposition "to" that speakers in other parts of the country would typically use in that sentence. Forms of Black English may include omissions of certain grammatical forms (e.g., the contracted "is" or "are"; the infinitive "to") and changes in grammatical form (e.g., "hisself" for "himself" "be" for "has been [continually]") in certain sentence contexts. These are normal forms within some versions of this dialect (Terrell & Terrell, 1993; Washington & Craig, 1994). However, not all speakers of Black English and other dialects use all the linguistic or pragmatic elements associated with the dialect. For example, Washington and Craig (1994) reported that young children within the same region may vary in their frequency of Black English forms and the types of forms that characterize their speech. Speech-language pathologists must be able to distinguish between linguistic variation that reflects a dialect and variation that signals a disorder and to treat those aspects that are attributable to the disorder alone. However, if a dialect speaker, who shows no sign of a language disorder, wishes to improve his or her use of standard English, a speech-language pathologist may provide such assistance (ASHA, 1983).

Children who speak more than one language may also show language differences that may be mistaken for a disorder. For example, the Navajo child in northeastern Arizona may be bilingual, using Navajo at home and English at school. Vocabulary development in each language may be restricted to the environment in which it is used. These children may appear to have limited lexical knowledge when tested in only one of their languages, but often have a large and rich vocabulary when both languages are considered. If a Navajo child moves to Los Angeles, his or her language *use* might be judged faulty by their non-Navajo listeners in the new city. Children in many parts of the world are multilingual, using a particular language for a specific situation. For most children, learning two or more languages (or dialects) in the preschool years is relatively easy given adequate experience with those languages. Some children, however, are unable to use any of the languages of their community proficiently.

Early Signs of a Language Disorder

Infants at Risk

Some infants are born with genetic conditions, illnesses, or disabilities that interfere with their development (Clark, 1994; Sparks, 1984). In Chapter 5, we saw that a great many genetic and acquired conditions may affect hearing, and consequently will alter the course of language development. Many other conditions, such as drug exposure (Johnson, Seikel, Madison, Foose, & Rinard, 1997), infection (Bent & Beck, 1994), low birth weight, and premature birth (Byrne, Ellsworth, Bowering, & Vincer, 1993), increase the risk that a child will experience language and learning difficulties. In some cases, serious illness itself may interfere with language development. Infants who require hospitalization will not receive the same stimulation from their parents as a healthy baby. Babies who are confined to a hospital nursery will have limited opportunities to explore and interact with the people and objects around them. Other infants have physical disabilities that interfere with normal development, including speech and language development.

A speech-language pathologist may work with the infant's family and the hospital staff to provide the infant with experiences that facilitate language development. In these cases, speech and language intervention often must be integrated with medical treatments, physical therapy, and occupational therapy. The speech-language pathologist and the audiologist are members of a multidisciplinary team, which may also include medical staff, rehabilitation staff, and social services. The team works closely with the infant's family to ensure that the parents and family understand their child's needs and how to best address them. When a child is born with an obvious disability, parent counseling and intervention for the child can begin right away. However, the impact of prematurity on language and academic disorders appears years later, as the child develops (e.g., Halsey, Collin, & Anderson, 1996). Therefore, parents and professionals may need to monitor progress throughout childhood.

Late Talkers

One group of children at risk for language disorders are toddlers who lag behind their peers in the ability to understand or produce words. These children have been referred to as "late talkers." In the research literature, late talkers are typically defined as young children (between approximately 16 and 30 months) whose language skills fall below 90 percent of their age peers. These are children who may be slow to acquire their first 50 words and slow to combine words into phrases. For example, Rescorla, Roberts, and Daahlsgard (1997) reported their group of late talkers had an average of 20 words at age 26 months, compared with their normal peers who had an average of 226 words. Furthermore, only one of their 34 late talkers was combining words into phrases. The parents of late-talking toddlers may also report that they seem to understand fewer words than would be expected for their age. Nonetheless, these children lack a history of hearing loss, cognitive impairment, or medical factors that would otherwise place them at risk for poor language development.

Investigators who have followed the development of late talking children have demonstrated that these children are at risk for continued language problems. Toddlers who are identified as late talkers tend to remain behind their peers over time (Rescorla et al., 1997; Thal, Bates, Goodman, & Jahn-Samilo,1997). However, what is true for the group is not necessarily true for all its members. In fact, some late talkers do "catch up" with their peers (Thal, et al., 1997; Ellis Weismer, Murray-Branch, & Miller, 1994; Rescorla et al., 1997). There is currently no clear consensus concerning what factors present at early ages might predict which children simply prove to be "late bloomers" versus which will manifest continued language difficulty. Some studies have suggested factors that predict language outcome include poor comprehension skills (Thal & Tobias, 1992), limited use of gestures for communication (Thal & Tobias, 1992; Thal et al., 1997), limited vocabulary (Fischel et al., 1989; Thal et al., 1997), and initial severity (Rescorla et al., 1997; Rescorla & Schwartz, 1990). In addition, the older a child is when identified as a late talker also appears to be predictive, with the younger children in the groups faring better than slightly older late talkers (Paul, 1993; Rescorla & Schwartz, 1990; Thal et al., 1997).

Late-talking toddlers are typically first identified by their impoverished vocabularies. However, for those late talkers who do not move into the normal range, a variety of language signs emerge over time. As we saw in Chapter 4, normally developing children acquire a corpus of single word utterances that they then begin to combine into two word utterances. From this point, children lengthen their phrases and eventually begin to produce more complex sentences. However, by age 3 or 4, children who were late-talking toddlers produced much shorter and morphologically and syntactically simpler phrases than their normally developing peers (Paul & Alforde, 1993; Rescorla et al., 1997). Interestingly, many of these late-talking toddlers moved into the normal range for their vocabulary skills (Rescorla et al., 1997). Kindergarten children who were late talkers were less proficient in relating a story in logical order than their normally developing peers (Paul, Hernandez, Taylor, & Johnson, 1996). By second grade, however, these children appeared to have caught up in terms of narrative ability. However, there were still other differences in expressive language skills between the late-talking group and their peers (Paul, Murray, Clancy, & Andrews, 1997).

These studies demonstrate the long-term sequelae associated with late-talking status as a toddler. However, we also saw that not all late-talking toddlers have a poor language outcome. Despite our imperfect ability to predict outcome, status as a "late talker" is sufficient to indicate risk for language disorder. The long-term risk warrants close monitoring of late-talking children so that those who go on to show clear signs of a language disorder may receive the earliest possible intervention (Thal et al., 1997).

Developmental Language Disorders

For many children with language problems, there is no obvious cause for the impairment. They do not have the physical characteristics that would signal the presence of a developmental syndrome. Likewise, their cognitive abilities are good, ruling out mental retardation as a cause for poor language skills. They hear normally and lack any sign of brain damage or disease that might lead to impaired language, but their language skills lag behind those of their peers. These children are said to have a **developmental language disorder**.

Developmental language disorder is actually an umbrella term that encompasses children with a wide range of language-related problems. Although the exact cause of these disorders is unknown, parents are often relieved to know that it does not appear to be related to rearing practices or the way they have talked to their child. Instead, the underlying cause appears to be biological. Current information suggests that the brains of language-disordered children develop differently from most people (Cohen, Campbell, & Yaghmai, 1989; Gauger, Lombardino, & Leonard, 1997; Plante, Swisher, Vance, & Rapcsak, 1991). This altered brain development may underly altered language development. Evidence of altered brain anatomy can also be found among the parents and siblings of these children (Plante, 1991; Jackson & Plante, 1997). Likewise, when one member of the family has a developmental language disorder, it is common that others do as well (e.g., Tallal, Ross, & Curtiss, 1989; Tomblin, 1989). The fact that both the biological and behavioral aspects of this disorder tend to cluster in families suggests that it may be inherited in some cases.

Children may have developmental problems with receptive language, expressive language, or both. Language deficits may encompass any or all of the components of language *form*, *content*, or *use* (see Chapter 4 for a review). In fact, we will see that a particular child's language difficulties may change over time. When language deficits occur in the absence of other handicapping conditions (e.g., cognitive, motor, sensory, emotional), the child is said to have a **specific language impairment**. To understand this disorder, let us look at the development of one child diagnosed with specific language impairment.

> Troy had difficulty with communication from a very early age. He was reportedly about 20 months before he used his first word. His parents became concerned when at age 2 he used few words, communicating instead largely by grunting and pointing. Despite his limited expression, both parents felt that he understood speech well for his age. Troy's pediatrician also noticed his slow language development and arranged for him to be evaluated by a speech-language pathologist.
>
> During his initial evaluation, Troy passed a hearing screening. His parents completed a questionnaire that surveyed cognitive, motor, self-help, and social skills. Their responses placed him well within normal limits for each of these areas. Troy was then given a formal evaluation of language skills that involved a series of simple activities to test receptive and expressive skills. He correctly pointed to pictures and followed commands appropriately for his age. His score for receptive language confirmed relatively normal skills in that domain. In contrast, his expressive score placed him in the first percentile, or below 99 percent of other children his age. He had great difficulty naming pictures and imitating words on request. He often used the same "word" /da/, to refer to a variety of pictures and objects. In addition, Troy had a limited number of sounds that he used spontaneously, relying mostly on stop consonant-vowel combinations in the words he attempted.

In Troy's case, early deficits involved vocabulary and phonology. These delayed communication skills were present despite the fact that he was developing normally in other areas. As we saw in our discussion of late talkers, such a delay is a risk factor for a developmental language disorder. However, not all children with a developmental language disorder are noticeably different from other children at this young age. For some, the first words emerge right on schedule for normal development, and a disorder only becomes apparent as the child fails to progress from words to sentences.

Troy was enrolled in a preschool program for children with specific language impairment at age three. His parents reported remarkable improvement from that time forward. In addition to his preschool class, his parents implemented a home program of language stimulation. This involved techniques for introducing new vocabulary and encouraging him to produce longer utterances. Troy's vocabulary expanded rapidly from 14 words to well over 100 words in five months. His phonological repertoire also expanded, so that he was producing many more of the sounds appropriate for his age. At age 3, he was occasionally combining words to form two-word utterances as well. His mother reported that Troy was showing fewer signs of frustration in his attempts to communicate, and that people outside of the family were having much less difficulty understanding his speech.

At age 4, Troy was using many two- and three-word phrases, with an occasional four-word phrase in spontaneous speech. However, he used few grammatical morphemes (e.g., verb tense markers, prepositions), which is very unusual for a child his age. At age 4 years, 7 months, the following conversation was recorded while he played with a toy fire station:

Troy: This the fireperson. This the bell (indicating the fire alarm).
Mother: Does the bell ring in an emergency?
Troy: No. The bell, it has . . . the car come out.
Mother: The cars come out when the bell rings?
Troy: (nods) The telephone do that too!

Not surprisingly, formal tests documented below normal expressive language skills at this time, including morphology and syntax. Although language form was still delayed, Troy showed great improvement in language content and use. He spoke readily in a variety of contexts and was able to use language for a variety of purposes (e.g., requesting, explaining, directing).

This pattern of differential impairment across language domains is fairly common during the preschool years. In addition, we observed a shift from the initial vocabulary deficit, which was apparent at age 2, to morphosyntactic deficits at age 4. This phenomenon is known as "growing into a deficit." We did not see morphosyntactic deficits early on simply because English-speaking children do not use syntax or morphology until words are combined into phrases. Therefore, we had to wait until Troy reached a developmental stage where these skills could be expected before evaluating whether they were impaired.

Some children with early language disorders ultimately achieve parity with their normally developing peers. For some of these children, this marks the end of their language difficulties. However, for others, this period is temporary and is referred to as a period of "illusory recovery" (Scarborough & Dobrich, 1990) because these children who appear to recover once again fall behind their peers as they progress through grade school. In addition to these children are others who continue to show signs of language deficits as they enter the school years. We saw this pattern with Troy.

Troy's speech and language skills were re-evaluated by the school speech-language pathologist when he entered first grade at 5 years 9 months. At that time, his early problems with phonology had almost completely resolved. His speech could be easily understood, and the only remaining errors were an occasional mispronunciation in conversation, and these involved only the late-acquired sounds of speech (see Chapter 3). However, his conversations consisted primarily of short, simple sentences. He continued to have difficulty with grammatical morphemes, making substitutions like "the paint guy" for "paint*er*" and "the more big one" for "bigg*er*" or omissions like "He run" for "He run*s*." Once again, formal testing documented poor language expression despite good overall comprehension. Both receptive and expressive vocabulary remained strong.

The school speech-language pathologist continued to see Troy twice a week for work on morphology. She also coordinated activities with the classroom teacher and Troy's parents to reinforce correct use of the morphological items that Troy was learning. This intervention was quite successful, and by the middle of second grade, Troy's conversational speech no longer contained obvious morphological errors. He was re-tested at this time because the school was considering his dismissal from therapy. However, his standardized test scores continued to indicate that his expressive language skills lagged behind his peers. Because he was keeping up in the classroom and was doing well socially, it appeared that his weak expressive language skills were not a handicapping factor at this time. The school decided to monitor his progress, but to discontinue direct services.

The school staff's decision to discontinue services for Troy is consistent with their mandate to provide services to children with *educationally handicapping conditions*. The public law (P.L. 94-142) that first mandated services in 1975 guaranteed a free and appropriate education for all children with educationally handicapping conditions. Speech and language disorders are among the disorders covered under this law and subsequent legislation (P.L. 99-457, Individuals with Disabilities Education Act [IDEA], discussed in Chapter 5). Because Troy was functioning well in the educational system, the school staff decided he was best served in the regular classroom with monitoring and consultative support by the speech-language pathologist. For Troy, this educational plan places him in the *least restrictive environment* in which he is capable of functioning.

Other children with more serious handicaps may require more educational support. This may include "pullout" services, in which the child leaves the classroom for brief periods of direct therapy, or special classrooms within the regular school, or even specialized schools for severely handicapped children. Each of these modes of intervention involves increasing restrictions on the child's environment because less time is spent with normally developing peers. The type and frequency of service each child receives may change over the years as the degree to which the child's disorder impacts educational progress changes. The type and frequency of the child's services are determined by a multidisciplinary team that includes parents, teachers, therapists, and others who can provide insight into a particular child's learning difficulties. This team develops an *individualized educational plan* (IEP) that specifies the level of services, who will provide the services, and what the goals will be.

Three years later, at age 10, Troy's skills were re-evaluated. This testing session revealed a shift in his language profile. Although his comprehension skills were previously a relative strength, comprehension skills had fallen below the average range at this time. This may well be another instance of "growing into the deficit" because these problems emerged at an age at which comprehension demands increase. This pattern of worsening comprehension, seen in Figure 7-1, was maintained into the teenage years. In fact, by age 14, his expressive skills exceeded his receptive skills. This impairment was significant because comprehension skills become increasingly important in the later school years. The sentences spoken by teachers are often longer and more syntactically complex than those heard in casual conversation. Students are expected to conduct multiple language tasks simultaneously, by listening to the teacher lecture, extracting the principal concepts, and encoding them as written notes. Comprehension becomes a learning tool, not just in listening to the teacher but also in reading. Reading comprehension is a major source of vocabulary growth and academic learning through the school years.

Troy's expressive skills showed only slight improvement relative to others his age on standardized tests (see Figure 7-1). Once again, as children reach an age where more complex use of language is expected, new deficits may appear. Consider his attempt to relate the plot of a movie during a conversation, recorded when Troy was 12 years old:

> "It was hilarious. He didn't put the . . . um . . . 'owies.' He only put the best 'owie.' No, that was the second best 'owie.' The first was when the rope that he went down was soaked in some kind of thing . . . that it makes fire go on . . . makes it go faster and they were on the rope and say 'Hey Harry, are you there?' No, that's Clorox, or something like that. (Speaks for a movie character.) 'Oh guys.' (sound effect of guys falling) 'Get up! Get up!' (sound effect of guys yelling and hand gestures.) Then there's like a bridge and they fall right through and they get covered with all kinds of . . . sticky stuff.

We can see a number of problems in this short sample. First, the story he is telling lacks the structure of a identifiable beginning, middle, and end. Characters are referred to without first being introduced to the listener (e.g., He didn't put the … um … "owies"). We hear pauses and revisions

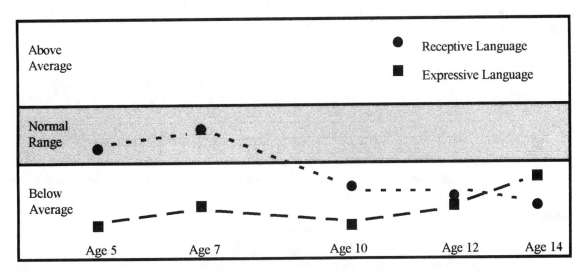

FIGURE 7-1   For children with developmental language disorders, the components of language can change over time. Here we can see receptive and expressive language skills shift over time in a single child relative to typically developing peers.

throughout. In addition, the use of sound effects and gestures suggested that he may have been having difficulty retrieving specific words to communicate his thoughts.

The ability to organize and sequence verbal information becomes increasingly important as a child progresses through school. In fact, Troy's written work shows many of the same characteristics that we see in the verbal sample above. In addition, he often makes the same morphological errors in written language that we saw in his spoken language at age 5. For example, at age 12 he wrote:

Mom caned the riped vejedetables.

I don't wan't any.

But the two dog eat it.

At this point, Troy's language difficulties were again interfering with his academic progress. His reading was slow, and he did not always glean as much meaning from reading as he should. His writing was messy, with many spelling errors, and the flow of thoughts did not always follow a logical sequence. Because his weak language skills were having the greatest impact on educational skills, the school staff considered providing services for a **learning disability**.

Many children, like Troy, who experience early language difficulties go on to have academic problems later in life. In fact, several skills that Troy had difficulty with are predictive of later reading problems. The presence of early language problems, including phonological problems, morphosyntax, and naming, and the impaired ability to think about the components of language, places a child at risk for later language problems (Bishop & Adams, 1990; Lewis & Freebairn, 1992; Menyuk & Chesnick, 1997; Snyder & Downey, 1997). Therefore, it is not surprising that many children identified during the school years as having a learning disability or **dyslexia** also have language difficulties (Catts & Kamhi, 1986; Pennington, Van Orden, Smith, Green, & Haith, 1990; Scarborough, 1990). In Troy's case, the diagnostic label used by the school changed, not because the underlying deficit changed, but because its impact on his life shifted from oral communication alone to include academics. Other children with early language difficulties may have few problems learning to read, and some children whose early oral communication skills were unremarkable may nonetheless show reading deficits later.

The long-term outcome of children with developmental language disorders is quite variable. Some will overcome the handicap of an early language disorder. Others may struggle with language in either the oral or written modalities for years. Even as adults, children with a history of language therapy may still show subtle, residual deficits on standardized measures (Tomblin, Records, & Freese, 1992). However, these language difficulties may or may not prove handicapping in the individual's everyday life. In fact, adults with a childhood history of language disorders appear no less satisfied with their quality of life than those without such a childhood history (Records, Tomblin, & Freese, 1992).

Disorders That Impact Language

Children experience difficulty with language for a variety of reasons. In the 1950s, the audiologist and speech-language pathologist emphasized the cause, or etiology, of the child's language disorder. With the growth of behavioral and operant psychology in the 1960s, however, emphasis switched from etiology per se to changing the child's behavior regardless of etiology. However, knowledge of etiology presents at least two primary advantages. The first is being able to address parents' desires to know "why" their child has a disorder (Aram, 1991). The second involves clinical management. The initial diagnosis can serve to orient the clinician to the likely behavioral strengths and weaknesses. Given a diagnosis of seizure disorder, for example, a clinician is alerted by the diagnostic category to examine receptive language skills. The same clinician, faced with a case involving dyslexia would be prepared to evaluate the potential impact of language on reading abilities. Although the diagnostic "label" does not predict with 100% accuracy any individual's true profile, it can orient the clinician to what the most salient problems may be. Let us take a look at a small selection of the many conditions associated with impaired language to see how language may vary with different developmental conditions.

Attention Deficit Disorder

Children with Attention Deficit Disorder (ADD) are characterized by inattention and impulsivity, with hyperactivity occurring in a subset of children with ADD. Children with ADD are highly distractable, finding it difficult to focus, sustain their attention, and direct their activities toward the task at hand. These signs occur in the absence of any frank neurological deficit or acquired disorder. Parents often report that the first signs appear in the preschool years, although children may not be referred for services until their difficulties cause them problems in school. Their difficulties with attention and impulse control are a significant handicap in the classroom, interfering with the ability to listen to directions and complete work assignments. It is not surprising, therefore, that most children with ADD have difficulty learning. The signs of ADD can persist throughout the childhood years, with an estimated two-thirds to one-half of individuals continuing to show signs in late adolescence (Claude & Firestone, 1995; McGee, Partridge, Williams, & Silva, 1991).

The distractability and impulsivity that interfere with school work are equally disruptive in games and conversations. Other children may view the ADD child as a troublemaker who breaks both rules and toys. Children with ADD often interrupt others who are trying to talk, shift from topic to topic without warning, and otherwise appear to have difficulties with the social aspects of language use. Other language problems may be a side effect of inattention. For example, children whose attention fluctuates may miss parts of what is said to them, mimicking a comprehension deficit. A subset of children with ADD also have co-existing speech and language disorders that are independent of attentional problems. For this reason, the American Speech-Language-Hearing Association (ASHA, 1997) recommended that speech-language pathologists and audiologists serve on multidisciplinary teams for the assessment of children with ADD.

The signs of ADD may be managed medically and behaviorally. Stimulant medications help some children by increasing their attention span and decreasing impulsive and hyperactive behaviors. Medication, even when beneficial, does not cure the disorder. Behavioral intervention is designed to provide the child with methods for staying on task and minimizing the effects of ADD in daily life. Some intervention techniques involve modifying the child's environment by providing routine and structure to support on-task behaviors. Rewards or recognition may also be effective in promoting appropriate behaviors. For older children, helping them to develop plans for monitoring their own conduct may be appropriate.

Autism

The term *autism* describes a developmental disorder that profoundly affects the child's interactions with other people and with the world. The earliest signs of the disorder include disturbed social interaction between the infant and its parents. Even as infants, these children do not seem to bond with or take comfort from others. They may seem content watching the movements of their hands or performing repetitive actions. A majority of children with autism fall into the mentally retarded range of intellectual functioning. However, not all cognitive domains are equally affected. Minshew, Goldstein, and Siegel (1997) tested autistic individuals whose IQ scores fell within normal limits (although many were lower than average) and found that these individuals' greatest deficits involved the ability to handle complex information processing in many forms (e.g., high-level language tasks, complex memory). Simple information processing systems and visual-spatial memory were relatively spared.

As children with autism grow, other aspects of disturbed communication become apparent. Some of these children acquire some early language skills, only to lose them during the preschool years. For others, language development is disturbed from the start. Dunn (1997) reviewed the characteristics of autistic language, which can include deficits in language form, content, and use. Common characteristics include poor language comprehension and poor pragmatic skills. In more severe forms of the disorder, expressive language characteristics may become more apparent. A complete lack of speech, or mutism, is most likely to occur when the signs of autism are most severe (Miranda-Linne & Merlin, 1997).

The language signs most typical of this disorder involve disturbances of language *use.* Individuals with autism frequently have disturbed prosody in spoken language. They may repeat the words of others (a characteristic called *echolalia*) or use stereotyped speech routines rather than the original and context-appropriate speech of normally developing children. For example, one child repeated the phrase "want juice please" over and over again as he spun in a circle. However, this was not an actual request for juice, but continued use of a phrase beyond the setting in which it was appropriate. The bizarre elements of their communication also extend to nonverbal pragmatics. For example, children with autism often have a flat facial affect and aberrant patterns of attention to people and objects and abnormal gaze during conversations (Lord & Pickles, 1996; Shields, Varley, Broks, & Simpson, 1996).

The bizarre social interactions of these children led early investigators to hypothesize that autism was the product of uncaring parents who failed to provide the emotional support children require (Kanner & Eisenberg, 1955). Later, more biological explanations of the disorder were offered (e.g., Rimland, 1964). Today, we have evidence of abnormal brain development in autistic individuals (e.g., Courchesne, Yeung-Courchesne, Press, Hesselink & Jernigan, 1988) and preliminary evidence of a genetic role in the disorder (Petit, Herlault, Martineau, Perrot, Barthelemy, Hameury, Sauvage, Lelord, & Muh, 1995) .

Childhood Aphasia

Children who were developing normally can lose language skills because of brain damage. This acquired language disorder is known as childhood aphasia. Aphasia in children can be caused by the same disease processes that cause adult aphasia (see Chapter 8). These include relatively focal trauma to the head, stroke, infectious disease, tumor, or seizures. Also similar to the adult form of aphasia, language deficits typically occur after damage to the brain's left hemisphere (Aram, Ekelman, Rose, & Whitaker, 1985; Cranberg, Filley, Hart, & Alexander 1987). We see one such case with Daniel:

Daniel was 4 1/2 years old when he began having daily headaches, which were soon accompanied by behavioral problems, and vomiting. He was taken to the hospital and received a brain scan. This revealed a large tumor in the left temporal-parietal area of his left hemisphere. He was immediately scheduled for surgery to reduce the tumor. On the morning following surgery, Daniel was unable to speak and showed signs of weakness on the right side of his body. A second brain scan showed that he had had a stroke, caused by bleeding of the middle cerebral artery, which damaged the language areas of the left hemisphere (see Chapter 2 for a review).

Within days, Daniel began talking, but his speech and language were not at the level they had been before he was hospitalized. Initially, his speech was slow and effortful, and he drooled intermittently. He had great difficulty attending to what was said and could only follow simple directions. A preschool test of general language abilities indicated low language skills compared with others his age. He had difficulty identifying pictures of words on a vocabulary test. Many times when speaking, he would substitute nonspecific pronouns for specific nouns (e.g., "push thing" for wagon; "the one" for any object). In addition, Daniel had difficulty on a test that required him to produce grammatical sentences to describe pictures. The speech-language pathologist worked with him three times a week until he was released from the hospital. He also arranged, upon release, to have Daniel enrolled in a preschool program for children with language disorders.

An estimated 3 in 100,000 children each year experience a stroke (NIDCD, 1991). When the stroke leads to aphasia, children show difficulty comprehending or using spoken language, despite normal intelligence. As in Daniel's case, children may initially be mute following brain damage, and as they recover, begin to show signs of fluent or nonfluent aphasia types (we will look at adult aphasia in Chapter 8). Children with fluent aphasia may use sentences with appropriate rate and intonation, but with jargon or nonsense words (Van Dongen, Loonen, & Van Dongen, 1985). Nonfluent aphasia is more commonly reported in children. These children use short, simple phrases and sentences. Like Daniel, they omit grammatical morphemes, creating the impression of telegraphic speech. Children may also have difficulty with reading and writing. Since reading, listening, and following directions are frequent school activities, it is not surprising that children with aphasia have academic difficulties (Cranberg et al., 1987). In contrast, language use is often well preserved. Language difficulties may resolve with time, so that the casual listener may be unaware that the child had experienced aphasia. However, language problems can persist and be documented with standardized testing years after the aphasia first appeared (Vargha-Khadem, O'Gorman, & Watters, 1985; Woods & Carey, 1979).

Traumatic Brain Injury

Each year, approximately 200 of every 100,000 children experience a traumatic brain injury (TBI) (NIDCD, 1991). TBI can be focal, as occurs after a penetrating or "open-head" injury (e.g., a gunshot wound), or diffuse, as the result of force applied without penetration of the skull (i.e., a "closed-head" injury). Most commonly, it involves some combination of focal and diffuse injury. TBI can be caused by any number of events, including motor vehicle accidents, in which the injury includes both diffuse damage from the brain moving within the skull as well as focal contusions where the brain contacts the skull. Other events that can produce a combination of diffuse and focal injury include rough shaking (e.g., shaken baby syndrome), falls, sports injuries, assaults, and pedestrian-motor vehicle collisions.

There is great heterogeneity among individuals with TBI. Some of this can be accounted for by differences in the nature and severity of the injury (Chapman, 1997). Other sources of heterogeneity are related to the child's pre-injury intelligence, health, and personality, as well as family and cultural factors. Among those at highest risk for severe injury are teenaged males, primarily due to driving accidents. Because of the widespread nature of the brain damage, the behavioral sequelae range far beyond language skills. This is illustrated by the following case:

> Gerard was a 17-year-old high school junior when he had his car accident. He was ditching his afternoon classes with three friends when he lost control of his truck and it went off the road, flipping over several times. The two boys in the back were killed and the third was paralyzed by the crash. Gerard was in a coma for two weeks with severe head injuries. When Gerard emerged from his coma, cognitive and linguistic deficits were apparent. He was highly distractible and easily overwhelmed by new information or situations. Memory testing indicated that his post-injury abilities were in the fifth percentile, or below the performance of 95 percent of the normative sample for the test. He also had great difficulty understanding both written and spoken language, needing substantial amounts of time to process information, and not always arriving at the correct interpretation. In contrast, his spoken language form and content appeared unaffected by his injury.
>
> His most noticeable communication deficit involved language use. Gerard's affect was flat and he failed to use the prosodic variations that conveyed emotion in his speech. Likewise, he did not seem to pick up on the nonverbal cues of others in conversations. His thinking had a concreteness that did not allow him to interpret jokes or sarcasm. This concrete thinking had pervasive effects on his daily life as well. He was unable to conceptualize the future or plan for it effectively.

Language difficulties after TBI are different from those associated with developmental language disorders. For example, many children with TBI may do comparatively well on standardized tests of vocabulary, morphology, and syntax (Biddle, McCabe, & Bliss, 1996; Chapman, Watkins, Gustafson, Moore, Levin, & Kufera, 1997; Ylvisaker, 1993). These tests tap knowledge gained prior to the injury. Communication breakdowns are more likely to occur in tasks that tap language in conversational or discourse contexts (Chapman, Levin, Matejeka, Harward, & Kufera, 1995; Chapman et al., 1997) or on language tasks that place particular demands on attention, information processing, and memory (Turkstra & Holland, 1988). Survivors also may have profoundly handicapping impairments in those abilities referred to collectively as executive functions (Ylvisaker, Szekeres, & Feeney, 1998). These functions include the ability to plan and organize behavior, make decisions taking multiple factors into account, and regulate one's own behavior. An important difference between those with TBI and those with developmental language disorders is that individuals with TBI are likely to have had a period of normal development and must begin a new life with an uncertainty about their post-injury skills and limitations (Ylvisaker, 1998). This may have a profound effect on their attitude toward therapy.

> For Gerard, therapy began in the hospital as soon as he was conscious and medically stable. This was a multidisciplinary effort, with a speech-language pathologist, physical therapist, and psychologist helping Gerard address the physical, cognitive, and emotional aftermath of his injuries. By the time he was well enough to resume school, he had missed most of his

junior year. The school provided a full-time classroom aide who took notes for him in class, organized his program of study, and helped him with assignments. The school's speech-language pathologist focused on improving Gerard's basic reading, helping him learn strategies for working within the limits of his impaired memory. Other activities included role-playing practice for various social and vocational situations to improve his poor pragmatics in these communicative contexts. Therapy was a challenge because Gerard did not acknowledge his language deficits and therefore did not see the point of the activities. Gerard also participated, although grudgingly, in a once weekly meeting with other teens who had sustained brain injuries.

The long-term profile of individuals with TBI is dependent in part on which abilities were already acquired and which were still developing at the age when the injury occurred. The full affects of the injury may not be apparent until months or years later (Chapman, 1997). As stated by Lash (DePompei, Blosser, Savage, & Lash, 1997), after traumatic brain injury "time reveals all wounds." For example we do not expect coherent, logical stories from 4-year-olds, but by 10 years of age incoherent storytelling would signal a deficit. When a brain injury is mild, the child may eventually return to normal or near normal functioning. However, when injuries are severe, the long-term outlook may be less positive.

Two years after his injury, Gerard was finishing high school, although his graduation was uncertain. His involvement in the school's TBI program focused on vocational training to prepare him for post-graduation life. However, he had been through four jobs in as many months, quitting each time because he was bored or felt the job was beneath him in some way. He drifted away from the teens who were his friends before the injury, and his social and pragmatic problems make it difficult for him to make new social contacts.

Mental Retardation

Language development is a complex task that depends, in part, on the development of other cognitive and social-adaptive skills. Slow development affects the way children with **mental retardation** learn about their world and the people and objects in it. Children who are slow in all aspects of development are frequently also slow in the acquisition of language skills. The *Diagnostic and Statistical Manual of Mental Disorders* (DSM-IV, APA, 1994) defines mental retardation by an intelligence quotient (IQ) of less than 70 on a standardized IQ measure along with significant deficits in adaptive functioning. Even when an IQ is low, an individual who shows no difficulty functioning in everyday life would not be considered to have mental retardation. The degree of mental retardation that any individual shows may vary considerably. DSM-IV recognizes four broad severity levels: mild, moderate, severe, and profound, which reflect a range, from individuals considered "educable" to those few who require life-long assistance.

There are many developmental conditions associated with mental retardation. Some of these are genetic (e.g., Down syndrome, Noonan syndrome, fragile X syndrome), some are due to exposures to toxins (e.g., fetal alchohol syndrome, lead poisoning), and for others the cause is unknown (idiopathic mental retardation). With this range of conditions included within the spectrum of mental retardation, it is not surprising that the language correlates can be quite variable. In general, however, children with mental retardation are slow to acquire communication skills. Even at the prelinguistic stage, some toddlers with retardation are less interactive and use fewer nonverbal forms of communication than normally developing children at ages. The onset of spoken words may occur at a later chronological age. General language ability in retarded children is frequently reported to be like that of younger, normally developing children.

As noted, however, this general profile may not apply to all conditions associated with mental retardation. Children with different types of mental retardation have more difficulty with certain areas of language development than others. For example, some children with Down syndrome appear to have particular problems with syntax and morphology (Stoel-Gammon, 1990). In contrast, children with Williams syndrome are unusually proficient in syntax and morphology, despite having poor semantic skills (Bellugi, Marks, Bihrle, & Sabo, 1988). Children with fragile X syndrome tend to have particular problems with verbal and nonverbal pragmatic skills (Scharfenaker, 1990). Within any group of retarded children, there is much individual variability in the acquisition of language skills. With guidance, retarded children can develop communication skills to the limits of their cognitive and social-adaptive potential.

Seizure Disorder

Childhood **seizures** can have many different underlying causes, or have no known cause at all. For many, a childhood seizure episode may cause considerable concern at the time, but have no long-lasting consequences. However, when seizures are severe and persistent, behavioral deficits, including impaired language, may follow. We saw one such case with Anita, who was diagnosed as having aphasia with convulsive disorder:

> Anita had been having seizures since 6 months of age. Management of those seizures included drug therapy and periodic monitoring of brain electrical activity. However, this was only partially successful. Anita spoke her first words at 18 months and speech-language development had been slow but steady since then. Following a particularly long generalized seizure at age 4, Anita lost her ability to speak and communication was reduced to slurred sounds and gestures. Although she regained some language skills after that episode, her language remained markedly impaired.
>
> At age 5, she was evaluated at a university clinic. At that time, she failed to respond when a pure-tone audiometric screening was attempted and she was scheduled for a full audiometric evaluation. The results for pure tones and speech awareness were considered borderline normal but response reliability was only fair. A parent questionnaire revealed a significant delay in all areas of development, including motor, social, and self-help skills. Formal language assessment was discontinued because Anita was unable to maintain her attention to the tasks and became frustrated. However, during an hour-long session with her mother, Anita used fewer than 120 words total. Most of her utterances were one or two words in length, and about half consisted of signed words. Speech was slow and effortful; words were sometimes slurred. Anita established attention very slowly and had difficulty maintaining it. This affected her comprehension, which was poor overall. Her mother used a number of techniques to facilitate attention and comprehension. She maintained a close proximity to her daughter. The mother touched her own lips before speaking to draw Anita's attention. The mother physically directed Anita's attention first to her face as she spoke and

then to the objects under discussion. She used short sentences and many repetitions to support the conversation. Occasionally, Anita echoed those repetitions back to her mother.

As we see in Anita's case, a prolonged period of seizure activity can lead to a deterioration of skills that were once evident. In fact, a change in language status, such as seen here, is a leading sign of an underlying neurological disturbance. In Anita's case, both language comprehension and expression were affected by seizure activity, as well as general functioning in nonverbal domains. In other cases of seizure disorder, receptive language abilities are far more impaired than expressive skills (Rapin, Mattis, Rowan, & Golden, 1977; Worster-Drought, 1971). Receptive abilities can be so severely impaired that the child behaves as if deaf. However, these children have normal hearing acuity, as established by an audiometric evaluation. No longer able to understand his or her own speech, the child may stop talking altogether, or speech may become garbled. However, language expression can continue if the child is introduced to signed language.

One subtype of seizure disorder is particularly associated with loss of language skills. Landau-Kleffner syndrome was first described as involving loss of language skills in children who had seizures (Landau & Kleffner, 1957). The seizure activity of these children typically involves both temporal lobes and is easily managed with medication. However, the language signs may persist even after the seizures are brought under control. Recovery of language is quite variable, ranging from a few weeks to many years (Mantovani & Landau, 1980).

Evaluation of Language Disorders

Evaluation of children with suspected language disorders takes many forms in order to accommodate the wide range of disorders that involve impaired language. The evaluation may address a number of questions of interest to the clinician and the parents. Does this child have a language disorder? Are there any factors that might account for the presence of a language disorder? How do the child's skills in various language domains compare to peers? If intervention is warranted, what aspects of language should be addressed? As we will see, components of the diagnostic process are tailored to address these types of questions.

Language Screening

Language screenings are designed to determine whether a child's language skills warrant a full evaluation. Screenings are relatively quick to administer and often sample a range of language skills that could potentially be impaired. They may be formal measures that have been administered to large groups of children who serve as a **normative sample**. Normative samples permit comparison of a single child's performance to a group of children who are of the same age. These children serve as a reference for the range of normal performance that can be expected. Other screenings may be informal in order to accommodate regional variations in language or dialect or to target skills of particular interest for a certain setting (e.g., conversational speech, reading readiness). Frequently, language screening is used as a cost-effective method of evaluating large numbers of children, most of whom will not have any difficulties with language skills. For example, a school district may routinely screen the language of all of their incoming kindergarten children. Only those children who fail the screening are referred for a full evaluation.

Because children who do not fail the screening receive no follow-up attention (unless referred later by a parent, pediatrician, or teacher), the screening must be highly sensitive to the presence of a language disorder. In diagnostic parlance, test **sensitivity** refers to the proportion of individuals who have a disorder and are also identified by a test as having the disorder. The flip side of sensitivity is test **specificity**, the rate at which a test correctly identifies children with normal skills. For a screening measure, low specificity means that the clinician must spend time and resources evaluating children who do not need their services. However, this is less serious than the consequences of low sensitivity. The major consequence of low sensitivity is failure to identify children who may truly need services.

Since language screening is applied to large numbers of children, most of whom are expected to fall within normal limits, a third calculation involving test sensitivity is used to evaluate the accuracy of screening measures. This is known as **positive predictive validity**. This metric takes into account the prevalence of the disorder in the population that the clinician is sampling from (e.g., all incoming kindergarteners). When a disorder is rare in the population as a whole, few children would be expected to fail the screening for that disorder, whereas the likelihood of finding children with a disorder will increase if it occurs frequently in the population. If a screening measure lacks positive predictive validity, children who are in need of help will not receive further evaluation and services may be delayed (at best) or denied altogether.

The Case History

The case history on a child is a way to gather background information that may be used for many purposes. The case history may be gathered through conversation with those who know the child best (usually the parents). In other cases, it may consist of a form that is completed prior to or during the initial evaluation. Many case histories include information concerning pregnancy, birth, and medical background. This information can be important for identifying potential causes for a language disorder. For example, if a mother reports having had rubella during her pregnancy, the clinician would be alerted to the possibility of a hearing loss, which sometimes occurs under those conditions. The clinician can then plan for either a hearing screening during the evaluation, or arrange a referral to an audiologist for a full hearing assessment if the child's hearing had not already been tested. Information concerning developmental and family history can help determine the degree of risk for a language disorder. As we saw in earlier sections, children who have developmental language disorders are very likely to have a family member who also has a language or learning disorder. In other cases, a parent who reports a change or cessation of language skills during the child's development would alert the clinician to explore the possibility of autism, seizure disorders, or disease processes that would impact previously normal development.

Sometimes a case history will also ask parents for more subjective information. Parents may be asked what led them to become concerned about their child's language development. They may report on what they see as their child's overall strengths and weaknesses. The parents' input may help identify those skills that, if remediated, would make the biggest improvement in their child's daily life. They may even be able to provide information on strategies that they have developed that seem to help their child the most. This type of information is invaluable for guiding subsequent therapy.

Observation

Important diagnostic information can be gathered simply through observation. Let us consider the following case:

> Charise was a speech-language pathologist who worked at a community clinic that handled referrals from the state's program for children with disabilities. She always made a point of meeting her clients in the lobby because, as she said, "I can always tell a lot about the way things are going to go on the walk from the front door to my office." One particular morning, she had a new referral of a child with a reported language delay. The child, a 2-year-old boy, came in hand-in-hand with his mother. He was a little overweight, and his belly peeked out beneath his t-shirt. When Charise dropped down to his eye level, he greeted her with a smile as she explained who she was. He had a round, pleasant face, with widespread, almond-shaped eyes, a broad nose, and full cheeks and lips. Overall, his face appeared soft, as if the underlying muscle tone might be low. He seemed social and he pointed and made short one- or two-word comments about the children's paintings that hung along the hallway. There was only one moment of difficulty when it came time to turn the corner and his eye caught something interesting in the opposite direction. He stamped his foot and sat down defiantly in the middle of the hallway. With a bit of cajoling, his mother got him back up and back on track. Once in the office, Clarise confirmed the presence of a language delay with formal diagnostic measures. She also made a referral to a medical geneticist. The facial features, low tone, and high weight, combined with a general immaturity, made her think that a genetic syndrome might be playing a role in this child's language problems. In fact, two months later, a follow-up report was received that confirmed a diagnosis of Prader-Willi syndrome, which involved a genetic abnormality involving chromosome 15.

In this case, the speech-language pathologist's initial observations contributed to this child's diagnosis. Observation is important at all stages in the diagnostic process. The speech-language pathologist may visit the child's home in order to get an idea of typical communication style within the family. A gross assessment of language functioning can be obtained by listening to a child's conversations. How the child plays can provide insight into the level of cognitive and social functioning. Classroom observations of school-age children can provide insight into the specific conditions that precipitate communication problems for the child. The speech-language pathologist may notice simple things that can greatly enhance a child's chances of success.

Formal Measures

There are literally hundreds of commercially available, formal measures for assessing children's language. These tests vary remarkably in their focus, quality, and suitability for a specific diagnostic purpose. One method that clinicians use to select among formal measures is to consider the information that they hope to gain by administering the test. Different formal measures are developed for different purposes. For example, clinicians who wish to compare a child's performance to that of other children that age will select a different test than if they wish to establish whether a child can use certain syntactic structures in various speaking tasks. The former purpose would require a **norm-referenced test**, and the latter would require a **criterion-referenced test**.

Norm-referenced tests allow comparisons between a child's performance and a group of children of similar age. Beyond this common feature, there is great variation among norm-referenced tests. Some measure narrow domains of language functioning. For example, one norm-referenced test may examine the number of words that a child recognizes; another will evaluate broader knowledge of word meanings. Some consist of a collection of subtests compiled into a battery that examines various components of language functioning. These may sample across language domains of phonology, morphology, syntax, and semantics in both receptive and expressive modalities.

Criterion-referenced tests are typically more narrowly focused than norm-referenced tests. These tests are used to compare a child's performance against a standard, or criterion, for behavior. Most college examinations, for example, are criterion-referenced tests, in that the instructor compares each student's performance against a standard for knowledge of the course content. Criterion-referenced tests may be informal, as when a clinician develops a series of "probes" that are meant to assess whether a child is able to use structures trained in therapy. Others are commercially available measures that sample language skills to determine a child's proficiency.

After consideration of the purpose for administering a test, the clinician will examine its technical qualities. First and foremost, the clinician should find evidence that a test can provide the types of information that are needed. For example, a clinician hoping to use a test to identify impairment should find evidence in the test manual of good sensitivity and specificity. If the clinician is hoping to document whether a child can use various syntactic structures, there should be evidence that children known to use those structures actually produce them when presented with the test items. Although authors may claim their test can be used for one or more assessment purposes, empirical evaluation of the claims may reveal otherwise (e.g., Merrell & Plante, 1997; Plante & Vance, 1994, 1995; Sturner, Heller, Funk, & Layton, 1993).

Given evidence that a test meets the clinician's purpose, its overall psychometric properties should be considered. These properties relate to standards for test development that enhance test **reliability** and **validity**. Reliability refers to the degree to which the test provides consistent information. Validity refers to the degree to which correct interpretations about an individual's behavior can be drawn from test results (Messick, 1989). An unreliable test is never valid, in that it gives different information each time it is given. However, high reliability does not ensure validity. A ruler whose inch markings are too closely spaced will provide the same mismeasurement every time—highly reliable, but not at all valid! Standards for the assessment of test reliability and validity have been detailed by the combined efforts of the American Educational Research Association, American Psychological Association, and National Council on Measurement in Education (AERA/APA/NCME, 1985).

Despite such standards, many tests of child language fall short of minimal psychometric criteria (e.g., McCauley & Swisher, 1984; Plante & Vance, 1994). Unfortunately, use of a psychometrically weak test can lead to erroneous conclusions, as we see in the following example:

Brendon was just 3 1/2 when he was first enrolled in therapy for a language delay. At that point, his mean length of utterance MLU was moderately low for his age (see Chapter 4 for a review of MLU). A standardized test of expressive language placed him below the first percentile for his age, which means that 99 out of 100 children his age could be expected to score higher than Brendon on that particular test. A single-word vocabulary test was also administered, and he did not pass enough items to show that he understood even the most simple words. By contrast, his hearing, motor, and cognitive development tested well within normal limits. Based on these results, he was enrolled in a preschool program for children with specific language impairments. A little over a year later (age 4 years, 10 months), his skills were retested using a different battery of tests. At that time, all skills were well within normal limits according to the test norms. It was concluded that Brendon had overcome his earlier difficulties and was dismissed from the preschool program.

Two months later (age 5 years, 0 months), his mother, still concerned about her son's language skills, enrolled him in a university-based research project for children with specific language impairment. His language was retested with a third battery of tests. This time, Brendon received expressive language scores and receptive vocabulary scores that were once again below the first percentile for his age. How could the appearing-disappearing-reappearing language deficits be explained? The lead researcher, a speech-language pathologist, consulted the normative tables for the tests Brendon received at age 4. She discovered that the test items were so difficult that most normal 4-year-old children could not pass them. Therefore, failure to pass any items on that test battery placed a child within normal limits of performance!

In Brendon's example, a psychometric weakness known as a basement effect interfered with valid interpretations of his language skills. A basement effect occurs when few items are passed by the children on whom the test is normed. Performance by these children is "in the basement." This effect typically occurs at the youngest ages for which norms are included and is only one of the potential psychometric problems that can involve the normative sample. Other psychometric weaknesses involve construction and evaluation of the test items, poor score reliability and validity, and even specification of who can administer the test and how it should be administered (AERA/APA/NCME, 1985).

A final consideration in test selection is the context in which the skill domains are tested. The same items can be passed on one test and failed on another, just based on the context in which those items appear (e.g., Merrell & Plante, 1997; Wiig, Jones, & Wiig, 1996). Sabers (1996) pointed out that "the way a test measures behavior may introduce measurement aspects not intended for the test." In fact, if the simplest linguistic elements are presented in strange or difficult contexts, children will fail those items long after they are able to use and understand the elements in everyday life. For example, a child who has been using "me" since the age of 2 years will not use it in the context "You would have liked me to see the painting" until many years later. Test items designed to measure language, for example, may in fact be a stronger test of memory if the child is required to hold multiple words in memory before composing an answer using those words. Sometimes, the overall context of the test is enough to influence the final skill. Wiig and colleagues (1996) demonstrated this when they developed a computerized version of one of their tests. They found that teens' performance differed significantly on the traditional and computer-based versions of the test, even though the items were identical. For these reasons, the content and context influence how the clinician interprets the test results.

Hearing Evaluation

As we saw in Chapter 5, hearing impairment can be an underlying cause for poor language development. Therefore, a pure-tone hearing screening is typically part of a language evaluation. If a child fails to respond during the hearing screening, a full audiological evaluation should be scheduled to rule out hearing loss as a contributing factor in the child's language difficulties.

Language Therapy

Approaches to language intervention are as diverse as the children who receive services. There is no "recipe book" of procedures or one-size-fits-all method that will work with all children. In fact, therapy methods that are successful with one child may or may not work well with another. As we saw above, children with different types of language disorders can vary considerably in terms of their language profiles. Furthermore, the child's age, cultural background, and family situation may greatly affect the type of intervention that is best for them. Therefore, language therapy tends to be highly individualized.

When we examine different intervention methods, we first consider what the therapy approach is intended to do for the child. Wilcox (1994) reviewed major approaches to intervention: prevention, remediation, and compensation. *Preventive* services may be provided to children at risk for language disorders. These children may be at risk because they are born with conditions associated with language disorders (e.g., mental retardation, genetic disorders). Other children may receive preventive services because they are showing early signs of communication delay (e.g., late talkers). In this case, services are intended to maximize the child's potential early in development so that the impact on language can be lessened or avoided. Examples of preventive services include preschool "head start" programs and other programs designed to enrich a child's early language and educational experiences.

Remediation involves correction of current deficits and is perhaps the most frequent form of therapy for children. When therapy is oriented toward remediation, the clinician typically has very specific goals (e.g., increase use of target sytactic structures, morphemes, vocabulary). The clinician then devises a program to teach these linguistic targets. *Compensation* involves the introduction of strategies that assist the child to manage the effects of the disorder, rather than eliminating its signs. Compensation is often used with conditions that are not completely correctable, such as brain injury or hearing loss. For example, in our case of seizure disorder, the mother's use of visual cues provided a strategy to aid comprehension. For older children and teens, the child may be responsible for use of the strategy. A teen with a learning disability, for example, may be taught how to use diagrams to summarize information from his lecture notes.

As we saw with the cases presented in this chapter, children with language disorders often have many areas of difficulty that could benefit from therapy. However, working on everything at once would be overwhelming for both the clinician and child. Therefore, the clinician may need to prioritize the areas of need and target these sequentially. Some goals receive priority because they offer the greatest potential for positive improvement in the quality of the child's life. For example, a program that provides a nonverbal child with more communicative functions (e.g., requesting, commenting) can reduce frustration for parent and child. A school-age child may benefit most from therapy that allows him or her to participate more fully in classroom activities. Occasionally, the goal that would make the greatest difference in the child's language is not necessarily one selected. For example, one mother of a severely handicapped child was interested in her child learning social routines (e.g., greetings, "please," and "thank you"), even though other more functional aspects of communication could have been targeted. Social communication was important to the mother because she saw it as a way for her child to have positive interactions with others.

Certain therapy goals may receive priority because they help the child progress to a higher developmental stage. Wilcox (1992) developed an intervention program designed to move infants and toddlers from preverbal gestures and vocalizations to the verbal stage of communication. For a late-talking toddler, increasing the number of vocabulary words is a prerequisite for acquiring phrases and sentences. For older children, the developmental sequence for morpheme acquisition may guide selection of therapy targets. A developmental focus can combine both remediation and preventative components. For example, Dale and colleagues described a treatment method that used storybook activities to facilitate language in preschoolers (Dale, Crain-Thoreson, Notari-Syverson & Cole, 1996). The immediate goal of this program was language facilitation. However, the treatment context of reading introduced preliteracy skills that are thought to contribute to reading success in later years.

Once the language goals are selected, the therapist must consider the structure used to train those goals. Naturalistic contexts have become very popular over the last decade. As a result, there has been an emphasis on home programs, classroom-based programs, and other intervention techniques that are incorporated into the child's daily life. For example, many programs have demonstrated that parents can be effectively trained to facilitate language development at home. Various programs have been used to teach parents to modify their speech and change how they respond to the child's attempts at communication (e.g., Eiserman, Weber, & McCoun, 1995; Gibbard, 1994; Girolametto, Pearce, & Weitzman, 1996). In fact, parent-administered programs can be as effective as clinician-administered programs, at least in the early stages of intervention (Eiserman et al., 1995; Fey, Cleave, & Long, 1997). Other programs emphasize remediation in naturalistic contexts (e.g., conversation, play) during which a clinician, parent, or teacher facilitates the learning of new linguistic forms as opportunities arise to do so within the interaction (Figure 7-2). This technique is sometimes called "incidental

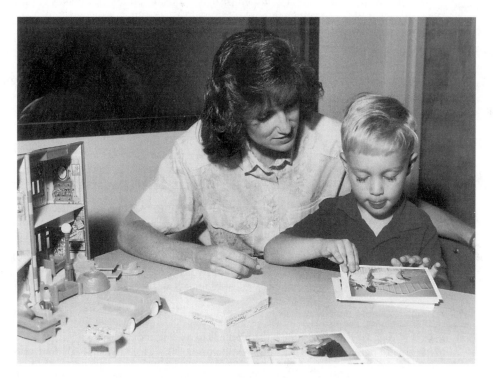

FIGURE 7-2 A speech-language pathologist works on storytelling using picture cards to help the child sequence information. (Courtesy of The University of Arizona, Department of Speech & Hearing Sciences)

teaching" because language instruction follows from natural interactions with the child. For example, a child may learn to use questions by learning to request toys, food, and other items encountered in his or her daily life. The effectiveness of naturalistic intervention can vary depending on the specific techniques used to facilitate language (e.g., Camarata, Nelson, & Camarata, 1994; Kaiser & Hester, 1994; Warren, Gazdag, Bambara, & Jones,1994) and the characteristics of the child (Yoder, Kaiser, & Alpert, 1991).

Some children need more structure than is afforded by naturalistic contexts because of the nature of their disorder. For example, a child with attention deficit disorder may prove too distractible in a completely naturalistic context to benefit from incidental teaching techniques. A teenager with a traumatic brain injury may not have deficits that involve conversational language per se, but may need help with aspects of communication that do not necessarily lend themselves to naturalistic intervention. Students who need assistance with language skills in the academic domain may use strategies that are explicitly taught. Finally, what is "natural" to one child may be completely unfamiliar to another. For example, in some cultures, a conversation between a child and an adult who is not a close relative is not at all natural. A clinician who uses such a "natural" context may be confronted with a child who will not talk at all under those conditions. In contrast, the use of computers as a tool for therapy may be natural for children who have been interacting with educational software programs from early ages. For these children, the high level of structure in a computer-based program may feel as natural as conversationally based therapy.

Effective therapy takes into account all of these considerations and makes adjustments to fit the needs of each child. The clinician may use a highly structured, compensatory-based approach with one child and a parent-administered, conversationally based approach with another. For a third child, the clinician may simply serve as a consultant to a classroom teacher who assists the language-disordered child with modifications of teaching activities and materials. This kind of flexibility allows therapy approaches to be tailored to each child's developmental stage and communicative needs.

Clinical Problem Solving

Becky is a 30-month-old girl who was brought to the clinic by her parents. They were concerned about her language development because she did not seem to use as many words as the other children at her preschool. Although Becky seemed quite interested in the toys and books in the clinic play room, she said few words and often seemed to substitute gestures for words. All of her verbal utterances consisted of single words, with no multiword combinations. She was in good health and, other than language, the parents did not have any other concerns about her development.

1. Is this child at risk for a language disorder? Why or why not?
2. What should be included in the initial evaluation of this child? What is the purpose for including each of these components?
3. Given the child's age and language level, what approach might therapy take?
4. What do we know about the long-term outlook for young children whose language lags behind their age-mates?

References

American Educational Research Association, American Psychological Association, and National Council on Measurement in Education (1985). *Standards for Educational and Psychological Testing*. Washington, DC: Author.

American Psychiatric Association (1994). *Diagnostic and Statistical Manual of Mental Disorders* (4th ed.). Washington, DC: Author.

American Speech-Language-Hearing Association (1997). Position Statement: Roles of audiologists and speech-language pathologists working with persons with attention deficit hyperactivity disorder. *Asha, 39*, 14.

American Speech-Language-Hearing Association (1983). Social Dialects. *Asha, 25*, 23–27.

Aram, D. (1991). Comments on specific language impairment as a clinical category. *Language, Speech, & Hearing Services in Schools, 22*, 84–87.

Aram, D.M., Ekelman, B.L., Rose, D.F. & Whitaker, H.A. (1985). Verbal and cognitive sequelae following unilateral lesions acquired in early childhood. *Journal of Clinical and Experimental Neuropsychology, 7*, 55–78.

Bellugi, U., Marks, S., Bihrle, A., & Sabo, H. (1988). Dissociation between language and cognitive funtions in Williams syndrome. In D. Bishop & M. Mogford (eds.), *Language Development in Exceptional Circumstances*. New York: Churchill Livingstone.

Bent, J.P., & Beck, R.A. (1994). Bacterial meningitis in the pediatric population: Paradigm shifts and ramifications for otolaryngology-head and neck surgery. *International Journal of Pediatric Otorhinolaryngology, 30*: 41–49.

Biddle, K.R., McCabe, A., & Bliss, L.S. (1996). Narrative skills following traumatic brain injury in children and adults. *Journal of Communication Disorders, 29*: 447–470.

Bishop, D., & Adams, C. (1990). A prospective study of the relationship between specific language impairment, phonological disorders and reading impairment. *Journal of Child Psychology and Psychiatry, 31*: 1027–1050.

Byrne, J., Ellsworth, C., Bowering, E., & Vincer, M. (1993). Language development in low birth weight infants: The first two years of life. *Journal of Developmental and Behavioral Pediatrics, 14*: 21–27.

Camarata, S.M., Nelson, K.E., & Camarata, M.N. (1994). Comparison of conversational recasting and imitative procedures for training grammatical structures in children with specific language impairment. *Journal of Speech and Hearing Research, 37*: 1414–1423.

Catts, H., & Kamhi, A. (1986). The linguistic basis of reading disorders: Implications for the speech-language pathologist. *Language, Speech, & Hearing Services in Schools, 17*: 329–341.

Chapman, S.B. (1997). Cognitive-communication abilities in children with closed head injury. *American Journal of Speech Language Pathology, 6*: 50–58.

Chapman, S.B., Levin, H.S., Matejka, J., Harward, H.N., & Kufera, J. (1995). Discourse ability in head injured children: Consideration of linguistic, psychosocial, & cognitive factors. *Journal of Head Trauma Rehabilitation, 10*: 36–54.

Chapman, S.B., Watkins, R., Gustafson, C., Moore, S., Levin, H.S., & Kufera, J.A. (1997). Narrative discourse in children with closed head injury, children with language impairment, and typically developing children. *American Journal of Speech Language Pathology, 6*: 66–76.

Clark, D.A. (1994). Neonates and infants at risk for hearing and language disorders. In K.G. Butler (Ed.), *Early Intervention I: Working with Infants and Toddlers*. Gaithersburg, MD: Aspen Publishers.

Claude, D., & Firestone, P. (1995). The development of ADHD boys: A 12-year follow-up. *Canadian Journal of Behavioral Science, 27*: 226–249.

Cranberg, L.D., Filley, C.M., Hart, E.J., & Alexander, M.P. (1987). Acquired aphasia in childhood: Clinical and CT investigations. *Neurology, 37*: 1165–1172.

Cohen, M., Campbell, R., & Yaghmai, F. (1989). Neuropathological abnormalities in developmental dysphasia. *Annals of Neurology, 25*: 567–570.

Courchesne, E., Yeung-Courchesne, R., Press, G., Hesselink, J.R., & Jernigan, T.L. (1988). Hypoplasia of the cerebellar vermal lobes VI and VII in infantile autism. *New England Journal of Medicine, 318*: 1349–1354.

Dale, P.S., Crain-Thoreson, C., Notari-Syverson, A., & Cole, K.(1996) Parent-child book reading as an intervention technique for young children with language delays. *Topics in Early Childhood Special Education,* *16*: 213–235.

DePompei, R., Blosser, J.L., Savage, R., & Lash, M. (1997, November). *Effective Long-Term Management for Youths with TBI.* Miniseminar presented at the annual conference of the American Speech-Language-Hearing Association, Boston, MA.

Dunn, M. (1997). Language disorders in children with autism. *Seminars in Pediatric Neurology, 4*: 86–92.

Eiserman, W.D., Weber, C., & McCoun, M. (1995). Parent and professional roles in early intervention: A longitudinal comparison of the effects of two intervention configurations. *Journal of Special Education, 29*: 20–44.

Ellis Weismer, S., Murray-Branch, J., & Miller, J.F. (1994). A prospective longitudinal study of language development in late talkers. *Journal of Speech and Hearing Research, 37*: 852–867.

Fey, M.E., Cleave, P.L., & Long, S.H. (1997). Two models of grammar facilitation in children with language impairments. *Journal of Speech and Hearing Research, 40*: 5–19.

Fischel, J.E., Whitehurst, G.J., Caulfield, M.B., & Debaryshe, B (1989). Language growth in children with expressive language delay. *Pediatrics, 82*: 218–227.

Gauger, L.M., Lombardino, L.J., & Leonard, C.M. (1997). *Journal of Speech, Language, and Hearing Research, 40*: 1272–1284

Gibbard, D. (1994). Parental-based intervention with preschool language-delayed children. *European Journal of Communication Disorders, 29*: 131–50.

Girolametto, L., Pearce, P.S., & Weitzman, E. (1996). Interactive focused stimulation for toddlers with expressive vocabulary delays. *Journal of Speech and Hearing Research, 39*: 1274–1283.

Halsey, C.L., Collin, M.F., & Anderson, C.L. (1996). Extremely low-birth-weight children and their peers. A comparison of school-age outcomes. *Archives of Pediatrics and Adolescent Medicine, 150*: 790–794.

Jackson, T., & Plante, E. (1997). Gyral morphology in the posterior sylvian region in families affected by developmental language disorder. *Neuropsychology Review, 6*: 81–94.

Johnson, J.M., Seikel, J.A., Madison, C.L., Foose, S.M., & Rinard, K.D. (1997). Standardized test performance of children with a history of prenatal exposure to multiple drugs/cocaine. *Journal of Communication Disorders, 30*: 45–72.

Kaiser, A.B., & Hester, P.P. (1994). Generalized effects of enhanced milieu teaching. *Journal of Speech and Hearing Research, 37*: 1320–1340.

Kanner, L., & Eisenberg, L. (1955). Notes on the followup studies of autistic children. In P.H. Hoch & J. Zubin (Eds.), *Psychotherapy of Childhood,* New York: Grune & Stratton.

Landau, W.M., & Kleffner, F.R. (1957). Syndrome of acquired aphasia with convulsive disorder in children. *Neurology, 7*: 523–530.

Lewis, B.A., & Freebairn, L. (1992). Residual effects of preschool phonology disorders in grade school, adolescence, and adulthood. *Journal of Speech and Hearing Disorders, 35*: 819–831.

Lord, C., & Pickles, A. (1996). Language level and nonverbal social-communicative behaviors in autistic and language-delayed children. *Journal of the American Academy of Child and Adolescent Psychiatry, 35*: 1542–1550.

Mantovani, J.F. & Landau, W.M. (1980). Acquired aphasia with convulsive disorder: Course and prognosis. *Neurology, 30*: 524–529.

McCauley, R.J., & Swisher, L. (1984). Psychometric review of language and articulation tests for preschool children. *Journal of Speech and Hearing Disorders, 49*: 34–42.

McGee, R., Partridge, F., Williams, S., & Silva, P.A. (1991). A twelve-year follow-up of preschool hyperactive children. *Journal of the American Academy of Child and Adolescent Psychiatry, 30*: 224–232.

Menyuk, P., & Chesnick, M. (1997). Metalinguistic skills, oral language knowledge, and reading. *Topics in Language Disorders, 17*: 75–87.

Merrell, A.W., & Plante, E. (1997). Norm-referenced test interpretation in the diagnostic process. *Language, Speech, & Hearing Services in Schools, 28*: 50–58.

Messick, S. (1989). Meaning and values in test validation: The science and ethics of assessment. *Educational Researcher, 18*: 5–11.

Minshew, N.J., Goldstein, G., & Siegel, D.J. (1997). Neuropsychologic functioning in autism: Profile of a complex information processing disorder. *Journal of the International Neuropsychological Society, 3*: 303–316.

Miranda-Linne, F.M., & Merlin, L. (1997). A comparison of speaking and mute individuals with autism and autistic-like conditions on the Autism Behavior Checklist. *Journal of Autism and Developmental Disorders, 27*: 245–264.

National Institute on Deafness and Other Communication Disorders. (1991). *National strategic research plan for balance and the vestibular system and language and language impairments* (NIH Publication No. 91-3217). Bethesda, MD: Author.

Paul, R. (1993). Patterns of development in late talkers: Preschool years. *Journal of Childhood Communication Disorders, 15*: 7–14.

Paul, R., & Alforde, S. (1993). Grammatical morpheme acquisition in 4-year-olds with normal, impaired, and late-developing language. *Journal of Speech and Hearing Research, 36*: 1271–1275.

Paul, R., Hernandez, R., Taylor, L., & Johnson, K. (1996). Narrative development in late talkers: Early school age. *Journal of Speech and Hearing Research, 39*: 1295–1303.

Paul, R., Murray, C., Clancy, K., & Andrews, D. (1997). *Journal of Speech and Hearing Research, 40*: 1037–1047.

Pennington, B.F., Van Orden, G.C., Smith, S.D., Green, P.A., & Haith, M.M. (1990). Phonological processing skills and deficits in adult dyslexics. *Child Development, 61*: 1753–1788.

Petit, E., Herlault, J., Martineau, J., Perrot, A., Barthelemy, C., Hameury, L., Sauvage, D., Lelord, G., Muh, J.P., (1995). Association study with two markers of a human homeogene in infantile autism. *Journal of Medical Genetics, 32*: 269–274.

Plante, E. (1991). MRI findings in the parents and siblings of specifically language-impaired boys. *Brain and Language, 41*: 52–66.

Plante, E., Swisher, L., Vance, R., & Rapcsak, S. (1991). MRI findings in boys with specific language impairment. *Brain and Language, 41*: 52–66.

Plante, E., & Vance, R. (1994). Selection of preschool language tests: A data based approach. *Language, Speech, & Hearing Services in Schools, 25*: 15–23.

Plante, E., & Vance, R. (1995). Diagnostic accuracy of two tests of preschool language. *American Journal of Speech-Language Pathology, 4*: 70–76.

Rapin, I., Mattis, S., Rowan, A.J., & Golden, G.G. (1977). Verbal auditory agnosia in children. *Developmental Medicine and Child Neurology, 19*: 192–207.

Records, N.L., Tomblin, J.B., & Freese, P.R. (1992). The quality of life of young adults with histories of specific language impairment. *American Journal of Speech-Language Pathology, 1*: 44–53.

Rescorla, L., Roberts, J., & Dahlsgaard, K.(1997). Late talkers at 2: Outcome at age 3. *Journal of Speech and Hearing Research, 40*: 555–566.

Rescorla, L., & Schwartz, E. (1990). Outcome of toddlers with expressive language delay. *Applied Psycholinguistics, 11*: 393–407.

Rimland, B. (1964). *Infantile Autism*. New York: Appleton-Century-Crofts.

Sabers, D.L. (1996). By their tests we will know them. *Language, Speech, and Hearing Services in Schools, 27*: 102–108.

Scarborough, H.S. (1990). Very early language deficits in dyslexic children. *Child Development, 61*: 1728–1743.

Scarborough, H.S., & Dobrich, W. (1990). Development of children with early language delay. *Journal of Speech and Hearing Research, 33*: 70–83.

Scharfenaker, S.K. (1990). The fragile X syndrome. *Asha, 32*: 45–47.

Shields, J., Varley, R., Broks, P., & Simpson, A. (1996). Social cognition in developmental language disorders and high-level autism. *Developmental Medicine and Child Neurology, 38*: 487–495.

Snyder, L.S., & Downey, D.M. (1997). Developmental differences in the relationship between oral language deficits and reading. *Topics in Language Disorders, 17*: 27–40.

Sparks, S.N. (1984). *Birth Defects and Speech-Language Disorders*. Boston: College Hill.

Stoel-Gammon, C. (1990). Down syndrome: Effects on language development. *Asha, 32*: 42–44.

Sturner, R.A., Heller, J.H., Funk, S.G., & Layton, T.L. (1993). The Fluharty preschool speech and language screening test: A population-based validation study using sample independent decision rules. *Journal of Speech and Hearing Research, 36*: 738–745.

Tallal, P., Ross, R., & Curtiss, S. (1989). Familial aggregation in specific language impairment. *Journal of Speech and Hearing Disorders, 54*: 287–295.

Terrell, S.L., & Terrell, F. (1993). African American cultures. In D.E. Battle (Ed.), *Communication Disorders in Multicultural Populations*. Boston: Andover Medical Publishers.

Thal, D.J., Bates, E., Goodman, J., & Jahn-Samilo (1997). Continuity of language abilities: An exploratory study of late- and early-talking toddlers. *Developmental Neuropsychology, 13*: 239–274.

Thal, D.J., & Tobias, S. (1992). Communicative gestures in children with delayed onset of oral expressive vocabulary. *Journal of Speech and Hearing Research, 35*: 1281–1289.

Tomblin, J.B. (1989). Familial concentration of developmental language impairment. *Journal of Speech and Hearing Disorders, 54*: 287–295.

Tomblin, J.B., Records, N., & Freese, P. (1992). Diagnosing specific language impairment in adults for the purpose of pedigree analysis. *Journal of Speech and Hearing Research, 35*: 832–843.

Tomblin, J.B., Records, N.L., & Zhang, X. (1996). A system for the diagnosis of specific language impairment in kindergarten children. *Journal of Speech and Hearing Research, 39*: 1284–1294.

Turkstra, LS. & Holland, AL. (1998). Working memory and syntax comprehension after adolescent traumatic brain injury. *Journal of Speech, Language, and Hearing Research, 41*.

Van Dongen, H.R., Loonen, M.C.B., & Van Dongen, K.J. (1985). Anatomical basis for acquired fluent aphasia in children. *Annals of Neurology, 17*: 306–309.

Vargha-Khadem, F., O'Gorman, A.M., & Watters, G.V., (1985). Aphasia and handedness in relation to hemisphere side, age at injury, and severity of cerebral lesion in childhood. *Brain, 108*: 677–695.

Warren, S.F., Gazdag, G.E., Bambara, L.M., & Jones, H.A. (1994). Changes in the generativity and use of semantic relations concurrent with milieu language intervention. *Journal of Speech and Hearing Research, 37*: 924–934.

Washington, J.A., & Craig, H.K. (1994). Dialectal forms during discourse of poor, urban, African American preschoolers. *Journal of Speech and Hearing Research, 37*: 816–823.

Wiig, E.H., Jones, S.S., & Wiig, E.D. (1996). Computer-based assessment of word knowledge in teens with learning disabilities. *Language, Speech, and Hearing Services in Schools, 27*: 21–28.

Wilcox, M.J. (1992). Enhancing initial communication skills in young children with developmental disabilities through partner programming. *Seminars in Speech and Hearing, 13*: 194–212.

Wilcox, M.J. (1994). Delivering communication-based services to infants, toddlers, and their families: Approaches and models. In K.G. Butler, *Early Intervention I: Working with Infants and Toddlers*. Gaithersburg, MD: Aspen Publications.

Woods, B.T., & Carey, S. (1979). Language deficits after apparent clinical recovery from childhood aphasia. *Annals of Neurology, 6*: 405–409.

Worster-Drought, C. (1971). An unusual form of acquired aphasia in children. *Developmental Medicine and Child Neurology, 13*: 563–571.

Ylvisaker, M. (1998). Traumatic brain injury in children and adolescents: Introduction. In M. Ylvisaker (Ed.), *Traumatic Brain Injury Rehabilitation in Children* (pp. 1–10) (2nd ed.). Boston: Butterworth-Heinemann.

Ylvisaker, M., Szekeres, S.F., & Feeney, T J. (1998). Cognitive rehabilitation: Executive Functions. In M. Ylvisaker (Ed.), *Traumatic Brain Injury Rehabilitation in Children* (pp. 221–270) (2nd ed.). Boston: Butterworth-Heinemann.

Ylvisaker, M. (1993). Communication outcome in children and adolescents with traumatic brain injury. *Neuropsychological Rehabilitation, 3*: 321–340.

Yoder, P.J., Kaiser, A.P., & Alpert, C.L. (1991). An exploratory study of the interactions between language teaching methods and child characteristics. *Journal of Speech and Hearing Research, 34*: 155–167.

Chapter *8*

Disorders of Language
in Adults

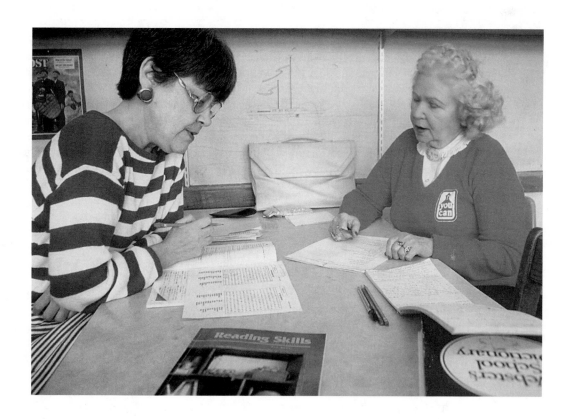

Preview

Language is well established by the adult years. Most adults have mastered the syntax and morphology of their primary language in both the spoken and written form, and language formulation and speech production occur with relatively little effort. Adult vocabularies continue to grow as life experience is gained, and adults may become more adept at the subtleties of language use. But for the most part, language knowledge and use are relatively stable with the exception of some minor word retrieval problems that occur with advanced age. In some adults, however, sudden or progressive damage to portions of the brain that are important for language and thought significantly disturb the ability to communicate. The extent and location of brain damage influence the resulting behavior so that various syndromes are associated with certain patterns of brain damage. Rehabilitation of adults with acquired communication disorders is challenging and rewarding work typically accomplished in partnership with the patient, clinician, and caregivers.

Normal language and cognition are dependent upon a healthy nervous system. Damage to portions of the brain that support language may result in an impairment of language referred to as **aphasia**. Because language centers are in the left hemisphere in most people, aphasia typically is associated with left hemisphere damage. Acquired language impairments may occur in children, as reviewed in Chapter 7, but aphasia is most often observed in adults. When the right hemisphere is damaged rather than the left, the resulting syndrome of cognitive and communication impairments is quite different from aphasia. In other cases, widespread or diffuse damage to both hemispheres may occur, as is frequently observed following traumatic brain injury (TBI). As discussed in Chapter 7, teenagers and young adults are at greatest risk for TBI, but older adults may suffer the cognitive and behavioral consequences of head injury as well. With advanced age, there is increased likelihood of progressive intellectual and linguistic decline associated with various type of dementia.

Aphasia

Aphasia is an acquired impairment of language. It results from damage to the language centers of the brain, typically in the left perisylvian region as reviewed in Chapter 2. The areas of damage or injury are called **lesions**. In the case of aphasia, an individual who had normal language suddenly finds those abilities lost or degraded. Speech-language pathologists in medical settings frequently participate in the evaluation and rehabilitation of individuals with aphasia.

> Mr. Wallace was a right-handed man who had a bachelor's degree in engineering and had retired after a distinguished career in the army. At age 67, he had a stroke in the left cerebral hemisphere. He did not suffer any physical impairment after the stroke, but his ability to communicate was markedly impaired due to aphasia. A conversational exchange with Mr. Wallace went as follows:

PB: Tell me about the work that you did.

Mr. Wallace: When I grew up in the army, this was my whole *fife, lar . . . light*. I was in the army, the army, and the war and everything else under the sun. Everything. And various coun, coun, coun, countries, and things in different places we went and in the armies. I was a colonel in the infantry. And I liked it. I was very fond of . . . I knew everybody in Westpoint. We all grown in our lives, grown up, and we were children. And we knew a lot of people and I think we were useful. And the people we work with. And so we did.

Mr. Wallace did not have trouble pronouncing words, nor was his speech hesitant or effortful, but his language certainly was lacking content. He seemed to have difficulty coming up with the words he needed to explain his thoughts. For example, it was obvious that Mr. Wallace intended to say, "When I grew up in the army, this was my whole *life*." But he did not say the word *life*. He first said the word *fife*, then he said a nonword *lar*, and finally he said an incorrect word, *light*. Mr. Wallace retained his life-long memories and did not have an impairment of his intellect, he had an impairment specific to language—he had aphasia.

It is important to appreciate that aphasia is an impairment of language, not simply a problem with speech production. Recall from Chapters 3 and 4 that language is a symbol system used to convey thoughts, whereas speech refers to the product of the articulatory movements. Language includes the words we speak and the rules that govern how words are combined to make utterances. Mr. Wallace had trouble coming up with the appropriate words and also had difficulty combining them into meaningful sentences. Although some of Mr. Wallace's words were pronounced incorrectly, this was not due to a speech problem; it was part of his language impairment—he could not come up with the word he wanted to say. His speech was actually relatively intact in that his words were well-articulated and easy to understand. Some individuals with aphasia *do* have difficulty articulating words, that is, they have speech problems that co-exist with their aphasia. We will discuss two groups of speech disorders associated with neurological damage, **dysarthria** and **apraxia of speech**, in Chapter 9.

Language is distinguished not only from speech, but also from thought. Patients with severe aphasia often demonstrate that they have relatively well-preserved thought processes. They retain their world knowledge, remember their life histories, and learn new things about what is going on in the world. Therefore, aphasia is not an impairment of general intellect as is observed in dementing diseases. It would be an oversimplification to suggest that individuals with aphasia possess all the cognitive abilities they had before the onset of their aphasia (see, e.g., Beeson, Bayles, Rubens, & Kaszniak, 1993; Murray, Holland, & Beeson, 1997), but it is the language impairment that is central to their communication problem.

Characteristics of Aphasia

The difficulty in coming up with words that was evident in Mr. Wallace's conversation is called **anomia**, which literally means "without name." Anomia is the hallmark of aphasia, that is, all people with aphasia complain of difficulty coming up with the names of things. The rambling emptiness of Mr. Wallace's conversation resulted from his anomia. He overused pronouns such as *thing*, *it*, and *we* rather than giving specific names of people, places, or things. Word retrieval problems are even more apparent when individuals with aphasia are asked to give the names of specific items. Individuals with aphasia may identify instances of anomia by saying something like, "oh, I can't think of the word for it," or they may describe the item that they cannot name. For example, to refer to the Veteran's Administration hospital, a patient said, "you know, the place where I met you . . . with all the soldiers and where we did those things with the tests." This sort of "talking around the word" is called **circumlocution**. While circumlocution is an indicator of word retrieval problems, it is also a very useful communication strategy to compensate for anomia. Not all individuals with aphasia can detect or correct their errors. It is also important to note that not all individuals with aphasia can speak as fluently as Mr. Wallace. For many individuals with aphasia, word finding difficulties exist in the context of hesitant, effortful speech.

Sometimes incorrect words or nonwords are produced in place of the desired word. Such errors are called **paraphasias**. Mr. Wallace's incorrect attempts to produce the word *light* resulted in several paraphasias. They can be whole word substitutions, such as *world* for *life*, single sound substitutions such as *fife* for *life*, or nonwords that are close or totally unrelated to the target word, such as *lar* for *life*. Such nonwords are also called **neologisms**, meaning "new words," but they have no meaning to the listener.

Fluent versus Nonfluent Aphasia

Mr. Wallace's speech output was considered fluent in that it had relatively normal prosodic variations of pitch, loudness, and stress. Although there were some hesitations due to word finding difficulties, the words flowed in a manner that sounded fairly normal. It was also articulated without excessive effort. The utterances were generally of normal length in terms of the number of words and there was some syntactic structure, such as the use of articles, prepositional phrases, and appropriate word endings, such as -ed. The fluent aphasia exhibited by Mr. Wallace is called **Wernicke's aphasia**, a type of aphasia that will be described in greater detail in a subsequent section.

Not all individuals with aphasia speak fluently. Those with nonfluent aphasia produce utterances characterized by effortful, hesitant speech that may be poorly articulated. Mr. Brown provides an example of a type of nonfluent aphasia called **Broca's aphasia**. He was a 36-year-old man who had a congenital malformation of his vascular system that required surgery when he was 31. The surgery was complicated by a hemorrhage that occurred in the region of the left middle cerebral artery and caused extensive damage to the language areas of his left hemisphere. He had weakness of the right side of his body and a significant nonfluent aphasia. Two years after his stroke we had the following conversation.

PB: What can you tell me about the stroke?

Mr Brown: Um . . . (sighs) . . . um . . . (sighs) . . . left . . . (gestures to right side of body) . . . right side . . . (shakes his head and sighs).

PB: And before your stroke, what did you do?

Mr. Brown: Um . . . resale sales (holds up 6 fingers).

PB: Six years?

Mr. Brown: No. Six . . . store . . . chain . . . California.

PB: Did you do sales?

Mr. Brown: No. No. This time . . . general . . . manager.

Mr. Brown's utterances were quite different from those of Mr. Wallace. He spoke mostly in single words and short phrases. Whereas Mr. Wallace had an excess of vague, empty words, Mr. Brown's words were almost all meaningful content words. This type of output has been called telegraphic speech because it is lacking the little functor words that are typically omitted when one sends a telegram. (In the old days people sent telegrams rather than e-mails, and you had to pay by the word.) The pauses and interjection of "um" give the impression that Mr. Brown is struggling to find and produce the words he wanted to say. The overall speech pattern is lacking normal prosodic variation, that is, there is not the normal melodic variation of pitch, loudness, and stress. The term **nonfluent** is used to capture the essence of this effortful, telegraphic speech pattern. It should not be confused with the term **disfluent**, which refers to the disruption of speech fluency that is observed in stuttering (see Chapter 10).

There is a logical neuroanatomical correlation of the fluent versus nonfluent distinction among individuals with aphasia. As shown in Figure 8-1, the primary motor area and the areas important for motor planning are located in the frontal lobe, which is anterior to the central, or Rolandic, fissure. Broca's area is a frontal lobe region important for the motor planning of speech movements (see Figure 8-1). Therefore, it makes sense that brain damage to those anterior regions of the left hemisphere

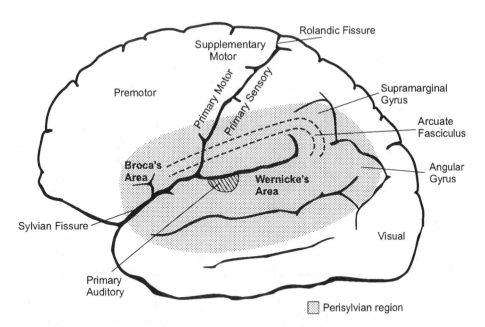

FIGURE 8-1 **A schematic drawing of the left hemisphere indicates the language centers in the perisylvian region. Note that the primary auditory area is actually hidden from view inside the Sylvian fissure; the arcuate fasciculus is a white matter pathway that is deep within the hemisphere. [Reprinted from Beeson, P. M., & Rapczak, S. Z. (1998). The aphasias. In P. J. Snyder & P. D. Mussbaum (Eds.), *Clinical Neuropsychology: A Pocket Handbook for Assessment* (pp. 403–425), with permission from American Psychological Association.]**

are likely to affect motor control and planning, and thus lead to a disruption of speech production like that observed in nonfluent aphasia. As observed with Mr. Brown, anterior lesions often damage the motor areas for the right arm and leg as well, so that individuals with nonfluent aphasia often have right-sided weakness, which is called right **hemiparesis**. Conversely, lesions that spare the anterior motor regions (i.e., that are posterior to the Rolandic fissure) are typically associated with fluent aphasia and no hemiparesis, as observed in Mr. Wallace. In general, anterior lesions are associated with nonfluent aphasia, and posterior lesions are associated with fluent aphasia. Large lesions that encompass both anterior and posterior regions would result in nonfluent aphasia because damage would include the critical anterior motor regions.

Beyond the distinction between fluent and nonfluent aphasias, classification systems have been used over the past century to distinguish identifiable aphasia subtypes. The Boston classification system is commonly used in North America (Goodglass, 1993; Helm-Estabrooks & Albert, 1991). This system includes the two aphasia types introduced thus far, Wernicke's and Broca's aphasia. In general the aphasia types reflect performance profiles that indicate (1) whether the aphasia is fluent or nonfluent, (2) whether auditory comprehension is relatively good or impaired, and (3) whether the ability to repeat sentences is preserved or impaired. Just as fluency characteristics offer some insight regarding lesion location, some inferences can be drawn from the status of auditory comprehension and verbal repetition abilities. An understanding of those processes is helpful before examining various aphasia types in more detail.

Auditory Comprehension

Auditory comprehension requires the extraction of meaning from spoken words and the processing of grammatical structures in connected utterances. Auditory comprehension problems are common in aphasia, but the degree of impairment can vary considerably. Some individuals have trouble understanding the meaning of single words and simple commands, such as when they are asked, "Show me the table." Others can respond to such simple requests, but have trouble when understanding is dependent upon careful processing of each word in relation to other words in the utterance. For example, the following verbal request would challenge most individuals with aphasia, "Do you want chicken or steak for dinner? Because if you want chicken, you need to get it out of the freezer."

Auditory comprehension is dependent upon information processing in the posterior, superior temporal lobe in the region called Wernicke's area, which is adjacent to the primary auditory region (Figure 8-1). Damage to Wernicke's area does not impair the ability to hear, but interferes with the understanding of spoken language. Lesions to Wernicke's area are considered "posterior," because they are posterior to the Rolandic fissure, and do not include the frontal motor regions. Mr. Wallace's stroke damaged Wernicke's area, and he had intermittent trouble understanding what was said in conversation. He also made errors on yes/no questions such as, "Do you eat a banana before you peel it?" Mr. Wallace's comprehension was assessed using a variety of tasks that included pointing to items in response to their name, simple and complex commands, yes-no questions, and more difficult tasks such as comprehending a paragraph read aloud.

Repetition

Although the ability to repeat what other people say is not a particularly important or meaningful use of language, it is a useful diagnostic task when examining for aphasia. The ability to repeat words, phrases, and sentences requires auditory processing by posterior regions of the left hemisphere as well as verbal formulation by the anterior regions of the left hemisphere. So, the ability to repeat sentences is a good test of the integrity of the entire left perisylvian region. Difficulty with verbal repetition can arise for several reasons. The attempts to repeat sentences by Mr. Wallace (with fluent aphasia) resulted in errors because of his auditory comprehension problems and his many paraphasic errors. Mr. Brown (with nonfluent aphasia) had trouble repeating sentences because he omitted the little grammatical words, just like he did in his conversational speech. Repetition can also be disrupted by damage to fibers that connect the posterior and anterior perisylvian regions. The **arcuate fasciculus** is a collection of nerve fibers that originate in the superior temporal lobe, course up and around the Sylvian fissure, and project to the frontal lobe (Figure 8-1). Damage to these fibers, as well as other posterior regions in the left hemisphere, disrupt repetition abilities even when Broca's and Wernicke's areas are spared (Damasio & Damasio, 1980). This type of aphasia in which repetition is significantly impaired is called **conduction aphasia**.

Relatively good verbal repetition is observed in some aphasias that result from brain damage that is on the periphery of the left perisylvian region, or from isolated lesions within the perisylvian region that do not devastate the input and output processes necessary for repetition. There is a relatively rare group of aphasia subtypes with surprisingly preserved ability to repeat sentences called the **transcortical aphasias**. Individuals with transcortical aphasia may have considerable difficulty speaking or understanding language, but despite these impairments, they can repeat fairly long sentences because the perisylvian region is relatively spared.

Summary of Neuroanatomical Principles Related to Aphasia

Several neuroanatomical principles have been introduced that highlight the relation between brain regions and language behaviors. Before summarizing those principles, it is important to remember that successful communication requires participation of many parts of the brain, and that damage to a particular area does not mean that *only* the damaged area is responsible for the impaired function. Also, it is known that people vary in terms of their precise brain organization. With those caveats in mind, the following generalizations can be made:

1. Large anterior lesions interfere with fluent speech production, so that nonfluent aphasia is associated with anterior lesions and fluent aphasias are associated with posterior lesions.
2. Lesions in and around Wernicke's area interfere with auditory comprehension, so that posterior lesions tend to be associated with poor auditory comprehension and anterior lesions may leave auditory comprehension relatively well preserved.
3. Lesions within the perisylvian region disrupt the ability to repeat sentences, but lesions on the periphery of the perisylvian region result in relatively preserved ability to repeat.
4. Lesions throughout the left hemisphere can disrupt naming abilities resulting in anomia, so there is no localizing value for anomia.

Aphasia Types

We have noted the general predictability of language performance based on lesion location and have suggested that patients with similar lesions tend to have similar language characteristics. Aphasia classification systems are useful for identifying such clusters of language behaviors. We will review the Boston classification system, which indicates aphasia type on the basis of fluency, auditory comprehension, and repetition abilities. Such classification systems are clinically useful, but not all individuals with aphasia will fit a specific type. In a large aphasia recovery study, Wertz and colleagues (1981) found that about 75% of the individuals with aphasia were classifiable by aphasia type, leaving 25% who were considered unclassifiable. In those cases, it is still useful to characterize the aphasia in terms of fluency, auditory comprehension, and repetition abilities.

Figure 8-2 shows the decision process for determining aphasia type, and the associated brain drawings are intended to depict a typical lesion location for each aphasia type. As shown, the nonfluent aphasias include damage to anterior portions of the brain, and the fluent aphasias are restricted to posterior lesions. As mentioned, however, there is considerable variation from person to person, so the predicted relations between lesion location and language behavior are not without many exceptions.

Broca's Aphasia

Broca's aphasia results from lesions affecting the posterior portion of the left inferior frontal lobe. These are considered anterior lesions because they lie anterior to the Rolandic fissure. When the le-

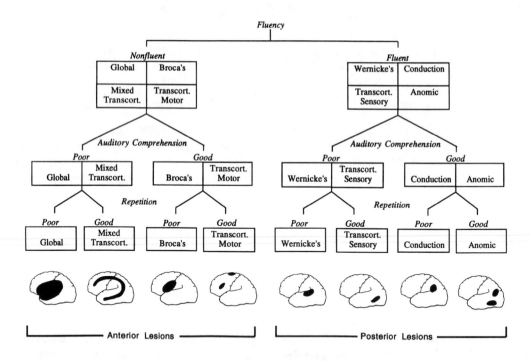

FIGURE 8-2   A decision tree used to guide the classification of aphasia type based upon fluency of spontaneous speech, auditory comprehension, and verbal repetition abilities. Schematic drawings of typical brain lesions associated with each aphasia type are included. Transcort. = transcortical. [Reprinted from Beeson, P. M., & Rapczak, S. Z. (1998). The aphasias. In P. J. Snyder & R. D. Mussbaum (Eds.), *Clinical Neuropsychology: A Pocket Handbook for Assessment* **(pp. 403–425), with permission from American Psychological Association.]**

sions are small and restricted to Broca's area, the individual may have Broca's aphasia for only a short time following the brain damage, and then recover to a more fluent aphasia. Persistent Broca's aphasia typically results from larger lesions that affect not only Broca's area but extend posteriorly to the anterior parietal lobe. An extensive anterior lesion often results in right hemiparesis as noted with Mr. Brown.

Broca's aphasia is a nonfluent aphasia characterized by slow, hesitant, telegraphic speech. Utterances are of reduced length, typically fewer than four words, and have little syntactic complexity. The utterances are mostly isolated productions of nouns with some adjectives and verbs, and they are notably lacking articles, prepositions, and other functors. Broca's aphasia is sometimes referred to as "motor aphasia" or "expressive aphasia," terms that highlight the observed production problems. Auditory comprehension is relatively well preserved for conversation, but breaks down when comprehension is dependent upon correct understanding of complex grammar or understanding of the little functor words. Repetition is limited to a few words. When asked to repeat full sentences, individuals with Broca's aphasia may simply repeat the content words. Reading and writing are also impaired in individuals with Broca's aphasia because the aphasia affects all language modalities.

Wernicke's Aphasia

Wernicke's aphasia is associated with lesions to the posterior superior portion of the left temporal lobe, an area important for auditory processing. Such posterior lesions typically spare the motor regions, so that individuals with Wernicke's aphasia rarely have hemiparesis. In contrast to Broca's aphasia, Wernicke's aphasia is characterized by fluent speech that is difficult to understand because it contains numerous paraphasias and is relatively devoid of content. In some cases verbal output is so disturbed that it is made up primarily of nonwords called neologisms that sound like jargon. This type of output is sometimes called **jargon aphasia**, and it is similar in some ways to the jargon of a child learning language because the prosodic variations may communicate agreement, disagreement, questioning, anger, and the like. The use of prosodic, or suprasegmental, variations to communicate, despite the absence of meaningful language, reinforces the point that individuals with aphasia still possess many cognitive abilities despite their language impairment.

Auditory comprehension is significantly impaired in Wernicke's aphasia, sometimes to the extent that the names of common objects are not recognized. This comprehension disturbance is highlighted in other terms used for the disorder: receptive aphasia and sensory aphasia. Another sign of impaired auditory processing is the failure to self-correct production errors. Repetition is severely impaired in Wernicke's aphasia due to poor auditory processing and production problems. Reading and writing are impaired in much the same way as auditory comprehension and verbal expression.

Conduction Aphasia

Conduction aphasia is associated with lesions in the left temporal-parietal region, particularly in an area that is immediately posterior to the Sylvian fissure called the supramarginal gyrus. As mentioned earlier, such a lesion disrupts the connection between the anterior and posterior language regions so that poor repetition of spoken utterances is a hallmark of this aphasia type.

Conduction aphasia is somewhat similar to Wernicke's aphasia in that the verbal output is fluent and paraphasias are common. Individuals with conduction aphasia have better auditory comprehension than those with Wernicke's aphasia, presumably because much of Wernicke's area is spared. It is not uncommon for individuals with conduction aphasia to attempt to self-correct their speech production errors, and frequently they are successful after several attempts. The self-corrections and hesitations associated with word-finding problems cause some disruption of the flow of speech, but the verbal output retains a sense of fluency in that articulation is accomplished with relative ease. Because the lesion spares the anterior motor regions, conduction aphasia typically is not associated with hemiparesis.

Anomic Aphasia

Anomic aphasia is characterized by word retrieval difficulty in conversation and in the context of naming tasks, with relative preservation of auditory comprehension and repetition abilities. Anomic aphasia can result from relatively isolated lesions in the posterior temporal-parietal region, but has also been associated with lesions throughout the left hemisphere. Some of the other aphasia types may evolve to anomic aphasia after a period of recovery if the extent of brain damage is not extensive. Therefore, the presence of anomic aphasia does not provide information about the location of the aphasia-producing lesion.

Transcortical Aphasias

There are three types of transcortical aphasia that share the common characteristic of remarkably preserved ability to repeat spoken utterances despite problems with self-generated language. As described earlier, transcortical aphasias are associated with lesions that spare the perisylvian region. They result from strokes that occur at the outer borders of the left hemisphere language zone (Figure 8-1). The transcortical aphasia types are distinguished from one another on the basis of fluency and auditory comprehension. **Transcortical motor aphasia** is nonfluent with relatively good auditory comprehension, so that it looks like Broca's aphasia with good repetition. It is associated with anterior borderzone lesions. **Transcortical sensory aphasia** is associated with posterior borderzone lesions; it is characterized by fluent output and auditory comprehension problems like Wernicke's aphasia, but repetition is preserved. **Mixed transcortical aphasia** is a rare syndrome that results from damage affecting both anterior and posterior regions of the perisylvian borderzone. Communication is severely impaired, but the patient is able to repeat full sentences, despite a lack of understanding of the meaning.

Global Aphasia

Global aphasia refers to severe language impairment affecting all domains. It is associated with large left hemisphere lesions that essentially damage the entire perisylvian region. In global aphasia, meaningful verbal output is typically extremely limited. In some cases, it is limited to repetitive utterances such as "one, two, three" or "I can see." In other cases, the utterances are repetitive jargon such as "nanna nanna nanna." Utterances that are repeated are called **perseverations**. It is worth mentioning that even individuals with significant global aphasia are capable of communicating wants, needs, and opinions if the listener provides a supportive communication environment.

Causes of Aphasia

There are about one million Americans with aphasia, and about 83,000 new cases of aphasia every year (Klein, 1995). It is a disorder most often associated with older age, with the average age for people with aphasia being about 67 years (Hier, Yoon, Mohr, Price, & Wolf, 1994). Stroke is the most common cause of brain damage resulting in aphasia. A **stroke**, also called a cerebrovascular accident, is an interruption of blood flow to the brain caused by blockage of an artery or the bursting of an artery (hemorrhage). When blood flow to brain cells is interrupted, they are deprived of oxygen, which ultimately results in cell death. Those brain cells do not regenerate, so the functions subserved by the damaged cells are impaired. Other causes of brain damage can also result in aphasia, such as traumatic accident, brain tumor, or infection.

It has long been known that in right-handed people, language problems tend to occur after damage to the left rather than the right hemisphere. It is damage to the left perisylvian region that typically results in aphasia. The major blood vessel that serves the perisylvian region is the middle cerebral artery; therefore, stroke affecting the left middle cerebral artery is the most common cause of aphasia (Benson & Ardila, 1996).

The onset of aphasia is typically abrupt but some etiologies may be associated with a slowly progressive onset. Brain tumors can cause slow onset of aphasia as they either infiltrate or compress critical language areas. **Primary progressive aphasia** is a relatively rare syndrome in which aphasia slowly develops in the absence of a documented neurological event (Duffy & Petersen, 1992).

Assessment of Aphasia

The initial evaluation of a person with aphasia may take place at their bedside while in an acute care hospital. Informal interaction with the patient allows observation of some aspects of verbal fluency, auditory comprehension, and word retrieval. A few structured tasks can further inform the speech-language pathologist of the patient's ability to understand spoken and written language, to repeat sentences, and to communicate by writing. The initial assessment goal is typically to characterize the nature of the impairment to appraise the functional abilities of the patient. A more comprehensive language assessment is typically deferred for a few days or weeks when the patient is able to sit at a table and tolerate the demands of sustained, structured interaction. However, the speech-language pathologist can be of considerable assistance to the patient and family during the first few days after the onset of aphasia as they seek to understand this strange disorder. Most importantly, the speech-language pathologist can facilitate successful communication with the patient and begin the process of training useful compensatory strategies to be used on a temporary or long-term basis.

Comprehensive language assessment is frequently accomplished by the use of standardized tests for aphasia. Some of the more commonly used aphasia tests are the *Western Aphasia Battery* (Kertesz, 1982), the *Boston Diagnostic Aphasia Examination* (Goodglass & Kaplan, 1983), and the *Aphasia Diagnostic Profiles* (Helm-Estabrooks, 1992). Most of these tests take an hour or less to administer. They sample language behaviors of varying difficulty and allow the examiner to create a summary profile of aphasia type and severity. There are many supplemental tests that may also be used to characterize patient performance, as well as informal measures constructed by the speech-language pathologist. Some protocols are specifically designed to examine the impact of the language impairment on everyday communication situations and are considered functional communication measures (Frattali, Thompson, Holland, & Ferketic, 1995; Holland, 1980). The overall goal of assessment is to document the current status of the patient and provide direction for the treatment plan.

Treatment for Aphasia

Individual Therapy

The goal for aphasia treatment is to maximize the recovery of impaired language functions, to assist in the development of alternative and compensatory communication strategies, and to help the patient adjust to the residual deficits (Rosenbek, LaPointe, & Wertz, 1989). There are countless approaches to achieving such goals. It is the responsibility of the speech-language pathologist to select an existing treatment approach or to design a unique approach that is appropriate for the specific patient. The treatment plan should take into consideration the nature and extent of the language impairment as well as the residual language and cognitive abilities. Treatment plans are influenced by additional factors such as the time post onset of aphasia, the patient's functional needs, motivation, and desires. Although the classification by aphasia type is useful to characterize the overall aphasia profile, it does not offer specific direction for treatment because individuals with the same aphasia type may differ in many ways.

There is a large body of literature to guide speech-language pathologists to appropriate treatment approaches for a particular set of symptoms (see, e.g., Chapey, 1994; Helm-Estabrooks & Albert, 1991; Holland & Forbes, 1993; Rosenbek et al., 1989); however, it is the patient's response to treatment that is the ultimate test of its effectiveness. The experienced clinician knows that a given treatment can be effective for patients with different impairments, and that patients with similar impairments may respond differently to the same treatment approach (Hillis & Caramazza, 1994).

When selecting or designing a treatment plan, the speech-language pathologist may approach treatment from several different perspectives. One approach is to stimulate the return of language abilities that are impaired but appear to have potential to improve or be restored. For example, the stimulation approach pioneered by Hildred Schuell employed the repetition of phrases and sentences to improve auditory comprehension and verbal production (Jenkins, Pabon-Jimenez, Shaw, & Williams Sefer, 1975). Many treatment protocols are designed to stimulate language by following a task hierarchy that elicits responses that are progressively more difficult for the patient to produce (some are reviewed in Helm-Estabrooks & Albert, 1991). The speech-language pathologist may determine what support or cues are necessary to help the patient respond correctly, and then systematically withdraw the support as the patient progresses. This approach incrementally shifts the burden from the clinician to the patient to achieve the desired response. When implementing a treatment plan, the speech-language pathologist is challenged to find the appropriate tasks that help the patient improve to a higher level of functioning. Whereas patients or family members may initially set their goals for completely normal language without any intermediate steps, the speech-language pathologist charts a realistic path that moves toward normal language but has many intermediate goals.

Some treatment approaches take advantage of residual abilities that can be used to substitute or compensate for impaired abilities. For example, a patient may be able to write a word, or part of a word, that he is unable to say. The use of writing to supplement spoken output may be an effective strategy; however, another possibility is that the written word may facilitate the spoken production of the word. Many individuals with aphasia are able to say a word if they hear the first sound or syllable of the word. This responsiveness to phonemic cueing (as it is called) can be particularly useful if the patient can learn to provide his own phonemic cue for the word. For example, a patient may write the word *popcorn*, and then cue himself that it starts with *puh*. In order to come up with the sound *puh*, he must first retrieve a word that he can typically produce. For example, the patient may be able to say *Pat* because that is his wife's name, so he looks at the word *popcorn*, and recalls that it starts just like *Pat*. By self-cueing with the sound *puh*, he is then able to say *popcorn*. The success of this approach was documented by DePartz (1986) and Nickels (1992). We have found that it not only works as a compensatory strategy for selected patients, but it serves as a means for them to ultimately regain the ability to produce the word without the cue. In other words, the strategy served to help the recovery of normal word retrieval.

Individual treatment plans may include several goals that variously address auditory comprehension, speech production, reading, writing, and gestural communication. As noted above, some tasks are directed toward more than one modality, such as speaking and writing. Therapy goals are selected so that they are appropriate for the particular patient and have immediate or eventual impact on their functional communication abilities. For example, the patient shown in Figure 8-3 participated in a writing treatment program that facilitated the return of his ability to write single words to communicate thoughts and needs that he was unable to say or gesture.

Group Therapy

Significant aphasia may result in social isolation and few opportunities to engage in conversation. Group therapy for individuals with aphasia provides a setting where conversation is facilitated and supported by the clinician, and patients can learn to maximize their communication skills (see Figure 8-4). In a small group of three to five individuals with aphasia, the speech-language pathologist can work with the patients to (1) facilitate successful communication despite their residual language impairment; (2) encourage communication using all modalities; and (3) teach and elaborate specific communication strategies (Beeson & Holland, 1995). In the small group setting, patients can learn from the clinician and from each other how to compensate for language difficulties. Alternative communication strategies including gestures, drawing, and writing are encouraged to supplement

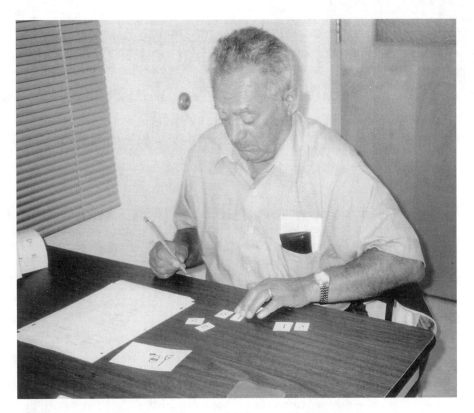

FIGURE 8-3 Individual therapy to improve writing for single words that includes arrangement of letters to spell the word and copy of the word. (Courtesy of The University of Arizona, Department of Speech & Hearing Sciences)

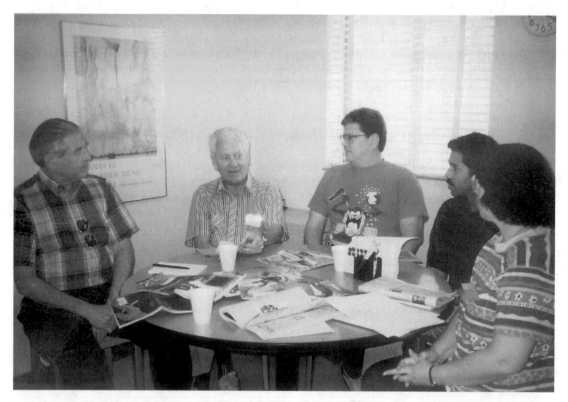

FIGURE 8-4   Group therapy for aphasia focuses on conversational language supplemented by writing and gestures. (Courtesy of The University of Arizona, Department of Speech & Hearing Sciences)

the spoken utterances of group members. Groups also can offer considerable psychological and social support for members as they adjust to their impairment. Many examples of structured and informal conversational activities have been reported in recent literature regarding group therapy (Elman, 1998; Kearns, 1994; Marshall, 1993; Springer, 1991), and there is evidence that some individuals with aphasia can continue to improve language abilities long after their strokes (Holland & Beeson, 1998).

Acquired Reading and Writing Impairments

As noted, most individuals with aphasia have difficulty reading and writing as well as listening and speaking, so that aphasia treatment frequently includes intervention in all language modalities. On relatively rare occasions, damage to the left posterior temporal-parietal region results in isolated impairments of reading and writing in the absence of aphasia. The speech-language pathologist is often involved in the assessment and treatment of these disorders. Pure **alexia**, also known as **alexia without agraphia**, is an unusual syndrome wherein the patient is able to write but cannot read. It is thought to result from a disruption of the visual input to the part of the brain that recognizes the word. The individual with pure alexia can see the words, and may even be able to identify the letters of the word, but fails to recognize the word as a whole. Many individuals with pure alexia compensate for their lack of word recognition by reading the individual letters aloud; when they hear the word spelled aloud, they can recognize the word. This letter-by-letter reading approach is useful, but painfully slow. One treatment approach to this problem is to practice reading and rereading a given passage, so that it becomes familiar, yielding improvement in reading rate on practiced text. Several clinical researchers have found that this approach results in increased reading rate for new material as well (Beeson, 1998; Moyer, 1979).

It is even more rare when reading and writing are both impaired despite the presence of relatively normal spoken language and auditory comprehension (Kirshner, 1995). This syndrome, called **alexia with agraphia**, is associated with damage to the inferior parietal lobe that affects the angular and supramarginal gyri (Figure 8-1). Treatment approaches for alexia with agraphia may incorporate strategies used for pure alexia as well those specifically designed to improve writing.

Right-Hemisphere Communication Disorders

Damage to the right hemisphere may result in some word retrieval difficulties similar to that observed in left-hemisphere damage, however, the prominent features of right-hemisphere damage (RHD) tend to be quite different from those associated with left hemisphere damage. Individuals with RHD may have a host of subtle impairments in their thought organization, mental flexibility, and their use of language that affect their ability to understand and communicate effectively (Myers, 1997; Tompkins, 1995). Although individuals with RHD typically understand the content of individual sentences, they often fail to understand the gist of the conversation; may not appreciate humor, figures of speech, facial expressions, and other nonverbal communication cues; and simply fail to keep up with natural give-and-take and shift of topic in conversation. These functions are referred to as extralinguistic aspects of communication, meaning that they are features other than the actual words used to speak. These problems sound rather vague and, in fact, individuals with RHD simply may be perceived as odd, or rude, or inattentive, rather than brain-damaged. Their change in cognitive and communication abilities is clearly evident to friends and family, however. One of the patients at our clinic, Mr. Rice, explained his perception of one of the effects of his right hemisphere stroke as follows:

> Taking turns in talking in conversation was very difficult . . . because I would interrupt and have something to say in the middle of the conversation and interrupt everything. Train of thought and everything else. I thought I had to jump in otherwise I'd lose what I was trying to say.

Mr. Rice was 66 years old when he experienced a right hemisphere stroke. One year after his stroke he still had weakness of his left arm and leg, but he could walk without assistance and communicated effectively. His speech was easy to understand but the prosody sounded somewhat flat, as if lacking emotion; even when he joked, his voice and facial expression were difficult to interpret. It was notable that Mr. Rice was able to provide some insight into the nature of his problem because many individuals with RHD do not recognize their problems.

Mr. Rice also experienced **left neglect**, in that he tended to orient his gaze away from the left and was relatively unaware of sensory input on the left side of his body and the left side of his visual field. Left neglect is relatively common following right-hemisphere damage, and it occurs even when there is no loss of sensory or motor function on the left side and no loss of vision on the left (Heilman, Watson, & Valenstein, 1993). These effects of brain damage have shown that the right hemisphere plays a special role in maintaining attention to the space around us, and our intrapersonal space as well. Left neglect may interfere with communication in that people to the patient's left are ignored, just as the left half of the page may be ignored when reading and writing. Myers (1997) suggested that neglect may be a significant contributor to the cognitive-communication impairment in a more general sense. Future research may help to clarify the relation between neglect and the behavioral profile associated with right-hemisphere damage.

Incidence of Right-Hemisphere Damage

Given the relatively subtle nature of the cognitive-communication problems associated with RHD, it is not surprising that the incidence and prevalence are not well documented. The American Heart Association (1992) reported that there were about 500,000 new strokes each year in the United States, with about half affecting the right hemisphere. Tompkins (1995) estimated that about half of RHD adults will have communication impairments, so we would estimate 125,000 new cases of right hemisphere-related communication impairments per year.

Assessment and Treatment

Assessment of the patient with RHD typically includes sampling language in conversational and picture description tasks, assessing the extralinguistic aspects of communication, and examining for evidence of neglect or attentional problems (Myers, 1997; Tompkins, 1995). Examination of extralinguistic deficits includes tasks such as interpretation of a story or a pictured scene that requires integration of the component parts into one main idea. Patients may be asked to give the meaning of figures of speech or to produce the appropriate prosodic variation for expressions to convey different emotions. They may also be asked to produce and understand narrative stories. All of these tasks share the common goal of probing comprehension and use of language in a flexible, abstract manner that comes naturally to most adults, but is clearly at risk with RHD. Numerous tasks can be used to examine for neglect, including a very simple request for patients to put a mark on a line to divide it in half. Individuals with left neglect often mark the center of the line off to the right of the midline because they do not perceive the leftmost part of the line. The ability to sustain attention is also assessed using tasks that increase from focused attention on one stimulus to divided attention to two stimuli. Some standardized tests are useful to structure the examination of the RHD patient (Pimental & Kinsbury, 1989).

Treatment for cognitive and communication deficits associated with RHD is challenging. It may be directed toward facilitating recovery of the underlying impairment or toward the development of compensatory strategies to overcome the problems. Greater understanding of the underlying causes of the communication deficits observed in RHD is needed, but it is currently assumed that the extralinguistic deficits are related to the features of neglect and inattention (Myers, 1997). For that reason, some treatment tasks are directed toward improving performance on attention tasks. For example, patients may be asked to listen or look for specific stimuli such as a particular number or word in the midst of other numbers or words (Sohlberg & Mateer, 1990). These types of attention tasks are also used with individuals with traumatic head injury because they also may have problems with attention. Tasks that are directed toward improving extralinguistic abilities may be similar to those used for assessment. After observing the patient's deficits, the speech-language pathologist may structure the language tasks in such a way that a hierarchy of cues provides support for the patient. As discussed in aphasia therapy, the clinician's goal is to assist the patient to make small sequential gains in the direction of normal performance. This may require providing feedback when the patient fails to produce or comprehend the extralinguistic features, such as prosodic variation to mark emotion, followed by a model of the appropriate response. The treatment goals are directed toward improved performance in a variety of settings and communication environments, not simply in the therapy room. This is true for all treatments for speech, language, and hearing disorders, but is especially relevant for the problems associated with RHD because they are often most evident during real-life communication.

Dementia

Dementia refers to an acquired, progressive impairment of intellectual function that is chronic and affects several aspects of mental activity including memory, cognition, language, and the processing of visual-spatial information (Bayles & Kaszniak, 1987; Cummings & Benson, 1992). Dementia may also result in changes in emotion or personality. It is distinguishable from temporary conditions that impair mental function such as confusional states that may last for a few hours or a few days, at most. The progressive intellectual decline in dementia is distinct from isolated, specific impairments such as aphasia due to focal brain damage. Numerous disease processes can cause the diffuse brain damage that results in dementia. As shown in Table 8-1, some dementing diseases produce predominantly cortical damage, other diseases primarily affect subcortical structures, and others have widespread affects. The characteristics of the dementia vary to some extent depending on the disease process.

TABLE 8-1   Various Causes of Dementia Based on the Occurrence of Cortical or Subcortical Dysfunction

Cortical Dementias
   Alzheimer's disease
   Pick's disease
Subcortical Dementias
   Parkinson's disease
   Huntington's disease
   Progressive supranuclear palsy
   Wilson's disease
   Binswanger's disease
   Human immunodeficiency virus
Dementia with Combined Cortical and Subcortical Lesions
   Multiple strokes
   Creutzfeldt-Jakob disease

Cortical Dementia

The most common type of cortical dementia is **Alzheimer's disease** (AD) (Cummings & Benson, 1992). With about four million Americans affected by AD, it accounts for almost half of all dementias. It is characterized by language, memory, and cognitive impairments that include poor judgment, difficulty with calculation, reasoning, and higher level thinking. Caregivers note that the early signs of dementia include memory and concentration problems including forgetting the location of things, poor recall for recent events, and trouble handling finances and performing complex tasks (Bayles, 1991). Speech is typically well articulated and fluent, and may have good grammatical structure, but the content is increasingly empty as the disease progresses. In the early stages, the language impairment may appear similar to anomic aphasia in that there are many instances of word-finding difficulties. In later stages, it may resemble transcortical sensory or Wernicke's aphasia. At the end stages there may be little verbal output at all.

Alzheimer's disease can be confirmed after death by the presence of specific brain changes observed if an autopsy is performed. For that reason, the diagnosis of AD prior to death is tentative, referred to as "probable" AD, based on the presenting symptoms and the exclusion of other causes of dementia. Criteria for the diagnosis of probable AD were agreed upon by the National Institute of Neurological Communication Disorders and Stroke (NINCDS) and the Alzheimer's Disease and Related Disorders Association (ADRDA) (McKhann, Drachman, Folstein, Katzman, Price, & Stadlan, 1984). Memory impairment is often the initial symptom of cortical dementia, however, in some cases the language decline may be the first sign. At our clinic, Mr. Dean brought his 67-year-old wife for an evaluation because her language "was becoming more and more confused," he said. Her speech was well-articulated and easy to understand, but it was devoid of meaningful content, and contained many perseverative thoughts. A report of a head scan indicated there was a generalized loss of brain substance, but there was no evidence of a stroke.

When shown a toy gun and asked to name it, Mrs. Dean said:

Mrs. Dean: This is to put. Um, you can put a thing inside the . . .

PB: Can you tell me the name of it?

Mrs. Dean: Well, it's supposed to be, to do. But that, that's musty. It's hard, when you're on the table and the table is dirty, I take the longer thing, like this this, and get the end. I don't, don't go by this thing. No, this I, see it always in my house. Oh here I can do this, I can do this. It goes if you go.

Mrs. Dean's verbal output sounded in many ways like an individual with aphasia. However there were some features of her behavior that were unlike those observed in aphasia. She showed anxiety and perseverative thoughts as she repeatedly asked where her husband had gone and how was she going to get home. Mr. Dean indicated during a private interview that his wife had become paranoid about her money. She no longer used the bank, but had begun stuffing money under the mattress at home. Six months following the interview, Mrs. Dean's neurologist observed that her behavior became increasingly bizarre, showing signs associated with frontal lobe damage, such as lack of inhibition and modesty. The neurologist rejected a diagnoses of primary progressive aphasia and Alzheimer's disease in favor of a working diagnosis of Pick's disease. Like AD, Pick's disease is a cortical dementia. In Pick's disease, brain changes occur primarily in the frontal and temporal lobes resulting in changes in personality that accompany the changes in intellect, memory, and language.

Like Alzheimer's disease, the diagnosis of Pick's disease is not actually confirmed unless the brain is studied after death.

Subcortical Dementias

Subcortical dementias are more likely to be associated with movement disorders than cortical dementias. They include dementia associated with syndromes such as Parkinson's disease and Huntington's disease. The motor problems affect speech production so that it is often difficult to understand, although language formulation may be relatively preserved. Memory and cognition are affected so that forgetfulness and slowed thought are typical. Subcortical dementia can also arise from multiple strokes affecting the deep gray or white matter in the brain, or from white matter diseases such as multiple sclerosis or the human immunodeficiency virus (HIV).

Dementias with Combined Cortical and Subcortical Lesions

Multiple strokes may damage both the cortical and subcortical structures in the brain resulting in multi-infarct dementia. Such vascular etiologies tend to have a stair-step decline with each stroke rather than the continual progressive decline observed in cortical and subcortical dementias. Individuals with multi-farct dementia, and those with other causes of combined cortical and subcortical lesions, experience communication problems related to speech, language, and cognitive impairments.

Prevalence

Approximately 16 to 21% of the population over the age of 65 has dementia, with 6% of those having a severe form (Cummings & Benson, 1992). The prevalence increases with age, so that approximately 3% of people 65 to 74 are affected, about 13% of those between 75 and 84, and somewhere between 16 and 47% of those over 85 years have dementia (Evans, Funkenstein, Albert, Scherr, Cook, Chown, Hebert, Hennekens, & Taylor, 1989; Kokmen, Chandra, & Shoenberg, 1988). The prevalence of dementia is expected to increase as the older segment of our population continues to grow in number.

Assessment and Intervention

A comprehensive neuropsychological examination of cognitive function is critical to the diagnosis of dementia and may be performed by a neuropsychologist. Several standardized rating scales are used to screen for dementia, such as the *Mini-Mental State Examination* (MMSE; Folstein, Folstein, & McHugh, 1975), which briefly evaluates whether a person is oriented by asking for his or her name, the date, and where they are. The MMSE also includes tasks that look at memory, general knowledge, communication, and the ability to copy a figure. Other scales rate the severity of dementia by using observational criteria, such as the *Global Deterioration Scale* (Reisberg, Ferris, de Leon, & Crook, 1982). The *Mattis Dementia Rating Scale* (Mattis, 1976) is a test of cognitive function that evaluates attention, initiation and perseveration, construction, conceptualization, and memory. A test battery that may be administered by the speech-language pathologist is the *Arizona Battery for Communication Disorders of Dementia* (ABCD; Bayles & Tomoeda, 1993), which provides examination of linguistic comprehension and expression, verbal memory, visuospatial skills, and mental status.

Speech-language pathologists are taking an increasingly active role in the care of individuals with dementia. Although dementia is an irreversible process, therapeutic approaches may be employed that maximize communication and cognitive performance. There are numerous sources of information regarding environmental and linguistic manipulations that positively influence the behavior of individuals with dementia (Bayles & Tomoeda, 1995; Glickstein, 1988; Lubinski, 1991). For example, communication performance can be improved by minimizing distractions and using familiar objects or pictures to stimulate recollections. Auditory comprehension may be improved with the use of simplified syntax and vocabulary. Memory demands can be minimized by making use of a memory book that contains biographical information, pictures of family and friends, and schedule information (Bourgeois, 1992).

The patient's performance profile on a test battery can be examined to determine the relative strengths and weaknesses of the individual with dementia. This information combined with observation and experimentation may help clinicians discover the cognitive, language, and environmental manipulations that minimize the effects of the dementia (Bayles & Tomoeda, 1995). It is often the role of the speech-language pathologist to develop a program that outlines strategies for communicating with specific dementia patients. The speech-language pathologist works with caregivers including family members and nursing home staff to implement the plan and thus provide consistent support to maximize the performance of the dementia patient. In the case of Mrs. Dean, it was apparent that her husband was exhausted by his failure to communicate successfully with his wife. He stated, "she can't even tell me what she wants to eat for dinner." One easy solution to that problem was discovered: If Mr. Dean wrote down three choices for dinner as he asked his wife what she would like, she was able to respond by pointing to one of the options. Other suggestions were made to Mr. Dean to adapt his communication style in such a way as to maximize his wife's ability to communicate.

In closing this chapter, we want to emphasize that acquired impairments of language and cognition may have profound implications for the lives of the affected individuals and their families. Patients may experience significant limitations on their daily activities and may greatly restrict their participation in society. Thus, speech-language pathologists who work with adults with acquired language disorders are not simply concerned with the acquired impairment, but with the consequences of that impairment. Evaluation and treatment approaches are sensitive to the specific needs of a given individual in their unique life situation.

Clinical Problem Solving

Mrs. Anderson was a 55-year-old woman who suffered a left-hemisphere stroke that resulted in aphasia. She was administered the Western Aphasia Battery (Kertesz, 1982) to sample her language abilities. As part of the test, she was asked to describe what was happening in a pictured scene of a man and a woman having a picnic near a lake. Her spoken response followed:

> Is family, um, picnic. And fish, and man is, um, oh, um reading, and, and, um lady is pouring and set, um, son is, is, ha . . . is, um, is, um, flying kite. And neighbor is fishing and neighbor is um, sailing, and boy is, um, playing in water, and man, and lady in, listen to radio. And daughter, I mean, dog, oh . . . oh . . . stave, is lady, is man, is stave, oh, stay. I don't know.

1. Would you classify Mrs. Anderson's aphasia as fluent or nonfluent?
2. In what lobe of the brain is the lesion most likely to be located? Why?

3. Mrs. Anderson had trouble repeating sentences longer than four words. Would you expect her lesion to be in the perisylvian region or outside the perisylvian region? Why?
4. Would you guess that Mrs. Anderson had right hemiparesis? Why, or why not?

References

American Heart Association. (1992). 1992 heart and stroke facts, quoted in medical news and perspectives. *Journal of the American Medical Association, 267*: 335–336.

Alzheimer's Association. (1995). *The Changing Face of Alzheimer Care: Proceedings of the 4th National Alzheimer's Disease Education Conference.* Chicago: Author.

Bayles, K.A. (1991). Alzheimer's disease symptoms: Prevalence and order of appearance. *Journal of Applied Gerontology, 10*: 419–430.

Bayles, K., & Kaszniak, A.W. (1987). *Communication and Cognition in Normal Aging and Dementia.* Austin, TX: Pro-Ed.

Bayles, K.A., & Tomoeda, C.K. (1993). *Arizona Battery for Communication Disorders of Dementia.* Tucson, AZ: Canyonlands Publishing.

Bayles, K., & Tomoeda, C. (1995). *The ABC's of Dementia.* Tucson, AZ: Canyonlands Publishing.

Beeson, P.M. (1998). Treatment for letter-by-letter reading: A case study. In Helm-Estabrooks, N., & Holland, A. L. (Eds.), *Approaches to the Treatment of Aphasia* (pp. 153–177). San Diego, CA: Singular Publishing Group.

Beeson, P.M., Bayles, K.A., Rubens, A.B., & Kaszniak, A.W. (1993). Memory impairment and executive control in individuals with stroke-induced aphasia. *Brain and Language, 45*: 253–275.

Beeson, P.M., & Holland, A.L. (1995). New technologies and intervention approaches: A new look at aphasia groups. *Topics in Stroke Rehabilitation, 2* (2): 85–88.

Benson, D.F., & Ardila, A. (1996). *Aphasia: A Clinical Perspective.* New York: Oxford University Press.

Bourgeois, M.S. (1992). *Conversing with Memory Impaired Individuals Using Memory Aids: A Memory Aid Workbook.* Gaylord: Northern Speech Services.

Chapey, R. (Ed.). (1994). *Language Intervention Strategies in Adult Aphasia.* Baltimore: William & Wilkins.

Cummings, J.L., & Benson, D.F. (1992). *Dementia: A Clinical Approach.* Boston: Butterworth.

Damasio, H., & Damasio, A. (1980). The anatomical basis of conduction aphasia. *Brain, 103*: 337–350.

DePartz, M. (1986). Re-education of a deep dyslexic patient: Rationale of the method and results. *Cognitive Neuropsychology, 3*: 149–177.

Duffy, J.R., & Petersen, R.C. (1992). Primary progressive aphasia. *Aphasiology, 6*: 1–15.

Elman, R. (1998). *Group Treatment of Neurogenic Communication Disorders: The Expert Clinician's Approach.* Boston: Butterworth-Heinemann.

Evans, D.A., Funkenstein, H.H., Albert, M.S., Scherr, P.A., Cook, N.R., Chown, M.J., Hebert, L.E., Hennekens, C.H. & Taylor, J.O. (1989). Prevalence of Alzheimer's disease in a community population of older persons: Higher than previously reported. *Journal of the American Medical Association, 262*: 2551–2556.

Folstein M.F., Folstein, S.E., & McHugh, P.R. (1975). Mini-mental state: A practical method for grading the mental state of patients for the clinician. *Journal of Psychiatric Research, 12*: 189–198.

Fratalli, C.M., Thompson, C.K., Holland, A.L., Wohl, C.B., & Ferketic, M.M. (1995). *ASHA Functional Assessment of Communication Skills for Adults.* Bethesda: American Speech-Language-Hearing Association.

Glickstein, J.K. (1988). *Therapeutic Interventions in Alzheimer's Disease.* Rockville: Aspen Publishers.

Goodglass, H. (1993). *Understanding Aphasia.* San Diego, CA: Academic Press.

Goodglass, H., & Kaplan, E. (1983). *Boston Diagnostic Examination for Aphasia.* Philadelphia: Lea & Febiger.

Halper, A.S., & Cherney, L.R. (1996). *Clinical Management of Right Hemisphere Dysfunction* (2nd ed.). Gaithersburg, MD: Aspen Publishers.

Heilman, K.M., Watson, R.T., & Valenstein, E. (1993). Neglect and related disorders. In K.M. Heilman and E. Valenstein (Eds.), *Clinical Neuropsychology* (3rd ed., pp. 279–336). New York: Oxford University Press.

Helm-Estabrooks, N. (1992). *Manual of Aphasia Diagnostic Profiles.* Chicago: Riverside.

Helm-Estabrooks, N., & Albert, M.L. (1991). *Manual of Aphasia Therapy*. Austin, TX: Pro-Ed.

Hier, D.B., Yoon, W.B., Mohr, J.P., Price, T.R., & Wolf, P.A. (1994). Gender and aphasia in the stroke data bank. *Brain and Language, 47*: 155–167.

Hillis, A. & Caramazza, A. (1992). The reading process and its disorders. In D.I. Margolin (Ed.), *Cognitive Neuropsychology in Clinical Practice* (pp. 229–262). New York: Oxford University Press.

Hillis, A.E., & Caramazza, A. (1994). Theories of lexical processing and rehabilitation of lexical deficits. In M.J. Riddoch & G.W. Humphries (Eds.), *Cognitive Neuropsychology and Cognitive Rehabilitation* (pp. 449–484). Hillsdale, NJ: Lawrence Erlbaum Associates.

Holland, A.L. (1980). *Communicative Abilities in Daily Living*. Austin, TX: ProEd.

Holland, A.L., & Beeson, P.M. (1998). Aphasia groups: The Arizona experience. In R. Elman (Ed.), *Group Treatment of Neurogenic Communication Disorders: The Expert Clinician's Approach*. Boston: Butterworth-Heinemann.

Holland, A.L., & Forbes, M. (Eds.). (1993). *Aphasia treatment: World Perspectives*. San Diego, CA: Singular.

Jenkins, J.J., Pabon-Jimenez, E., Shaw, R.E., & Williams Sefer, J. (1975). *Schuell's Aphasia in Adults: Diagnosis, Prognosis and Treatment* (2nd ed.). Hagerstown, MD: Harper & Row.

Kearns, K.P. (1994). Group therapy for aphasia: Theoretical and practical implications. In R. Chapey (Ed.), *Language Intervention Strategies in Adult Aphasia* (3rd ed, pp. 304–318). Baltimore: Williams & Wilkins.

Kertesz, A. (1982). *Western Aphasia Battery*. New York: Grune & Stratton.

Kirshner, H.S. (1995). Alexias. In H. S. Kirshner (Ed.), *Handbook of Neurological Speech and Language Disorders* (pp. 277–293). New York: Marcel Dekker.

Klein, K. (Ed.) (1995). *Aphasia Community Group Manual*. New York: National Aphasia Association.

Kokmen, E., Chandra, V., & Shoenberg, B. S. (1988). Trends in incidence of dementing illness in Rochester, Minnesota, in three quinquennial periods, 1960–1974. *Neurology, 38*: 975–980.

Lubinski, R. (1991). (Ed.) *Dementia and Communication*. Philadelphia, PA: B. C. Decker.

Marshall, R. (1993). Problem focused group therapy for mildly aphasic clients. *American Journal of Speech-Language Pathology, 2*: 31–37.

Mattis, S. (1976). Mental status examination for organic mental syndrome in the elderly patient. In L. Bellak & T.B. Karasu (Eds.), *Geriatric Psychiatry* (pp. 77–121). New York: Grune & Stratton.

McKhann, G., Drachman, D., Folstein, M., Katzman, R., Price, D., & Stadlan, E. M. (1984). Clinical diagnosis of Alzheimer's disease. *Neurology, 34*: 939–944.

Moyer, S.B. (1979). Rehabilitation of alexia: A case study. *Cortex, 15*: 139–144.

Murray, L.L., Holland, A.L., & Beeson, P.M. (1997). Accuracy monitoring and task demand evaluation in aphasia. *Aphasiology, 11*: 401–414.

Myers, P.S. (1997). Right hemisphere syndrome. In L.L. LaPointe (Ed.), *Aphasia and Related Neurogenic Language Disorders* (2nd ed., pp. 210–225). New York: Thieme.

Nickels, L. (1992). The autocue? Self-generated phonemic cues in the treatment of a disorder of reading and naming. *Cognitive Neuropsychology, 9*: 155–182.

Pimental, P.A., & Kinsbury, N.A. (1989). *Mini-Inventory of Right Brain Injury*. Austin, TX: Pro-Ed.

Reisberg, B., Ferris, S.H., de Leon, M.J., & Crook, T. (1982). The global deterioration scale for assessment of primary degenerative dementia. *American Journal of Psychiatry, 139*: 1136–1139.

Rosenbek, J.C., LaPointe, L.L., & Wertz, R.T. (1989). *Aphasia: A Clinical Approach*. Austin, TX: Pro-Ed.

Sohlberg, M.M., & Mateer, C.A. (1990). *Attention Process Training*. Austin, TX: The Psychological Corporation.

Springer, L. (1991). Facilitating group rehabilitation. *Aphasiology, 6*: 563–565.

Tomkins, C. A. (1995). *Right Hemisphere Communication Disorders: Theory and Management*. San Diego, CA: Singular Publishing Group.

Wertz, R.T., Collins, M.J., Weiss, D., Kurtzke, J.F., Friden, T., Brookshire, R.H., Pierce, J., Holzapple, P., Hubbard, D.J., Proch, B.E., West, H.A., Davis, L., Matlvitch, V., Morley, G.K., & Resurreccion, E. (1981). Veteran's Administration cooperative study on aphasia: A comparison of individual and group treatment. *Journal of Speech and Hearing Research, 24*: 580–594.

Chapter 9

Disorders of Articulation

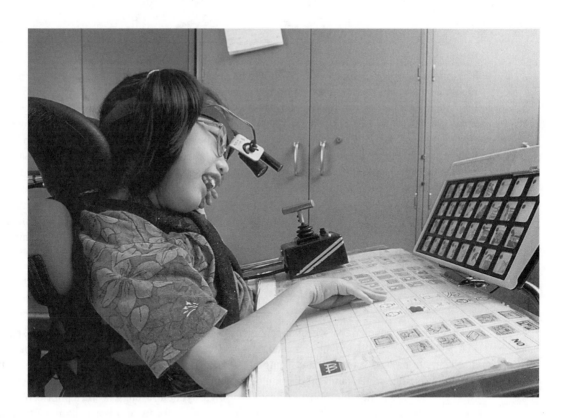

Preview

Disorders of articulation affect both children and adults. Sound errors may range from a mild lisp to nearly unintelligible speech that results from many sound substitutions, omissions, and distortions. Childhood articulation problems may be caused by structural abnormalities such as a cleft palate, but are more frequently related to faulty phonological processes. Some adults show the residual signs of a childhood articulation disorder. In others, articulation disorders result from damage to the central nervous system. Brain damage may produce the slurred or labored speech of dysarthria, the unpredictable articulation errors of apraxia, or even the complete loss of speech in cases of mutism. In evaluating the wide range of articulation disorders, the speech-language pathologist must recognize the factors that cause and maintain the disorder. Intervention typically includes behavioral therapy, alone or in combination with medical management.

The emergence of spoken words is one of the most important milestones in a toddler's life. We commonly hear from excited parents who report hearing the word "papa" or "mama" in the babblings of their child well before the child is using theses sounds as true words. As long as the baby's word attempt contains sufficient phonemes to be recognized, the listener accepts it as the target word. In the first three years of life, parental concern focuses on the emergence of new words, new combinations of words, and communication, rather than on the precision of articulation. If the young child's speech can be understood, there is usually little concern about articulation. During the preschool years, children's articulation improves and approximates adult sound production. However, some children persist in using immature patterns of speech, often interfering with their ability to make themselves understood. In the case of acquired articulation disorders, an adult may begin to make speech errors following an illness or injury. Persistent articulation errors in either adults or children may warrant concern.

Types of Articulation Errors

In Chapter 2, we studied the speech mechanisms required for the production of normal speech; and in Chapter 3, we considered the consonants, vowels, and diphthongs of English speech patterns. We also learned that spoken words are strung together in connected speech. We say these sounds very rapidly. It is often in the rapid production of sounds required for normal speech that articulatory errors become most noticeable. Whether heard in a single syllable, a single word, a phrase, or sentences, such errors are known as **misarticulations**. There are four forms of misarticulations: **omission errors** (*fi'* for *fish*), **substitution errors** (*fith* for *fish*), **distortion errors** (a lisped sh in *fish*), and **addition errors** (*fisha* for *fish*). The reader will note that throughout this chapter, the phonemic designation of an utterance uses the // markers, whereas phonetic transcriptions that reflects actual the actual speech production uses the [ ] (Grunwell, 1981).

Omissions

When speakers omit sounds from words, their speech is difficult to understand. Consider the following exchange between a 28-month-old boy and his father:

Dad: Look at all that stuff!

Child: I bri a boo. A bir boo.   (I bring a book. A bird book)

Dad: (Looks at book.) Is it a bird book?

Child: I ge thi un, you ge tha un.   (I get this one, you get that one.)

Dad: Oh. Ok, I get this book about shells.

Child: I a pi un.   (It's a pink one.)

Dad: It's a pretty pink shell.

As we can see, it is difficult to tell what this child is saying from his words alone. If not for the father, who provides a running translation, we might not know what this child was actually saying.

Although omissions may occur anywhere within a word, they are more often observed in the final position. A particular sound or a whole class of sounds may be omitted. Occasionally, a young child will leave all endings off words. Shriberg (1980) noted that the omission of consonants, known as a syllable-simplification process, is a natural part of phonological development. In some children, simplification processes can lead to the omission of an entire syllable, which is what occurs when the young child says *nana* for *banana* or *amblance* for *ambulance*. In each case an unstressed syllable has been omitted from the word. These omissions of either sounds or syllables occur frequently in the speech of toddlers and become less common as the child grows. However, when a 4-year-old child persists in making sound omissions, or an adult begins to produce them after years of normal speech, these omissions signal an articulation disorder.

Substitutions

Along with omissions, substitutions are a common articulation error in young children. Preschool children often substitute one phoneme for the target phoneme, with a certain logic or predictability. In many cases, the incorrect sound is similar to the target sound in terms of the place and manner of articulation and voicing characteristics of the sound (see also Chapter 3). For example, the child who says, *I tee the wabbit* has used two common substitutions heard in the speech of young children with articulatory errors of substitution. Like the /s/ in *see*, the substituted /t/ is a voiceless sound that is made near the same spot in the front of the mouth; the /w/ has many production similarities to the target sound /r/ that it replaces. In other cases, the incorrect sound shares similarities with other sounds within the word. For example, when a child says *bate* for *bake*, the /t/ replaces /k/ because /t/ is produced forward in the mouth, closer to where /b/ is produced. This is a case of progressive, or forward, assimilation, because a sound at the beginning of the word (the /b/ in *bake*) influenced the production of a later sound, the /t/ for /k/ in this case. Regressive, or backward, assimilation occurs when sounds following the target phoneme influence its pronunciation as when a child says *guck* for *duck*.

Until children acquire a particular sound of the adult phonemic system, they often replace it with a sound they have some success in making. Many of the substituted sounds are ones that are acquired by children at earlier ages than the target sound. For example, if 4-year-olds cannot say an /s/, they might well substitute a sound that they can say, such as /t/. Substitution is perhaps the most common articulatory error in the child who demonstrates a general developmental phonological disorder.

Distortions

As we saw in Chapter 3, the production of a sound must be relatively close to the target to be perceived by listeners as correct. Slight variations of a sound that still sound like the target sound are acceptable allophones, but marked variation in sound production is classified as a distortion. In a distortion error, the target sound is produced with some change of the sound, although not enough to be classified as a substitution or an addition. One of the most common distortions and among the easiest to identify is the lateral lisp, in which the target /s/ or /z/ phonemes sound slushy (the /s/ or /z/ sounds as if it has an unvoiced /l/ as part of its production).

To record distortion errors correctly, the International Phonetic Alphabet includes a number of **diacritics** (modified phonetic symbols) used to describe the distorted error (Shriberg, 1980). For example, the mark for a lateralized lisp is [^]; so the word *sun* said with such a lisp would be transcribed as [ŝʌn]. A retroflex error, marked as [ͅ], would note the production of a sound when the tongue is curled back too far toward the pharynx; in this case, the word *sun* is heard as [ʂʌn]. Distortion errors can be seen in both children and adults who have disorders of articulation.

Additions

A fourth type of articulatory error involves an addition of a sound. We might hear an individual with an addition error saying *boata*, phonetically transcribed as [botə]. In other cases, an extra vowel may be inserted between the two consonants of a consonant blend (e.g., *galass* for *glass*). As in these examples, the addition error is often an unstressed /ə/. Unlike other types of articulation errors, addition errors are not typically seen as a part of normal development. They can occur when an individual adds a voicing dimension to a word or is unable to stop the flow of air (voiced or voiceless) at the end of it. Occasionally, an individual with a disorder such as cerebral palsy or other physical disability affecting motor control will make voicing additions.

Articulation Disorders in Children

It is often difficult to isolate a specific cause of articulation problems in children. The great majority of young children who have difficulties pronouncing words basically do not differ emotionally, mentally, or physically from their age-peers. In most cases of developmental articulation disorders, children's success in communicating is limited by their ability to make themselves understood. Their pattern of articulation errors may make them sound younger than they are. This type of articulation disorder would be classified as a developmental phonological disorder, probably related to central nervous system factors that are yet unknown. Disorders of speech articulation affect 10 to15% of all preschool children. About 6% of school age children have a speech disorder (Office of Scientific and Health Reports, 1988).

Phonological Disorders

Some children's poor articulation skills are not readily attributable to structural abnormalities. Parents become concerned when their child's speech seems to lag behind their playmates. For some children, speech articulation errors are limited to just a few sounds. In other cases, articulation errors are so numerous that the young child's speech is nearly impossible to understand.

When a child is referred for an articulation disorder, a speech-language pathologist will attempt to characterize the child's sound errors. Some children will mispronounce only a few sounds, such as /r/, /l/, or /s/. Since children tend to master these sounds relatively late (4 years old or older), the speech-language pathologist may recommend a "wait and watch" approach. Intervention may be limited or deferred while the child is given a chance to self-correct articulation through normal maturation. For school-age children, even a few sounds produced in error is unusual. A 10-year-old boy's lisped /s/ rarely interferes with his ability to communicate his ideas. It can, however, negatively affect the way other children view him (Hall, 1990). Such children are typically candidates for therapy and are often quite motivated to correct their speech.

For many children, the problem is not limited to a few consistently misarticulated sounds. More often, the speech-language pathologist finds errors on many of the consonant sounds. These errors may at first glance seem inconsistent. Certain consonants may be correctly produced in a few words, whereas in others they are omitted, distorted, or replaced with another consonant. A careful examination of these speech-sound errors almost always reveals a pattern. For example, when a child says *Tuta too my tir* for *Susan took my shirt*, the errors might be classified in the two ways shown in Table 9-1. Substitution errors are shown by writing the error sound followed by a slash (/) and the target sound. Omitted sounds are noted by an aminus (-) sign.

When the sound errors are listed individually in Table 9-1, we notice that the child is inconsistent in the use of the /t/ sound. The child uses it correctly when attempting the word *took* but substitutes it for each /s/ in *Susan* and /ʃ/ in *shirt* and omits it altogether at the end of *shirt*. This use would be puzzling if we concentrated only on the individual sound errors. However, all these errors, plus those not involving /t/, can be accounted for by two general patterns, or **phonological processes**. The substitutions of /t/ for /s/ and /ʃ/ are all examples of a process called stopping, in which a stop

TABLE 9-1 Examples of Sound Errors in Children's Speech

	Individual Errors	Phonological Processes
Attempted statement: Susan took my shirt.		
Child's statement: Tuta too my tir.	Initial t/s t/ʃ	Stopping
	Medial t/s	Stopping
	Final -n -k -t	Final consonant deletion

consonant (e.g., /t/, /d/, or /g/) is substituted for a continuant (/s/, /f/, or /v/). All the errors of omission occur on the final consonant, indicating a process of final consonant deletion. Many phonological processes are seen in normally developing children, but persist in children with phonological disorders.

A phonological profile of children who are brought to the attention of a speech-language pathologist can be obtained by examining the features that co-occur with phonological disorders (Ruscello, St. Louis, & Mason, 1991; Shriberg, Kwiatkowski, Best, Hengst, & Terslic-Weber, 1986). About two-thirds of the children referred for services for phonological disorders are boys, the majority of whom have a history of ear infections that may have affected their hearing at some time. Frequently, there are signs of general neuromotor problems. These children may be described as "clumsy," with many of them showing mild signs of muscle weakness and incoordination. Frequently, a developmental language disorder co-occurs with the phonological disorder. Difficulty with language production is more common than problems with language comprehension. Half of the children with phonological problems also have difficulty learning to read. Problems with academics may persist long into the school years, even after speech is no longer an obvious impairment (Shriberg & Kwiatkowski, 1988). Sometimes, a family history of phonological as well as other speech-language disorders can be documented for these children (Lewis, 1990).

The phonological approach to articulation disorders recognizes that the child has some difficulty in mastering the adult phonology of the language. In his or her attempts to use language, the child in effect makes systematic simplifications of the phonology. From this point of view, children with a phonological disorder continue to use a simplification process beyond the time when others their age use them. Because children's errors are systematically related to these phonological processes, articulation therapy concentrates more on eliminating the processes than on treating individual sound errors. Robbie is one such child.

At age 4, Robbie was brought to a university speech-language clinic by his concerned parents. The parents, most other family members (including three older siblings), and neighbors had difficulty understanding him. He was found to have normal hearing, normal cognitive ability, and normal speech mechanisms at the time of the speech evaluation. His articulation errors were abundant. In the initial position of a word, he could correctly say m, p, b, t, d, n, and he correctly said m, p, b in the medial position. He produced no final consonants correctly. Most of his consonant errors were actually omissions (he left the sounds out completely), although he made a few consonant substitutions (substituting another sound for a target sound): t/k, d/g, t/f, b/v, t/θ. Of the twenty-five English consonants, he said only six of them correctly; most of his vowel sounds were produced correctly. His overall attempts at conversation were restricted to two- or three-word utterances, many of which were not intelligible. He appeared to limit his mean length of response to two or three words as a conscious gesture to accommodate his listeners; he apparently had learned that if he said more than that, no one would understand him.

Because Robbie could say six consonants correctly in the initial position, a phonological approach to his problem focused on making him aware that many words had consonant endings that he could say. At the start of therapy, the stop consonants that he could produce correctly (/p/, /b/, /t/, /d/) were presented at the beginning and the end of a word. The phonological approach was to teach him the place in a word to say the sound. In therapy, he was soon able to produce most of the six target sounds (the ones he could say at the evaluation) at both the beginning and the end of a word, such as *pop, top, mop, Bob, tub, mom, Pam* (his sister), and so forth. Saying two words in a rapid series, in which the last consonant of the first word and the first consonant of the second word were the same, such as *mom-mop*, seemed to facilitate the production of the omitted consonant in the medial position. Later therapy sessions included working on phonetic sounds that Robbie should have been making correctly; not only was production practiced in therapy, but also some phonological instruction was included, providing him with the rules for applying his newly acquired sounds.

Probably the majority of young children with developmental articulation problems can profit from a phonological-process approach in therapy. Some children show isolated, residual errors, even after the more general processes have been corrected. These children seem to know the phonological rules of production but may have learned a faulty muscular pattern for producing a particular sound. They may require additional therapy with a focus on the individual sound in error.

Anomalies of the Oral and Facial Structures

Various acquired or genetic abnormalities of the facial skeleton can cause severe articulation problems. Many of these facial abnormalities are part of a broader pattern of anomalies that are known collectively as a **syndrome**; that is, a certain number of predictable features (e.g. skeletal anomolies, distinctive facial features, motor involvement, cognitive difference) co-occur. For example, a child may be classified as having the Berry-Treacher Collins syndrome, characterized by a lack of mandible-facial growth, a downward slanting of the eyes, a notching of the lower eyelid, and microtia (a lack of external ear development). This syndrome in genetic in origin and may often be observed in several members of the same family. Extensive and repeated plastic surgery is usually successful in minimizing the oral-facial abnormalities that characterize Berry-Treacher Collins syndrome. A syndrome is usually named after the physician(s) or other professional who first described the group of signs that co-occurred in their patients. Other syndromes, such as fetal alchohol syndrome, are named for the factors that cause the condition. Besides oral-facial abnormalities, problems in communication may be part of the symptom complex that includes hearing loss, language delay, mental retardation, or problems in speech articulation.

Sometimes we see children in speech-language clinics who were born with facial or tongue muscles that lack neural innervation. One girl, age 8, was unable to smile because the necessary facial muscles had no innervation; by extensive neuro- and plastic surgery, some of the nerve fibers used in opening the jaw were transplanted to innervate the muscle fibers used in smiling. The operation was successful, giving her a smile and enough functional control of her lips to improve her faulty articulation.

Occasionally, tongue problems may contribute to articulation difficulty. Another structural problem of the tongue is that it may appear to be too large (macroglossia) or too small (microglossia). Macroglossia, seen with certain developmental syndromes, has been thought to contribute to poor articulation. At one time, tongue reduction surgery was recommended for these children, but follow-up studies have failed to document improved articulation (Lynch, 1990). Sometimes the tongue appears to be too large because it is riding forward in the mouth and protruding, possibly because of abnormalities in the back of the oral cavity, such as enlarged tonsils. In other cases, a forward tongue carriage may be the result of low oral muscle tone and inadequate neural innervation of the tongue muscles. These types of problems will be discussed as part of the physiological problems observed in dysarthria later in this chapter.

A tight lingual frenulum is another feature of the tongue that has been blamed for articulation problems. The lingual frenulum is the small band of tissue on the base of the tongue's underside. When it is too tight, forward and upward movement of the tongue tip is restricted. In rare cases, this could interfere with the production of sounds, like /l/, for which the tongue tip must be elevated. This condition is sometimes called tongue tied. When protruded, the tongue will often appear to be heart-shaped, indented at the tip. Most "tongue tied" children, however, experience no difficulty with articulation. In the rare case when this condition interferes with speech articulation, some parents may elect to have the lingual frenulum clipped by a surgeon. However, this practice is declining because the necessity of surgical intervention in these cases is open to question.

Dental abnormalities have also been blamed for articulation problems. Shelton and colleagues (Shelton, Furr, Johnson, & Arndt, 1975) looked closely at the influence of various dental abnormalities on improvement in articulation therapy, concluding that even children with severe malocclusion could learn to articulate normally. Severe malocclusions, as seen in underbite or overbite, may or may not have an effect on articulation. Sometimes the orthodontic correction of malocclusion, the wearing of braces or bands, will interfere with tongue precision, creating a possible articulation problem. Such problems are temporary, and the child usually learns to adjust speech movements to accommodate the orthodontia.

Tongue Thrust

Several generations of Americans have been evaluated and treated for **tongue thrust** as part of an orthodontic management program. Children with tongue thrust use an unusual sequence of oral movements when swallowing. The tongue pushes forward against the anterior teeth (particularly the upper incisors). This forward tongue movement while swallowing has led some to refer to tongue thrust as reverse swallowing. The forward tongue movement is accompanied by high tension in the muscles controlling lip movement, which is needed to prevent the tongue from protruding as it pushes forward during swallowing. This abnormal and inefficient pattern of swallowing tends to make children with tongue thrust messy eaters. In addition, the frequent forward pressure of the tongue forces the teeth out of alignment. For this reason, many orthodontists are reluctant to fit a child with braces until the tongue thrust habit has been overcome. This problem frequently requires direct intervention with special procedures know as **myofunctional therapy**, the development of optimal intraoral tongue postures (Barrett & Hanson, 1978).

Some children with identified tongue thrust also have an associated articulation disorder, most commonly heard by others as a lisp because the anterior sibilants (particularly /s/ and /z/) are mispronounced. Speech-language pathologists who have been trained in myofunctional therapy techniques may choose to treat the articulation disorder and tongue thrust simultaneously. When there is tongue thrust but no articulation disorder, the speech-language pathologist may elect to administer myofunctional therapy to correct abnormal tongue and lip postures and movements (ASHA, 1991).

Cleft Lip and Palate

Many oral-facial abnormalities contribute to problems in the physical production of sounds. **Cleft lip and cleft palate** are oral-facial malformations that typically have severe impact on developing normal articulatory skills. Cleft lip and palate result when facial tissues do not fuse normally during fetal development. McWilliams, Morris, and Shelton (1990) wrote concerning the **incidence** of cleft palate, "A safe, conservative estimate appears to be approximately one in every 750 live births" (p. 11). Of these children, about 25% have unilateral or bilateral clefts of the lip only; about 50% have unilateral or bilateral clefts of both the lip and the palate; the remaining 25% have clefts of only the palate (Fogh-Anderson, 1942). In summarizing clinical demographic data over time, the 1942 Fogh-Andersen data seem to hold up well.

Clefts of the lip may appear on either side of the "cupid's bow" of the upper lip. The malformation may involve as little as a notch along the upper lip to an opening that extends to the nostril on the side of the cleft. Clefts of the lip may be unilateral or bilateral. Clefts within the oral cavity appear along the suture lines that join the bones within the roof of the mouth. Two of these suture lines run between the incisors on either side of the maxilla and converge toward the front and center of the hard palate, behind the alveolar ridge. Clefting along these lines may be unilateral or bilateral and often is accompanied by a cleft lip. Bilateral clefts, as seen in Figure 9-1, can isolate the

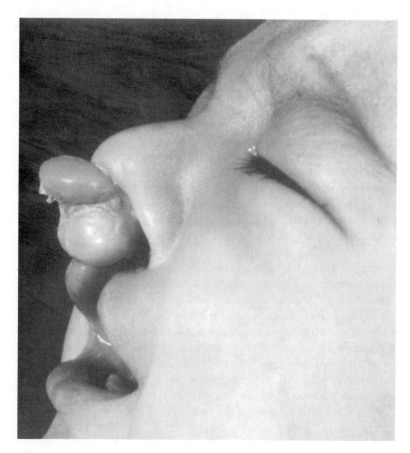

FIGURE 9-1   A newborn with a bilateral lip and palatal cleft with upper lip and premaxilla attached to the nose. Surgery will be initiated within the first few weeks of life to begin to repair the defect. (Courtesy of The University of Arizona Medical Center)

premaxilla so that it hangs outside the mouth at the base of the nose. Beyond the point where the two bone sutures converge on the hard palate, a single suture line continues on to the end of the hard palate. Clefts can also appear along this midline suture. Clefting can also occur along the soft palate, behind the hard palate. These clefts also run along the midline and may be narrow or wide.

Most cleft lips can be well repaired today through plastic surgery. It is rare for a cleft lip to have a lasting, permanent effect on articulation. Rather, the high success rate of plastic surgery ensures that the baby born with a unilateral or bilateral cleft lip will eventually develop a functional lip, a more normal appearance, good mobility, and be quite capable of normal articulatory function. The successful management of cleft palate usually requires the combined efforts of a cranial-facial team, which may include a plastic surgeon, otolaryngologist, orthodontist, prosthodontist, audiologist, speech-language pathologist, psychologist, and social worker (see Chapter 12 for an example of one such team). In most major population areas, these specialists meet regularly as a team to discuss and plan the overall management strategies required for a particular child with these lip or palate malformations. The team works closely with both the child and the family, planning the sequence of treatment. In the case of the cleft lip, focus is given to both cosmetic improvement and adequacy of function. Family counseling can begin the day the child with a cleft lip and palate is born. It is important to establish early that with the right surgery, dental management, speech and voice training, the child's problems will become less apparent. A more normal appearance and normal function are typically realistic goals. In many cases, a series of surgeries are required to fully repair a cleft palate. The initial surgery may be followed by the fitting of a prosthodontic appliance, or *obturator*. An obturator is a bulb that fits into the unrepaired portion of the cleft. It is attached to a dental appliance that resembles a retainer that might be worn after completing orthodontia.

A child with a cleft palate, even when the cleft has been surgically closed, may still experience difficulty with velopharyngeal closure. *Velopharyngeal insufficiency* occurs when complete oral and nasal cavity separation is not possible. The opening between the cavities permits airflow to escape through the nose and contributes to excessive nasal resonance. This can contribute to distortion of high intraoral consonants, such as stops, fricatives, and affricates. In some cases, the range of consonants that a child uses may be restricted as the child substitutes one class of sounds (e.g., stop consonants) for another set that is difficult for the child with an open cleft to produce (e.g., fricatives) (Harding & Grunwell, 1996). Velopharyngeal insufficiency also contributes to feeding and swallowing problems, allowing liquids and soft foods to escape into the nasal cavities. The physical correction (surgical-prosthodontic) of velopharyngeal insufficiency is the primary management focus. Sometimes, after soft-palate surgery or in some children with short palates, we see inadequate velopharyngeal closure because of too large a gap between the velum and the pharyngeal walls. In sketch A of Figure 9-2, the velopharyngeal gap is closed with an obturator; in sketch B, the velopharyngeal opening has been closed surgically by an inferiorly based pharyngeal flap. Feeding and speech training, including voice therapy designed to reduce hypernasality, will have little effect until the structural inadequacy has been corrected.

The articulation errors of a child with a cleft palate are primarily related to the structural problems and altered control of the oral musculature. A cleft palate, with associated velopharyngeal insufficiency, allows air to escape through the nasal cavity at inappropriate times during speech. When air leaks through the nasal cavity, it lowers the air pressure within the oral cavity, which interferes with the production of voiceless consonants such as /s/, /tʃ/, or /f/. Children with cleft palate can raise intraoral pressure by increasing the rate of airflow (Laine, Warren, Dalston, Hairfield, & Morr, 1988).

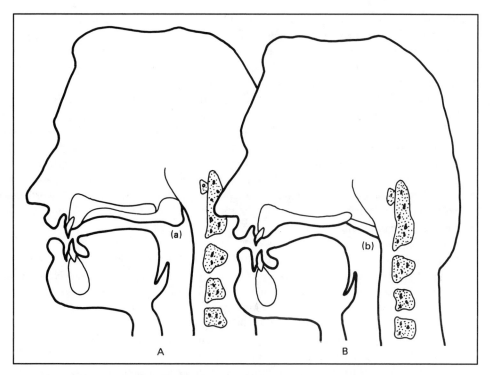

FIGURE 9-2   Two approaches for correcting velopharyngeal inadequacy. In sketch A we see an obturator bulb (a) in place; in sketch B we see an inferiorly based pharyngeal flap (b) from the posterior pharyngeal wall across to the velum.

This action helps build intraoral pressure but also forces more air through the nasal cavity, which leads to problems with hypernasality. The difficulties with sound production may also affect word acquisition in the young child. For example, children learning their first 50 words show preferences for words that begin with nasal sounds and tend to substitute nasals for sounds produced in the center of the oral cavity (Estrem & Broen, 1989). The speech-language pathologist can evaluate velopharyngeal function and determine whether it is adequate for normal speech. It may be that surgery or prosthetics can provide the opportunity for normal function, but the child must learn to use this capability during speech. The speech-language pathologist may help the child learn to produce sounds in ways that minimize or eliminate distortions or hypernasality.

Developmental Dysarthria and Apraxia

Although structurally based and phonological articulation disorders account for the majority of cases in children, a few children exhibit signs of speech disorders typically associated with brain damage in adults. These are children with signs of developmental dysarthria or apraxia of speech. Children identified as having developmental dysarthria typically have abnormal muscle tone in facial muscles, which may be worse on one side than the other. Low muscle tone may result in a soft, somewhat drooping facial expression. Muscle tone that is abnormally high may produce a taut appearance or contribute to facial distortions and grimaces. Some children may have trouble with drooling or eating. Children with dysarthria have difficulty producing rapid speech or nonspeech movements. Affected children typically are late in acquiring their first words. As they grow older, their speech often remains very difficult to understand. Dysarthria may be associated with conditions such as cerebral palsy (see below), but may also occur in the absence of a more pervasive disability.

Children with developmental apraxia of speech are somewhat more difficult to identify. Often, they lack the more apparent motor signs that characterize developmental dysarthria. Apraxia has been defined as an impairment in the ability "to program, combine, and sequence the elements of speech" (Jaffee, 1984, p. 166). A child with a pure apraxia of speech would demonstrate relatively normal comprehension of language but be unable to imitate a simple spoken word, despite having no muscular weakness or paralysis. A case presentation of a 6-year-old girl with apraxia of speech illustrates the problem:

> Esme was a friendly and enthusiastic 6-year-old who was enrolled in a public school kindergarten. From her first day, it was apparent that her speech skills were well below average. Esme was nearly impossible to understand. Her kindergarten teacher was also concerned about Esme's language skills. The kindergarten program was largely built around language arts, and Esme had difficulty participating in many of the classroom activities. The kindergarten teacher asked the school's speech-language pathologist to observe Esme in the classroom. The speech-language pathologist noted that Esme was rarely understood by her teacher or classmates and often showed signs of frustration and distress while trying to communicate. Immediate intervention was needed.
>
> The speech-language pathologist contacted Esme's mother to obtain permission to see Esme for a formal evaluation and for therapy. Esme's mother confided that her child had been evaluated once before. At the age of 2, Esme had been seen at the county's developmental disabilities center because she had not yet started to speak. At that time, based on her poor motor and speech development, she was diagnosed as mentally retarded. Her mother was so distressed at this diagnosis that she refused all preschool services and refused to release the records of that diagnosis to anyone. She was sure her child was bright and was afraid Esme would be stigmatized and held back by a diagnosis of retardation. Instead, the mother kept Esme at home and spent a great deal of time taking her on field trips and engaging in other creative activities with her. The mother waited until Esme was 6 to enroll her in kindergarten, hoping that the extra year would give her a developmental advantage to compensate for her poor communication. Although her mother remained wary of therapists and special education professionals, she agreed after some discussion to allow the speech-language pathologist to see the child again.
>
> Esme's formal evaluation revealed that she rarely pronounced any words correctly, even when speaking only single words. She often made sound errors on the initial sounds in words and omitted the ending altogether. Her sentences tended to be short, with an average of three words per sentence. A battery of language tests indicated that her receptive language skills were slightly above average and her expressive language skills were poor.

During subsequent therapy sessions, Esme made slow and inconsistent progress. The speech-language pathologist began noticing signs suggesting that Esme may have had more than the typical phonological disorder. She sometimes showed facial tension while speaking. Once, when trying to imitate the speech-language pathologist, she used her fingers to move her tongue in position to say a [d] sound. Sometimes she would reach for a card and grab the wrong one while telling herself "no!" These behaviors suggested problems with sequencing and executing movement. The speech-language pathologist made a diagnosis of developmental apraxia of speech. Esme's mother was convinced, after much counseling, to take the child back to the developmental disabilities center so that she could be evaluated by a physical therapist. The physical therapist confirmed that Esme had a mild limb apraxia in addition to apraxia of speech. With this information, the mother, school staff, and therapists met to discuss how classroom materials and procedures could be modified to minimize the effects of Esme's apraxia. The speech-language pathologist provided a teacher inservice on the expected impact that Esme's apraxia would have on her academic progress, including writing, test taking, and oral skills.

Apraxia of speech is more of a phonetic problem than an overall language problem; however, apraxia creates a marked discrepancy between receptive language and the ability to express language through speech. Often the affected children are forced to struggle at the single-word level. Even when they can produce multiword sentences, their speech lacks the normal prosody. Preschool children with apraxia require intensive individual therapy as well as language-based intervention in which efforts are made to encourage the development of a variety of communication skills.

Cerebral Palsy

Some children who display motor impairment early in their lives, often from the time of birth, have **cerebral palsy**. This is not a disease per se but rather a term used to label a number of motor-sensory conditions that result from damage to or imperfect development of the central nervous system. According to McDonald and Chance (1964), about three in every 1000 newborns could be classified as having cerebral palsy. This neurological impairment may occur before birth, during birth, or during the first three years of life. Therefore, there is often motor delay in many aspects of the child's life: crawling, sitting, standing, walking, chewing-swallowing, self-feeding, and talking. The finer the required motor skill, such as talking, the more likely the child will have a problem. In cerebral palsy, the motor deficits may be grossly divided into four types:

Spasticity. **Spasticity** is characterized by simultaneous contraction of both primary and antagonistic muscles, producing severe tightness and hypertonicity. Speech prosody is often interrupted by respiratory and voice breaks. Articulation is often severely defective.

Athetosis. **Athetosis is** characterized by a series of involuntary contractions, with flailing of extremities and much facial grimacing. There is marked variability in hypertonicity. Lack of respiratory control causes a monotonic voice, often lacking sufficient loudness. There are many phonemic distortions.

Mixed. This type of cerebral palsy represents a mixture of both tight spasticity and flailing athetosis, sometimes called tension athetoid.

Ataxia. **Ataxia** is characterized by a lack of balance, with severe problems in coordination of movements. Motor behavior is hypotonic. Ataxic speech sounds like the slurred, arhythmical speech of someone inebriated.

The motor speech problems of the cerebral-palsied child can be classified as a type of dysarthric speech. Dysarthria also occurs in adults who suffer brain damage and is discussed in greater detail below. Cerebral palsy implies a motor disorder of speech that is developmental in nature. If the condition is severe, the affected child enjoys few normal developmental experiences, and a marked delay in speech. The treatment of the dysarthria for the cerebral-palsied child, therefore, may be quite different from that of one who acquires dysarthria after normal speech patterns have been established.

Often the cerebral-palsied child is so physically active with muscle contractions or unstable head and trunk posture that speaking appears almost impossible. Therefore, the child must first develop some postural control and some control of extraneous movements before work can begin on the fine motor control required for speech (Mysak,1980). For example, learning to sit erect (with or without support) and keeping the mouth in a controlled, closed position are often prerequisite behaviors for attempting speech (Boone, 1972). The speech-language pathologist working with the cerebral-palsied child coordinates the speech-language program closely with other treatment specialists, such as the orthopedic surgeon, the physiatrist (a physician specializing in physical or restorative medicine), the physical therapist, the occupational therapist, and the special educator.

Articulation therapy is often coordinated with feeding training. Speaking ability and chewing and swallowing competence are often related to control of aberrant oral reflexes (Love, Hagerman, & Taimi 1980). For example, helping the child develop enough control of the mouth to open and shut it with volition would be a most helpful motor skill to establish before working on speech sounds per se. Once gross motor control has been developed, the mildly to moderately involved child may profit from articulation therapy that uses many of the traditional therapy approaches. For some severely involved cerebral-palsied children, articulate speech is not a realistic goal; for these children, some form of nonvocal communication system must be introduced. A manually or electronically operated communication board has been found to be an effective alternate communication system. The child has several items (e.g., pictures, objects, symbols) mounted on a board and selects the appropriate one by indicating with a hand, a foot, or perhaps a head-stick or headlight mounted on a helmet, or by eye gaze. With the improvement of electronic assistive devices, it is possible to activate stimulus selection by electronic switches attached to the chest, arm or leg. Eye movements have been used to activate stimulus panels on some electronic boards (Broen, 1981; Coleman, Look, & Myers, 1980). Thanks to modern technology, there are assistive communication devices available to meet the basic communication needs of the most severely handicapped cerebral-palsied child.

Hearing Loss

We learned in Chapters 2 and 5 the importance of the hearing mechanism in the development of normal communication. Human communication is primarily an oral-aural interaction. A conductive or sensorineural hearing loss can seriously impair the aural reception of language. Some young children with articulation delay have had a series of middle-ear infections, each of which caused a temporary hearing loss. As discussed in Chapter 5, hearing loss is a frequent cause of a developmental communication problem (articulation and language). Some children simply cannot hear certain phonemes. When children lack the ability to hear spoken sounds, it is difficult for them to learn to produce them. Common causes of hearing loss and its effect on speech sound development are described at length in Chapter 5.

Evaluation of Childhood Articulation Disorders

Articulation Screening

Most articulation screening programs are used in the public schools, particularly in kindergarten and the first few elementary grades. Such programs are typically set up in the fall, and all new children in the particular school district (kindergarten and other grades) meet with the speech-language pathologist for a brief screening. The screening might focus on naturalistic dialogues with the children to observe their articulation and their overall language function, voice quality, and speech fluency. Unfortunately, many young children are reticent about talking to a "stranger," making a natural conversation impossible. Therefore, it is usually necessary to structure the screening so that a maximum amount of information can be obtained from a relatively brief speech sample.

It should be noted that certain speech sounds are stressed in the screening program—usually those that young children typically mispronounce throughout the early years. Perhaps the most common articulation errors identified during screening programs are distortions and substitutions for /s/ and /z/ and the common w/l and w/r substitutions. The focus of the screening program is to identify the children who misarticulate, not to identify the reason for the problem or study the possible phonological-simplification processes involved. Ideally, the screening test should identify those children who will outgrow their problem with maturation and those with articulation problems who need remediation. Unfortunately, speech-language pathologists in the schools sometimes find that identifying children who "need" therapy does not necessarily satisfy the parents who want their 5-year-olds who make an /r/ substitution to begin therapy, whether the screening test indicates a need or not. More and more often, screening programs are heavily supplemented by teacher and parent referrals to the speech-language pathologist for a full speech evaluation.

Articulation Evaluation

Articulatory precision in the production of the phonemes of a language naturally facilitates communication. Formal articulation evaluation may begin by engaging the child (or adult) in a real conversation. The conversation may be between the client and other children, between parent and child, or between clinician and child. This may involve discrete observation of a school-aged child at home, on the playground, or in the classroom. Other children may be seen in a clinic testing suite (which often looks like playrooms for young children) that have observation mirrors permitting the clinician to observe the child in as natural a communication setting as possible. A conversation during spontaneous play will often reveal how the child actually talks outside of the testing situation. With an older child, an actual conversation about topics of interest will reveal the communicative ability, offering information about articulation proficiency as well as about voice, language, and fluency.

The experienced and well-trained speech-language pathologist is able to observe the child's productions systematically and make a useful summary statement based on the observations relevant to the articulatory adequacy, specifying type and number of errors, place of error, and so forth. It is possible, however, that observation of play and conversation will not reveal all of the client's articulatory errors, nor will conversation alone provide the diagnostic information that a more structured evaluation will include. Therefore, the evaluation is likely to include conversational speech and more formal testing.

Audiometric Testing

Audiometric testing, at least as a screening measure, should be part of every articulation evaluation. As we saw in Chapters 5 and 6, various levels of hearing loss can have devastating effects on phonology. The child's ability to perceive the sounds of words is an important part of the evaluation. Therefore, an audiometric testing may include evaluation of speech sound reception and discrimination levels.

Oral Peripheral Evaluation

A oral peripheral evaluation provides the speech-language pathologist with information relative to the adequacy of oral structure and function. As discussed earlier in this chapter, sensory losses, structural defects, and faulty movements of the articulators can all contribute to faulty articulatory production. An oral peripheral examination form (see Figure 9-3) lists the clinician's judgments about various structural areas of the vocal tract and how well they may function. The particular form pictured has been completed for an adult man with normal articulation who has a voice problem (Boone, 1982). The slight departures from normal described for this man apparently do not contribute in any way to faulty articulation. His ability to produce rapid alternating movements for speech (oral **diadochokinesis**), like other parts of the peripheral oral examination, was within normal limits.

The advantage to the speech-language pathologist of using a form to summarize the data from the oral examination probably lies in the need to be complete and systematic. The form, in effect, provides a checklist for each part of the oral mechanism in terms of its structural and performance adequacy. For the patient with dysarthria or a major structural defect (such as a cleft palate), a more detailed and supplementary examination would be required.

Articulation Inventory

Many commercially available articulation tests provide the clinician with a ready inventory of speech sounds. Most tests can identify not only the actual sounds produced incorrectly but also the place in the word where the error occurs (initial, medial, or final position) and the type of error (omission, substitution, distortion, or addition). A typical articulation inventory will provide the type of information found in Figure 9-4. This form shows the results of a single-word articulation test given to 5-year-old Katie, who demonstrated a number of speech-sound errors. This form shows how the errors may be described individually as substitutions (e.g., p/f) or omissions (e.g., f) in the initial (I), medial (M), or final (F) position in the word. In the column labeled Phonological Process, errors are ascribed to one of three phonological processes used. *Stimulability* testing and deep testing would follow the formal articulation test to see whether, under the special conditions of those tests, the incorrect sounds could be produced correctly. Both types of testing will be discussed shortly. A phonological-process evaluation (considered later in the chapter) might follow, particularly if stimulability and deep testing were unsuccessful in eliciting correct phonemic productions.

ORAL PERIPHERAL EVALUATION

	Structure	**Function**
Lips	Symmetry *normal* Scarring *none*	Pursing *normal* Smiling *normal* Close lips, puff out cheeks *normal*
Teeth	Alignment *slight overjet* Gap or Missing Teeth *none*	
Tongue	Scarring *none*	Moves side to side *normal* up and down *normal* in and out *normal*
Hard Palate	Vault Height *normal* Vault Width *normal* Scarring *none*	
Soft Palate	Symmetry *normal* Scarring *none*	Lifts on "ah" *normal* Symmetry of movement *normal*

Diadochokinesis:		
Pa (20 repetitions)	*4*	seconds
Ta (20 repetitions)	*5*	seconds
Ka (20 repetitions)	*5*	seconds
PaTaKa (20 repetitions)	*4*	seconds

FIGURE 9-3   An oral peripheral evaluation form.

Phonological Process Analysis

As young children develop beyond their early consonant-vowel productions in an attempt to match adult articulation models, they engage in a process of simplification. As Dunn (1982) wrote, "The term phonological process, however, is frequently used as a way to describe the systematic simplifications observed in child speech" (p. 147). The articulatory productions of young children who make articulation errors are systematic and seem to be the result of the same processes that normal children use (Ingram, 1981). Some common phonological processes are found in Table 9-2. It would appear, however, that children with articulatory errors persist in using simplification processes beyond the time when their age-peers use them (Grunwell, 1980). To test a child's use of phonologic processes, it is important to have a method of identifying the different processes that are used, control for the number of times a process is sampled, and identify the actual number of times that it has occurred. Several such tests are commercially available, particularly for young children who show developmental articulation disorders.

ARTICULATION TEST				
Name: Katie		**Age:** 5.0 years		
SOUND **ITEM**	**I**	**M**	**F**	**PHONOLOGICAL PROCESS**
p pencils, zipper, cup	✓	✓	-/p	Final consonant deletion
m matches, Christmas, drum	✓	✓	-/m	F.C.D.
n knife, Santa, gun	✓	✓	-/n	F.C.D.
w window	✓			
h house	✓			
b rabbit, bathtub	✓	✓	-/b	F.C.D.
g gun, wagon, flag	✓	✓	-/g	F.C.D.
k cup, chicken, duck	✓	✓	-/k	F.C.D.
f fishing, telephone, knife	p/f	p/f	-/f	F.C.D., Stopping
d duck, window, bed	✓	✓	-/d	F.C.D.
ŋ finger, ring		g/ŋ	-/ŋ	F.C.D., Stopping
j yellow	✓			
t telephone, bathtub, carrot	✓	✓	-/t	F.C.D.
ʃ shovel, fishing, brush	t/ʃ	t/ʃ	-/ʃ	F.C.D., Stopping
tʃ church, matches	t/tʃ	t/tʃ	-/tʃ	F.C.D., Stopping
l lamp, yellow, squirrel	w/l	w/l	-/l	F.C.D., Liquid Simplification
r rabbit, carrot, car	w/r	w/r	-/r	F.C.D., Liquid Simplification
dʒ jumping, pajamas, orange	d/dʒ	g/dʒ	-/dʒ	F.C.D., Stopping
θ thumb, bathtub, bath	t/θ	-/θ	-/θ	F.C.D., Stopping
v vacuum, shovel, stove	b/v	b/v	-/v	F.C.D., Stopping
s scissors, pencils, house	d/s	t/s	-/s	F.C.D., Stopping
z zipper, scissors	d/z	d/z	-/z	F.C.D., Stopping
ð this, feather	d/ð	d/ð		Stopping

FIGURE 9-4   Articulation test results for Katie, age 5 years. Items adapted from the *Goldman-Fristoe Test of Articulation* (Goldman & Fristoe, 1986) and the *Khan-Lewis Phonological Analysis* (Khan & Lewis, 1986).

TABLE 9-2   Phonological Processes

EXAMPLES

Natural Phonological Processes	Adult Word	Child Word
Syllable-Simplification Processes		
Deletion of the final consonant	ball	"ba__"
Deletion of the unstressed syllable	away	"__way"
Cluster reduction	stop	"__top"
Assimilation Processes		
Regressive (backward) assimilation	doggie	"goggie"
Progressive (forward) assimilation	television	"televivion"
Substitution Processes		
Stopping—fricatives are replaced by stop-plosives	shoes	"tood"
Fronting—palatal and velar sounds are replaced by alveolar sounds	bake	"bate"

Used with permission of Prentice Hall. From L.D. Shriberg. Developmental phonological disorders, in *Introduction to Communication Disorders*, ed. T. Hixon, L. Shriberg, and J. Saxman (Englewood Cliffs, NJ: Prentice Hall, 1980).

Distinctive Feature Analysis

Each phoneme (consonant and vowel) has one or more **distinctive features**, or production characteristics, that distinguish it from other phonemes. When analyzing articulation errors, the features of the incorrect sound are compared with those of the adult-model sound, in the hope that a particular feature error may be identified and corrected.

Two examples of a feature error are substituting a voiceless production for a voiced production, such as /t/ for /d/ (the voicing feature) and using a /t/ for a /k/ (a placement feature). If one were to make a feature-contrast analysis between two phonemes, it might resemble the one in Table 9-3. A distinctive-feature list has been included and is applied to the consonants /s/ and /t/, which are two

TABLE 9-3   A Distinctive-Feature Analysis Between /s/ and /t/

Feature	/s/	/t/	
High	-	-	
Back	-	-	
Low	-	-	
Anterior	+	+	
Coronal	+	+	
Voice	-	-	
Continuant	+	-	differ
Stop	-	+	differ
Nasal	-	-	
Strident	+	-	differ

sounds often confused by young children (who usually substitute the /t/ for /s/). We see that all phonemes share seven common features (no wonder the simpler /t/ is often used instead of the more complex /s/). The two consonants differ from each other in only three ways. For some clients, distinctive feature analysis identifies commonalities among sound errors that can be targeted for therapy.

Severity Estimation

Sound inventories and the analysis of speech sound errors are important prerequisites to selecting therapy goals. However, these forms of analysis do not always reflect the overall severity of a client's problem. For example, consider the speech of the following two children:

Maria: He go bi tee (he's got big teeth). Bu i no a he (But it's not a he). I a she! (It's a she!)

Joseph: I see a amblance (I see a ambulance). Let me see. I see an elphant (I see an elephant).

Both of these children have one phonological process that describes their speech errors. Maria tends to delete final consonants, and Joseph shows a pattern of weak syllable deletion. Although both children's errors can be described with a single process, Maria is much more difficult to understand than Joseph. This illustrates that knowledge of specific error types does not always provide an accurate insight concerning overall severity. Kent, Miolo, and Bloedel (1994) reviewed the wide variety of available methods for estimating the overall intelligibility of speech. They noted that these measures tend to emphasize different aspects of speech analysis. A clinician may select among measures that emphasize phonetic contrasts, phonological error patterns, whole word identification in isolation or in connected speech, or measures that require listeners to rate how well speech can be understood. Some of these measures were developed with the characteristics of a particular type of articulation problem in mind (e.g., speech associated with hearing impairment, dysarthria, phonological disorders). Therefore, the clinician's decision concerning which measure to select may reflect the type of client he or she needs to evaluate and even the types of speech sound errors the client shows (Kent et al., 1994; Shriberg, Austin, Lewis, McSweeny, & Wilson, 1997).

Stimulability

An important part of the articulation evaluation is to see how well the client can produce incorrect sounds when they are presented by the clinician as repeated auditory, visual, and tactile models. This is known as *stimulability*. For those children who can correct their sound errors when given visual, auditory, or tactile cues, the prognosis for correction is much better than for those who cannot. After the formal articulation test is completed, the speech-language pathologist selects several incorrect sounds to determine if the client is stimulable for that sound.

    Stimulability testing can occur at several levels. The higher the level at which the child is able to produce the sound correctly, the easier it is to correct the production of the sound. At the highest level, the clinician may ask the child to say a mispronounced word over again by prompting, "Can you say that better?" If the child does not self-correct the articulation, the clinician might ask the child to repeat the word after a model is given. If the child's attempt is incorrect, the clinician might draw attention to visual cues to aid articulation by instructing the child to "watch how I say it." If the addition of visual cues is not effective, the clinician might ask the child to produce a misarticulated sound in a consonant-vowel combination, like *la-la-la*. If necessary, visual and tactile cues may be added to help the child. These steps are taken to determine what capacity the child has for producing the sound and how much support and cueing the child needs to do so.

Language Testing

The majority of children with defective articulation appear to have a functional problem that may be classified as a phonological disorder. Locke (1983) wrote an excellent article explaining the treatment of speech-sound disorders, in which he noted, "It seems we need a single, generic term for disorders involving the sounds of a language. Rather than invent a new word, my own practice has been to call them *phonological disorders* since the sounds of a language are properly a part of its phonology" (p. 340). A phonologic problem may be a sign of an overall language difficulty. At the time of the articulation evaluation, the speech-language pathologist should certainly determine the overall adequacy of the child's vocabulary usage and recognition, syntax, and morphology.

Certain phonological processes may interfere with the clinician's ability to assess a child's morphology. For example, processes such as weak-syllable deletion and final-consonant deletion will eliminate many of the bound morphemes in English. Other processes, such as stridency deletion, simulate a more restricted morphological problem by eliminating the plural and possessive /s/. Often, comparing phonological and morphological testing can help distinguish a true difficulty with morphology from the effects of the phonological disorder on the form of spoken language. Because phonological disorders frequently co-occur with other language difficulties, many clinicians routinely include one or more language measures in their assessment.

Older children with isolated articulation defects, such as the persistence of a lateral lisp, are less likely to have an associated language problem. Rather, the child exhibits a phonetic problem related to executing speech movements with the precision required for production of the adult model. Similarly, the adult patient who acquires an articulation problem (perhaps due to dysarthria or even from a loose denture) is unlikely to exhibit an associated language problem.

Articulation Therapy for Children

Let us now consider several approaches to articulation therapy. Speech-language pathologists work with children (and adults) with articulation disorders in many ways. Earlier in the chapter, many possible causes of faulty articulation were reviewed. We could probably find as many advocates of particular approaches to therapy as there are causes of a problem. Causation, which is difficult to identify, can rarely be treated directly as a first step in the management of an articulation problem. That is, if a hearing loss were identified as a possible cause of a developmental articulation problem in a child, correction of that loss (sometimes possible in a conductive loss) will not magically cure the faulty articulation. It may still be necessary to make the child aware of the desired target behavior, work directly to modify the articulation, and develop strategies for generalization of the newly acquired pattern into everyday speech.

The most effective speech-language pathologists working with articulation disorders may be those who are familiar with different approaches and employ the one most appropriate for the individual with the defect. The least effective clinicians, in our opinion, use the same remediation steps for all their clients. The diagnostic evaluation data should provide the information needed to plan individualized treatment. Let us consider briefly what is done in articulation therapy, dividing the topic in two: acquisition training and generalization training.   ·

Acquisition Training

Helping the child or adult acquire target sounds is a common goal of all forms of articulation therapy. Many informal approaches and published programs attempt to accomplish this goal. Therapy programs are typically tailored to meet the individual needs of each client and may incorporate a variety of different techniques. We will examine a few of these techniques here.

A *semantic* approach to articulation therapy emphasizes the changes in meaning that sometimes accompany phonological errors. For example, children who substitute /t/ for /s/ will say *tail* when they mean *sail*. Likewise, children who delete all final consonants will say *toe* and *knee* for *toad* and *need*. If the clinician creates situations in which there is a need to do so, the children will learn to use final consonants to distinguish between the two words. For example, if they are playing "Go Fish" with picture cards and ask for *tail* they will get the picture of a dog's tail, even if they meant *sail*. Many children need only a few examples of these minimal pairs before they are able to produce the target sounds in additional words (Elbert, Powell, & Swartzlander, 1991). The semantic method serves to alert the children to the fact that there is a difference between what they are saying and what they should be saying, and that this difference is important. This method does not require children to think about the sounds themselves, an advantage for young children, who have little awareness of sounds as units smaller than words.

Some clients will not benefit from a semantic approach. They may see the differences in meaning between their sound errors and the correct production but be unable to produce the sound correctly without additional assistance. A *cross-modality* approach may provide that assistance. Cross-modality approaches utilize sensory information to facilitate correct articulation. For example, a client and clinician may face a mirror while the clinician demonstrates the target sound. The client may then attempt to repeat the sound while monitoring his or her movements visually in the mirror. In another case, a clinician may rub a child's alveolar ridge with a mint so that the child can "taste" where the tongue belongs for /t/ and /d/. Or clients are instructed to put their hand over their larynx to feel the difference between /s/ and /z/. This additional sensory input can be an effective way for adults or children to monitor their performance.

For some sounds there are few available cues that the client can see or feel. Sometimes it is possible to take advantage of the *coarticulatory context* to promote correct sound production. Coarticulatory context refers to the fact that the sounds preceding and following a phoneme will influence the way that phoneme is produced. For a phoneme like /r/, for which there are few visual cues, coarticulatory context can help in learning correct production. For example, the /g/ and /k/ in /gr/ or /kr/ blends require a high, back tongue carriage, which carries over to facilitate a correct production of /r/. Once this correct tongue placement is established in blends, it can be used in words with other sound combinations.

These different techniques can be used in conjunction with behavioral techniques. Many behavior-modification programs are commercially available for children with articulation disorders. They offer a number of attractive therapy materials designed to make the learning task interesting and fun for the young child. As a first step, the speech-language pathologist establishes a baseline of what the child is able to produce. For example, a particular target sound is selected, and the number of productions the child is able to say correctly, either spontaneously or by prompting, is established as the child's general proficiency for that sound. The treatment program for that sound then begins, following the systematic presentation of a particular program. The child is given an occasional prompt (a helping suggestion) to aid in production tasks, and as the typical program progresses, the clinician fades out support (doing less and less). A particular sound is usually taught to a particular success level (percentage correct); for example, the child who makes an /r/ error must produce that sound correctly 80% of the time before going on to the next (usually more difficult) task in the program.

Operant conditioning techniques can be integrated with articulation therapy. The goal of correct articulation for certain sounds (or classes of sounds) may be broken down into stages. An initial goal may be an approximation of the sound as it occurs at the beginning of words. When the client has mastered this step, closer approximations may be required until correct productions are made. Clients are rewarded for these closer and closer approximations. Rewards may be tangible or intangible. Very young children or mentally retarded individuals might receive a treat or tokens for meeting their goals. Other children may be rewarded by taking their turn in an articulation "game." For many older children and adults, articulatory and communicative success is frequently its own reward.

Generalization

If clients have learned the correct pronunciation of the /r/ sound, it does them little good if they can produce it only in /gr/ blends or only in the therapy setting. The goal of articulation therapy is for clients to be able to use the newly corrected sounds in all words and in all situations. When clients are able to transfer their newly learned articulation skills to untrained words and new settings, we say that they are demonstrating generalization of articulation skills. Generalization does not always occur automatically. The therapist should incorporate activities that promote generalization into the therapy program.

Generalization goals may be broken down into categories, such as generalizations to other sound contexts, to different speaking tasks, and with different speaking partners. In some cases, the therapist may be able to find a few words in which the client is able to correctly produce the target sound. Generalization then involves transferring this limited skill to greater numbers of words (Prather & Whaley, 1984). For example, the client may lateralize the /s/ (air escapes over the sides of the tongue) in /sl/ blends but produce /st/ blends accurately. In this case, the therapist may present /sl/ blends in conjunction with /st/ blends to facilitate generalization. If the target sound is never produced correctly, the therapist may select a small set of words that begin with the target sounds for initial training. When these are mastered, the therapist may incorporate new words containing the target sounds into the therapy sessions. This set of words is expanded to include words with the target sounds in the medial and final position. The therapist may also include combinations of sounds within words that are more difficult for the client. Different words will be included in each session to promote generalization to new words.

Single-word responses can be expanded into short phrases and sentences. Sometimes a standard carrier phrase can be used initially to facilitate articulation in longer utterances. For example, a group of children might play a game of twenty questions in which each child asks, "Is it a . . . ?" to find out what card the therapist holds. Older children and adults can practice articulation while reading sentences and short passages. The use of carrier phrases or reading tasks allow clients to practice their articulation skills without having to concentrate on the content of the message. As articulation skills become increasingly automatic, the clinician will incorporate conversational tasks into the therapy session.

As therapy progresses, children and adults become increasingly adept at monitoring their articulation during the therapy session. This self-monitoring process appears to relate to the client's ability to generalize articulation skills (Shriberg & Kwiatkowski, 1990). Outside of the therapy session, clients are typically more concerned with the content of their speech than their articulation. To promote generalization to other settings, the therapist may enlist the cooperation of others. For a child, the therapist may provide parents with tips for facilitating correct articulation at home. Teachers may monitor articulation in the classroom. A peer may be enlisted for activities outside the therapy setting. McReynolds (1982) writes that bringing other people into generalization sessions as critical listeners will sometimes accelerate generalization; however, she notes that we must caution others "not to overdo their help, so that the person does not become overly self-conscious about the problem" (p. 136). Generalization occurs primarily in a practice atmosphere. Individuals should be treated gently when they make mistakes and given realistic positive reinforcement when they produce sounds well.

Acquired Articulation Disorders in Adults

Adults who have developed normal speech and language abilities give little attention to their articulation processes when they speak. The motor patterns for speech are well established and relatively automatic under most circumstances, however, adults may acquire structural or neurological impairments that disrupt their articulation abilities. Treatment of such impairments differs from treating developmental articulation disorders because adults may need to change their articulation patterns, and formerly automatic processes may need to become more intentional.

Articulation Impairments due to Structural Impairments

Structural changes of the articulators can result from traumatic damage or surgical removal of all or portions of the larynx, tongue, jaw, teeth, or lips. Removal of the larynx results in the dramatic loss of the laryngeal voice and is discussed in Chapter 11. In some cases, portions of the tongue must be surgically removed because of cancer. The procedure is called a **glossectomy**, and it may be either partial or total, depending on the extent of the disease. Articulation is a challenge without the tongue; recall from Chapter 2 that many of the sounds of English are differentiated by movements of the tongue. The speech therapy goal following glossectomy is to adjust the placement of the remaining articulators to produce the most intelligible speech possible. There are many subtle adjustments that can be made to approximate speech produced without the tongue. For example, the sound /t/ normally requires the tongue to touch the alveolar ridge, just behind the teeth, but in the absence of the tongue, the patient might touch the lower lip behind the front teeth in a manner that stops and then releases the airflow. Because the manner of production is still a plosive and it is produced at the alveolar ridge, the listener may be tricked into thinking they heard a /t/. In fact, it is typically easier to understand the speech of a glossectomy patient if you do not look at the mouth, where some surprising articulatory placements are being made.

In some cases, structural changes of the articulators can be compensated for by specially designed artificial replacements, such as a prosthetic tongue and jaw (Arcuri, Perlman, Philippbar, & Barkmeier, 1991; Leonard & Gillis, 1982, 1983). The artificial tongue does not move, but fills in the gap resulting from tongue removal. This improves the speaker's ability to use the remaining articulators to overcome the changes in the oral structures. Some speakers adapt to their new anatomy by making appropriate articulatory adjustments. When therapy is needed, the speech-language pathologist works with the patient to come up with the most satisfactory approximation of sounds that are in error due to structural changes. In some cases the rate of speech must be slowed to allow the necessary time to articulate in a manner that is different from lifelong speech patterns.

Motor Speech Disorders

The most commonly acquired articulation disorders in adults are due to neurological impairments that affect the motor control for speech. They are collectively referred to as motor speech disorders and include the disorders of dysarthria and apraxia of speech. As we saw earlier in this chapter, these disorders can occur in children as well. When they occur in adults, they are typically caused by damage or dysfunction of the motor control centers in the central or peripheral nervous systems, or both. The disturbances may affect any or all aspects of speech production, including respiration, phonation, resonance, and articulation.

Dysarthria

The dysarthrias are a group of motor speech disorders caused by weakness, paralysis, slowness, incoordination, or sensory loss in the muscle groups responsible for speech. The muscle weakness and poor control typically result in imprecise articulation, so that speech is difficult to understand. The sounds may be distorted or involve the substitution of an incorrect sound. The specific characteristics of dysarthria tend to reflect the location of the damage to the nervous system, so that certain clusters of symptoms have been associated with certain diseases (Duffy, 1995). Some of the causes of dysarthria are stroke, Parkinson's disease, Huntington's disease, amyotrophic lateral sclerosis (Lou Gehrig's disease), and cerebellar diseases. In addition to imprecise articulation, other symptoms include hypernasality because of poor motor control of the soft palate; disturbed voice quality including harsh or breathy voice because of poor control of the larynx; and abnormal prosody because of poor control of the variations of pitch, loudness, and timing. If motor control is so severely impaired that no understandable speech can be produced, it is called **anarthria**.

Apraxia

Apraxia of speech differs from dysarthria in that there is no muscle weakness, paralysis, or incoordination but there is impaired ability to plan the movements for speech production. Thus, apraxia of speech has been referred to as an impairment of the motor planning for articulation. Speech is difficult to understand because of substitution errors, sound repetitions, and some inappropriate sound additions. The errors are often inconsistent, so that repeated attempts at the same word come out differently on each attempt. Apraxia of speech often co-occurs with the language impairment of aphasia, and in those cases it is difficult to separate the speech and language disorders. However, apraxia of speech can exist independently of aphasia, so that language formulation, reading, and writing are unimpaired, but speech production is disturbed (Duffy, 1995).

Treatment of Motor Speech Disorders

The goal for the management of motor speech disorders is to improve communication. This can be accomplished through therapy designed to improve the intelligibility, naturalness, and efficiency of speech production, but may also be achieved by the use of assertive devices. There are excellent resources that provide treatment approaches specific to particular syndromes (Duffy, 1995; Moore, Yorkston, & Beukelman, 1991; Square-Storer, 1989; Yorkston, Beukelman, & Bell, 1988). Treatment may be directed toward the restoration of normal speech production processes or the compensation for impaired motor control. In some cases, adjustments need to be made to overcome the impairment. For example, Parkinson's disease often results in a dysarthria that is characterized by imprecise articulation, decreased loudness, and flat prosody. A treatment approach called the Lee Silverman Voice Treatment trains patients to increase the effort that they exert while speaking by adjusting their loudness. With increased loudness, the Parkinson patients also increase their articulatory precision and thus remarkably improve their speech intelligibility (Ramig, Countryman, Thompson, & Horii, 1995).

Although the symptomatology of apraxia and dysarthria differs, there are similarities in some of the behavioral treatment approaches appropriate to these speech disorders. For both types of disorders, treatment is designed so that there is an orderly progression of treatment tasks and extensive drill to reestablish and stabilize the motor movements. For example, a treatment continuum for apraxia of speech begins with the clinician saying the target word, followed by the patient and clinician producing the target together. If the patient correctly produces the response simultaneously with the clinician, then the clinician reduces support by mouthing the word along with the patient, and ultimately the patient produces the response to a question, without support from the clinician (Wertz, LaPointe, & Rosenbek, 1984). In cases where speech production is not adequate for everyday communication, augmentative communication devices may be appropriate.

Augmentative Communication Systems

Some adults and children have physical limitations so severe that oral speech may not be an attainable goal. For these individuals, alternate methods must be found for communication. These range from a simple signaling device, like the call bell on a bedside nightstand, to sophisticated electronic devices that are tailored to the client's individual needs. The speech-language pathologist's challenge is to find the combination of features in a communication device that best matches the client's needs and abilities. A child who can identify pictures, but cannot yet read, may start with a picture board that includes objects and actions common to his daily life (see Figure 9-5). An adult who can read may do well with an electronic device that can produce both synthetic speech and written output (see Figure 9-6).

Before a device can be selected, an initial assessment of the client's abilities must be obtained, often through the coordinated efforts of a variety of professionals such as audiologists, vision specialists, psychologists, speech-language pathologists, and physical and occupational therapists. These individuals contribute information concerning the client's sensory, motor, cognitive, and language abilities. This evaluation is designed to determine the client's limitations as well as strengths that might be used for communication. For example, an individual with limited visual acuity may do better with simple line drawings than with glossy photos. An individual with severe cerebral palsy may

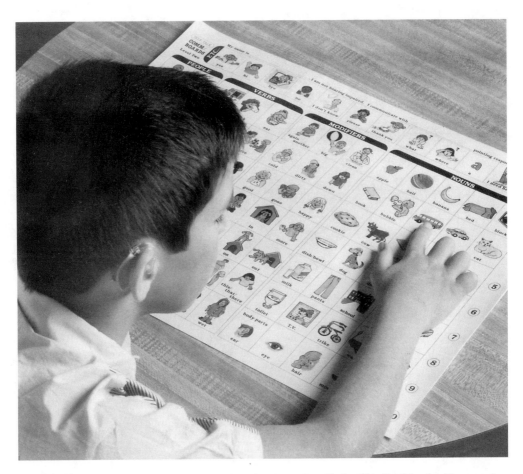

FIGURE 9-5   A child uses a communication board, called self-talk. (Used with permission of Communication Skill Builders, San Antonio, TX)

have sufficient control of eye movement, head movement, or even foot movement, to allow the use of certain switches with an electronic device. Perhaps different devices are needed to allow the child or adult to communicate from different positions, such as sitting in a wheelchair or lying on the floor or in bed. The devices selected must be able to accompany the client and be usable whenever the client needs to communicate.

The decision about how the child or adult will communicate is closely related to what information will be communicated. Communication involves a code that is passed from sender to receiver. For normal speakers, this code is oral language. For a patient who is recovering from surgery that removed the larynx, the code might be written language. For a child who cannot write, the code might be a symbol system. For a child of more limited language or cognitive abilities, pictures might be used. In selecting the code, both the client's abilities and the people they need to communicate with

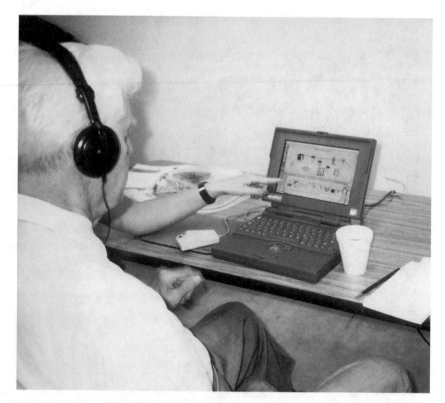

FIGURE 9-6 An adult uses the Lingraphica® (Tolfa) system to communicate recent events in his life. (Courtesy of The University of Arizona, Department of Speech & Hearing Sciences)

must be considered. It makes no sense to train clients to expert levels with a new symbol system, for instance, if their families, teachers, and classmates prefer not to learn this new symbol system to communicate with them.

After one or more communication systems are selected, training is vital for developing successful communication. Training is geared toward the client's developmental level and daily needs. For a toddler, it may mean starting with toys and activities that develop turn-taking skills and communicative intent. For a school-aged child, it might include the use of language for academic purposes as well as for interpersonal communication. For the adult, the goal may be to reestablish communication that has been affected by illness or injury. Training often involves trial and error on the part of both the client and the clinician. Imagine the dilemma of the clinician who must try to adapt a communication system to meet the particular needs of the client before the client has the means of communicating those needs. Imagine the frustration of the client who must wait until the clinician figures it out!

A client with the desire and means to transmit a message is still only half of a successful communication. Communication requires other people. Family members often receive direct training on how to use and maintain augmentative devices, but the client is also likely to encounter others who have never seen an augmentative device. Unfortunately, some people may not want to take the considerable time and effort involved in communicating through an alternative system. Communication is inevitably slower and is often less accurate. It can be tiring for both the sender and receiver. However, for many nonverbal individuals, the basic need to interact with other people provides the motivation and reward for the effort involved. This can clearly be seen in the case of Mr. Moser.

Mr. Moser had been a high-school science teacher until he suffered brain damage at the age of 43. An artery at the base of his brain was thin-walled and weak. Eventually, this section of the artery ballooned out, forming an aneurysm, which eventually burst. Immediate surgery was able to halt the bleeding but not before sections of his brainstem and cerebellum were damaged. When he recovered from surgery, he was left with a variety of permanent deficits.

Damage to the auditory tracts in the brainstem cause a rare form of an acquired auditory disorder. Although he could hear sounds and tell when two sounds were different, Mr. Moser could not attach meaning to what he heard. Consequently, he could not understand spoken language, although he could understand written language quite well. Damage to the motor tracts running through the brainstem and cerebellum left him confined to a wheelchair. He suffered from ataxia of movement. When he would reach for objects, his hands and arms would waver back and forth. He would frequently over- or undershoot his reach for the object he wanted. His speech was similarly affected. His voice was a monotone and low in pitch. He spoke with great effort, and his face often contorted as he struggled to get out the words. He spoke only when asked specifically to do so.

Because of his difficulty in producing the movements needed for speech and his inability to monitor his speech through audition, he became mute. In place of speech, he relied on an electronic communication system that allowed him to type in a message that was displayed on a small screen. Messages were typed with an ever-wavering index finger, one letter at a time. When he wished to convey a longer message, which he frequently did, the device printed the message on paper. His laboriously produced messages revealed his intelligent, inquisitive, and outgoing personality. Armed with his communication system and a large amount of persistence and charm, Mr. Moser was able to interact with others through written language.

Clinical Problem Solving

Kiesha, age 6, was brought into our research lab to participate in a language study. While she was there we taped the following conversation:

Kiesha: Hey, Piget (Piglet)!

Dad: There he is. You found him. There's Piglet.

Kiesha: Shhhhh.

Dad: Oh, is it because he's sleeping?

Kiesha: Kaiet (quiet)!

Dad: Ok, I'll be quiet. Are they all asleep?

Kiesha: We da he seep (Where does he sleep?)

Dad: What are they doing?

Kiesha: Let's make 'em seep (sleep). He's at home.

Dad: Who's this guy.

Kiesha: Gover (Grover). And Ernie. Cookie Monser (Cookie Monster).

1. Does this speech sample indicate an articulation disorder? Would you feel the same if the child had just turned 3? (To review normal development, consult Chapter 3).
2. Using Table 9-2, can you identify any phonological processes among the sound errors? Remember that identification of a phonological process requires evidence of a pattern that affects more than one individual sound.
3. What factors would you need to rule out as causes of these speech errors before considering therapy?
4. Which therapy approaches might you consider for remediation in this case? Which would not be appropriate? Why?

References

Arcuri, M.R., Perlman, A.L., Philippbar, S.A., & Barkmeier, J.M. (1991). The effects of a maxillary speech-aid prosthesis for the combined tongue and mandibular resection patient. *Journal of Prosthetic Dentistry,* 65(6): 816–22.

ASHA. (1991). The role of the speech-language pathologist in management of oral myofunctional disorders. *Asha,* 33, (Suppl. 5): 7.

Barrett, R.H., & Hanson, M.L. (1978). *Oral Myofunctional Disorders* (2nd ed.). St. Louis: Mosby.

Boone, D.R. (1972). *Cerebral Palsy.* New York: Bobbs-Merrill.

Broen, P., ed. (1981). *Language, Speech and Hearing Services in the Schools* (Special issue on nonvocal communication), 4:12.

Coleman, C., Look, A., & Myers, L. (1980). Assessing no-oral clients for assistive communication devices. *Journal of Speech and Hearing Disorders,* 45: 515–526.

Duffy, J.R. (1995). *Motor Speech Disorders: Substrates, Differential Diagnosis, and Management.* St. Louis, MO: Mosby-Year Book.

Dunn, C. (1982). Phonological process analysis: Contributions to assessing phonological disorders. *Communicative Disorders,* 7: 147–163.

Elbert, M., Powell, T.W., & Swartzlander, P. (1991). Toward a technology of generalization: How many exemplars are sufficient? *Journal of Speech and Hearing Research,* 34: 84–87.

Estrem, T., & Broen, P.A. (1989). Early speech production of children with cleft palate. *Journal of Speech and Hearing Research,* 32: 122–119.

Fogh-Anderson, P. (1942). *Inheritance of Harelip and Cleft Palate.* Copenhagen: Busck.

Goldman, R., & Fristoe, M. (1986). *Goldman-Fristoe Test of Articulation.* Circle Pines, MN: American Guidance Service.

Grunwell, P. (1980). Developmental language disorders at the phonological level. In F.M. Jones (Ed.), *Language Disability in Children.* Lancaster, PA: MTP Press.

Grunwell, P. (1981). *The Nature of Phonological Disability in Children,* New York: Academic Press.

Hall, B. J.C. (1990). Attitudes of fourth and sixth graders towards peers with mild articulation disorders. *Language, Speech, and Hearing Services in Schools, 22*: 344–340.

Harding, A., & Grunwell, P. (1996). Characteristics of cleft palate speech. *European Journal of Disorders of Communication, 31*, 331–357.

Ingram, D. (1981). *Procedures for the Phonological Analysis of Children's Language*. Baltimore: University Park Press.

Jafee, M.B. (1984). Neurological impairment of speech production: Assessment and treatment. In J. Costello (Ed.), *Speech Disorders in Children*. San Diego: College-Hill Press.

Khan, L., & Lewis, N. (1986). *Khan-Lewis Phonological Analysis*. Circle Pines, MN: American Guidance Service.

Kent, R.D., Miolo, G., & Bloedel, S. (1994). The intelligibility of children's speech: A review of evaluation procedures. *American Journal of Speech-Language Pathology, 3*, 81–95.

Laine, T., Warren, D.W., Dalston, R.M., Hairfield, W.M., & Morr, K.E. (1988). Intraoral pressure, nasal pressure and airflow in cleft palate speech. *Journal of Speech and Hearing Research, 31*: 432–437.

Leonard, R.J. & Gillis, R. (1983). Effects of a prosthetic tongue on vowel formants and isovowel lines in a patient with total glossectomy (an addendum to Leonard and Gillis, 1982). *Journal of Speech & Hearing Disorders, 48* (4): 423–6.

Leonard, R.J. & Gillis, R. (1982). Effects of a prosthetic tongue on vowel intelligibility and food management in a patient with total glossectomy. *Journal of Speech & Hearing Disorders, 47*(1): 25–30.

Lewis, B.A. (1990). Familial phonological disorders: Four pedigrees. *Journal of Speech and Hearing Disorders, 55*: 160–170.

Locke, J. (1983). Clinical phonology: The explanation and treatment of speech sound disorders. *Journal of Speech and Hearing Disorders, 48*: 339–341.

Love, R., Hagerman, E., & Taimi, E. (1980). Speech performance, dysphagia and oral reflexes in cerebral palsy. *Journal of Speech and Hearing Disorders, 45*: 59-75.

Lynch, J.I. (1990). Tongue reduction surgery: Efficacy and relevance to the profession. *Asha, 32*: 59–61.

McDonald, E.T., & Chance, B. (1964). *Cerebral Palsy*. Englewood Cliffs, NJ: Prentice Hall.

McReynolds, L.V. (1982). Functional articulation problems. In G.H. Shames and E.H. Wiig (Eds.), *Human Communication Disorders: An Introduction*. Columbus, OH: Charles E. Merrill.

McWilliams, B.J., Morris, H.L., & Shelton, R.L. (1990). *Cleft Palate Speech* (2nd ed.). Philadelphia: B.C. Decker.

Moore, C.A., Yorkston, K.M., & Beukelman, D.R. (Eds.). (1991). *Dysarthria and Apraxia of Speech*. Baltimore, MD: Paul H. Brookes.

Mysack, E. (1980). *Neurospeech Therapy for the Cerebral Palsied* (3rd ed.). Totowa, NJ: Teachers College Press.

Office of Scientific and Health Reports (1988). *Developmental Speech and Language Disorders: Hope Through Research* (NIH Publication No. Pamphlet 88–2757). Bethesda, MD: National Institute on Neurological and Communication Disorders and Stroke.

Prather, E., & Whaley, P. (1984). Articulation training based on coarticulation. In H. Winitz (Ed.), *Treating Articulation Disorders: For Clinicians by Clinicians*. Baltimore: University Park Press.

Ramig, L.O., Countyman, S., Thompson, L., & Horii, L. (1995). A comparison of two intensive speech treatments for Parkinson disease. *Journal of Speech and Hearing Research, 39*, 1232–1251.

Ruscello, D. M., St. Louis, K.O., & Mason, N. (1991). School-age children with phonologic disorders: Coexistence with other speech/language disorders. *Journal of Speech and Hearing Disorders, 34*: 236–242.

Shelton, R.L., Furr, M.L., Johnson, A., & Arndt, W.B. (1975). Cephalometric and intraoral variables as they relate to articulation improvement with training. *American Journal of Orthodontics, 67*: 423–431.

Shriberg, L. (1980). Developmental phonological disorders. In T.J. Hixon, L. Shriberg, & J. Saxon (Eds.), *Introduction to Communication Disorders*. Englewood Cliffs, NJ: Prentice Hall.

Shriberg, L., Austin, D., Lewis, B.A., McSweeny, J.L., & Wilson, D.L. (1997). The percentage of consonants correct (PCC) metric: Extensions and reliability data.

Journal of Speech Language and Hearing Research, 40, 708–722.

Shriberg, L.D., & Kwiatkowski, J. (1988). A follow-up study of children with phonologic disorders of unknown origin. *Journal of Speech and Hearing Disorders, 53:* 144–155.

Shriberg, L.D., & Kwiatkowski, J. (1990). Self-monitoring and generalization in preschool speech-delayed children. *Language, Speech, and Hearing Services in Schools, 21:* 157–170.

Shriberg, L.D., Kwiatkowski, J., Best, S., Hengst, J., & Terselic-Weber, B. (1986). Characteristics of children with phonological disorders of unknown origin. *Journal of Speech and Hearing Disorders, 51:* 140–161.

Square-Storer, P. (Ed.). (1989). *Acquired Apraxia of Speech in Aphasic Adults.* Salisbury, UK: Lawrence Erlbaum Associates.

Wertz, R.T., LaPointe, L.L., & Rosenbek, J.C. (1984). *Apraxia of Speech in Adults: The Disorder and Its Management.* Orlando, FL: Grune & Stratton.

Yorkston, K.M., Beukelman, D.R., & Bell, K.R. (1988). *Clinical Management of Dysarthric Speakers.* Boston, MA: College-Hill Press.

C h a p t e r 10

Disorders of Fluency

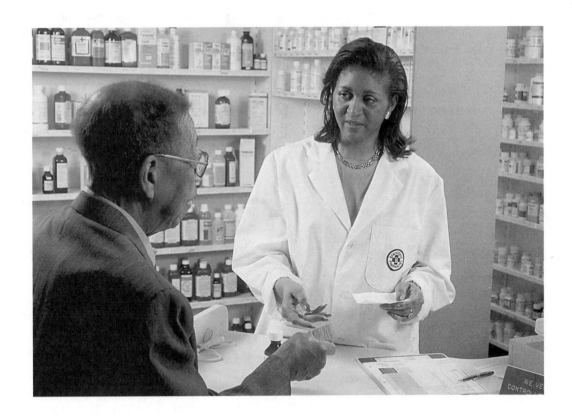

Preview

The area of fluency and fluency disorders has been one of the most dynamic areas within the profession of speech-language pathology. Principal among disorders of fluency is the phenomenon of stuttering. The various definitions of stuttering reflect a wide range of perspectives that experts have brought to bear in trying to understand this disorder of communication. Indeed, developmental, familial, psychological, neurological, and motoric factors all appear to interact in cases of stuttering. Although stuttering is the most common fluency disorder, there are other disorders characterized by changes in fluency. We will briefly consider disruptions of fluency associated with cluttering and cases of acquired stuttering in adults.

When Abraham[1] was about 3 years of age, his mother noticed that his sentences did not always flow smoothly. Sometimes he would repeat the same word several times before he was able to get the rest of the sentence out. There were pauses mid-sentence. In fact, at times Abraham sounded quite disfluent. This concerned both of his parents because they each had a family history of stuttering. The mother's brother had stuttered during most of his childhood, although he was described as completely fluent as an adult. The father's sister began stuttering as a child and continued to stutter into adulthood. The parents did not want Abraham to struggle to communicate the way their siblings had, and they were naturally concerned when Abraham seemed to go through periods when he was particularly disfluent. At age 3 years, 3 months, we had the following conversation with him:

Author: What's Wishbone?

Abraham: Um, he's one of the shows that I watch. He's a dog. The story of Wishbone is really . . . um, really a show.

Author: He's a dog. And he has his own show?

Abraham: No, there's a . . . there's a boy in it.

Author: What do they get to do?

Abraham: They do everything. But only in the shows, they get to do . . . I don't know.

[*Abraham notices the barnyard toys and goes to them.*]

Author: Let me see what's in this barn. There's a lot of animals in here.

Abraham: Yeah, I . . . [silence]

Author: All right. Well, there's a cow. And there's a baby cow. That's a . . . that's a brown cow.

---

[1]We have followed the speech and language development of Abraham in Chapters 3 and 4.

Abraham: No, that's a white cow. That's called . . . that's called . . . These two are cows.

Author: Oh yeah? What kind of cows?

Abraham: Black ones and white ones.

Author: Black ones and white ones. And this is a dog.

Abraham: This is . . . This is a dog.

Author: Do you think he's a sheep dog?

Abraham: Nooo.

Author: Do you think he's a cow dog? Does he have to watch out over the cows?

Abraham: [*Nods in agreement.*]

Author: Well, I've got some hay. [*Picks up a cow.*] Do you think he's a hay eater?

Abraham: Yes he is. I'll put hay on his . . . in his . . . in his . . . .in there so he can't eat anything.

[Abraham puts animals in the hay loft.]

Author: Now we have two cows in the hay.

Abraham: Is this one the . . . .the . . . the . . . the baby one?

Author: I don't know. Its kind of small. Maybe he is a baby one.

During this brief conversation, we were able to observe a number of interruptions in the flow of communication. These included whole word repetitions ("the . . . the . . . the . . . the baby one"), phrase repetitions ("This is . . . this is a dog."), and interjections ("um"). However, Abraham seemed completely unfazed by his disfluencies. His focus was on the toys and our play, and he was probably unaware of his own speech patterns. Notice, too, that Abraham was not the only one to show speech repetition. The author repeated part of a sentence ("That's a . . . that's a brown cow.") during the conversation as well. In fact, everyone experiences a minor interruption in the flow of speech at some time or another. Differentiating between "normal" disfluencies and stuttering is an ongoing challenge to those working in the area of fluency disorders.

It is not always easy to identify an episode of disfluency that characterizes stuttering unequivocally from an episode that is a momentary lapse of fluency. This is particularly true in the case of young children. As young children are learning to put together sentences, it is very common to hear them make false starts (I . . . he did it!), revise mid-sentence ("He's in . . . he's on T.V."), hesitate over the next word to come ("I want . . . juice."). We often get the sense that these interruptions in fluency have more to do with the child's partial grasp of the language than any struggle making the words come out. Likewise, we frequently hear a child who is so excited that word or phrase repetitions come pouring forth ("Mommy! Mommy! Mommy! Mommy! Mommy! Can I, can I, can I have one?!). For most children, these episodes reflect normal development, rather than the onset of stuttering. In fact, for Abraham, this proved to be the case. As he continued to develop speech and language skills, the episodes of disfluency decreased. By 4 1/2, no one, including his parents, had any concerns about his speech fluency.

Normal Disfluencies versus Stuttering

Conture (1990) noted that deciding who is and who is not stuttering is a relative, rather than an absolute decision, in that there is no behavior that children who stutter display that normal children *never* exhibit. Although normally developing children (and adults on occasion) sometimes experience breakdowns in these speech parameters, there is a much more normal flow of speech than is observed in a child who stutters. For example, normal children, such as Abraham, may repeat words or phrases at the age of three. However, by the age of 4½, normal children usually repeat utterances only when they wish to emphasize something (Curlee, 1980).

Early Signs of Stuttering

Although no method is foolproof for identifying the young child who will persist in stuttering, a number of behavioral signs are considered to be "red flags" for stuttering (see Table 10-1). In the case of stuttering, speech is frequently characterized by changes in duration, rate, and rhythm, with frequent interruptions of smooth fluency from sound to sound and from word to word. One distinction that has been suggested involves the unit of speech on which the disfluency occurs (Andrews, Craig, Feyer, Haddinott, Neilson, & Howie, 1983; Wall, 1988). The type of speech unit in which the individual is most likely to produce normal disfluency is the word, phrase, or sentence; those who stutter are most likely to do so on single sounds and syllables. A child showing normal disfluency may say "I want . . . I want it," whereas a child who stutters may say "I wwwwwwant it." The frequency of disfluent episodes is also different for children with normal disfluencies and for those who stutter. Wingate (1962) found that nonstuttering children seldom make repetitions for more than 3% of their total speech utterances; children who stutter were found to have a frequency of syllable disfluencies ranging from 7 to 14%.

The signs of stuttering are not restricted to interruptions of speech. Children who stutter are also likely to differ from their peers in facial movements accompanying episodes of disfluency. Conture and Kelly (1991) reported that young children who stutter could be differentiated from nonstuttering children by the types of facial behaviors they exhibit. For example, children who stutter were likely to look away, blink their eyes, raise their upper lip, or press their lips together during periods of dis-

TABLE 10-1   Signs Often Associated with Normal and Stuttered Speech

Normal disfluencies	
Word repetitions	I like that . .that book.
Phrase repetitions	I want a . .I want a big one!
Sentence repetitions	Watch me! Watch me! Watch me!
Hesitations	He took . . . my juice.
Interjections	We, um, got to go too.
Stuttering	
Syllable repetitions	We saw a vi-vi-vi-video.
Sound repetition	I g-g-g-got it from school.
Sound prolongations	Wwwwwwait for mmmme.
Sound blocks	[starts word but no sound comes out]
Nonspeech behaviors	[e.g., blinks, facial tension, limb movement]

fluency, whereas their fluent peers showed these behaviors less frequently. Stuttering children may show signs of struggle or tension while attempting to speak, whereas children with normal disfluencies typically seem unaffected by the disfluent episode.

Several investigators (Schwartz, Zebrowski, & Conture,1990; Yairi & Ambrose, 1992) have examined the earliest signs of stuttering by studying the behaviors of young children whose parents reported that stuttering had begun recently (within the previous 12 months). Yairi and Ambrose interviewed parents concerning the age of their children and the characteristics of their disfluent speech when stuttering began. Parents reported that their children were sometimes quite young, between the ages of 20 months to 5 years of age, when stuttering was first recognized. Just under half of the parents reported that their children began to stutter suddenly, whereas other parents remembered the onset of stuttering as evolving gradually over the course of several weeks. Schwartz and colleagues recorded the speech of such children on videotape to assess the behaviors associated with the earliest stages of stuttering. The investigators reported that the disfluencies of these children frequently included sound prolongations (33 to 60% of all disfluent episodes). They also frequently exhibited nonspeech behaviors, such as eye movements or eye closings during disfluent episodes. Somewhat surprisingly, the stuttering behaviors of children who were at the younger end of the age range did not differ remarkably from those at the older end. Although prolongations were somewhat more frequent for children who had been stuttering longer, the authors emphasized that there were more similarities among the behaviors of children at different ages than differences.

The signs that suggest the onset of stuttering, as opposed to developmental disfluencies, can vary between children and even within a single child. However, we have seen that there are some signs that signal that a child is struggling with more than just the normal disruptions of fluency that all children sometimes experience. These signs can be seen in the case of a young boy who was brought to the clinic for a fluency evaluation.

Jackson was 6 years old when he was first seen in the clinic. His mother brought him in because "he stutters." She reported that he started stuttering two years before, but that she had always assumed that he would grow out of it. Now that Jackson was in school, however, she was concerned that other children were teasing him. She had already noticed that Jackson seemed aware that his speech was different from other children. She reported that he sometimes got frustrated when trying to talk. As far as she knew, no one in her family had ever stuttered, and she couldn't recall anyone having had any kind of developmental problems at all.

When we talked with Jackson, it was apparent that his speech showed more than the typical amount of disfluency. In fact, sometimes it seemed as if he could hardly get his thoughts out. His speech was frequently disrupted by sound prolongations and blocks, when no sound came out at all. During these episodes, his mouth seemed to lock into a tense position from which he was unable to break free. His brows knit together; sometimes he would blink or contort his face until the disfluent period passed and speech resumed its normal flow. When asked why his mother brought him to the clinic, he replied "I-i-i-t's . . . because I t-t-t-t-t . . . alk . . . I can't talk."

In contrast to his fluency, a formal assessment of his language showed average to above average skills. Likewise, when he was not stuttering, he did not show problems with speech articulation. An examination of his oral mechanism (see Chapter 9) revealed normal structure, muscle tone, and nonspeech movement. Likewise, he could repeat nonsense words and say entire sentences in a sing-song cadence, which indicated he possessed the physical mechanisms to support normal speech.

Persistent Stuttering

A majority of the children who show early disfluencies will eventually develop fluent speech. However, some children will not. Yairi and colleagues reported that children destined to recover from early stuttering-like behaviors may initially show more disfluencies than children who continue to be disfluent. However, the children who recover begin to show reductions in their number of disfluencies within the first year after stuttering-like disfluencies began. In contrast, children who failed to recover were relatively stable in their rate of disfluency (Yairi, Ambrose, Paden, & Throneburg, 1996). Although there is a chance that some of these children will recover still later in childhood, they are at risk for struggling with fluency throughout their lives. Let us look at the case of one such man:

> Mr. Andrews, age 32, has stuttered since childhood. Although he had received therapy several times, he continued to show a variety of stuttering signs. His stuttering consisted primarily of silent blocks, during which his mouth and face contorted as he struggled to break free. Occasionally, he would also experience part-word repetitions, where the first sound of a word was repeated over and over. He had recently contacted the clinic because he thought that his stuttering was preventing him from advancing in his career as fast as he thought he could. He expressed, "T————-eam work is very important in my c-c-c-c-company, and I knnnnnnnnow that the others would rather not have me on the team b————-cause of my stuttering. When I present m——y ideas, they d—————on't take them as ssssseriously." He reported that he was able to speak fluently "most of the time" after his last experience with therapy in high school. However, to maintain fluency, he felt he had to concentrate harder on how he was speaking than on what he was actually trying to say. Over time, his disfluency slipped back to pre-therapy levels. He was willing to try again to reduce his stuttering severity.

Adults who stutter may continue to show some of the same characteristics of childhood stuttering. They may continue to produce sound repetitions and prolongations, along with silent interruptions, called blocks, in the flow of speech. "Secondary" characteristics of stuttering, which may have been present during childhood, may be more pronounced. These characteristics include facial tension, facial contortions, and extraneous movements during the stuttering episode. In addition, these adults typically have had years of frustration with their difficulty in communicating ideas with the ease that comes naturally to others. This frustration can become as problematic as the actual episodes of fluency breakdown.

It is not uncommon for nonstuttering individuals to stereotype those who stutter with a variety of negative traits, including being anxious, tense, insecure, or nervous (Kalinowski, Lerman, & Watt, 1987). Indeed, several studies have examined physiologic correlates of stress and found evidence of increased levels of stress and anxiety among those who stutter (Blood, Blood, Bennet, Simpson, & Susman., 1994; Weber & Smith, 1990). The question remains whether stuttering results from internal stress and anxiety, or if those traits are a consequence of repeated negative experiences with communication. Several studies suggest that the latter is the case. For example, Miller and Watson

(1992) reported that their subjects who stuttered were no more anxious overall than nonstuttering subjects. However, the two groups differed in terms of their attitudes toward communication, with attitudes worsening with increased stuttering severity. Craig (1990) showed that adults who stutter were significantly more anxious during a communication task than control subjects prior to treatment for stuttering. After reducing their level of disfluency through treatment of stuttering behaviors, anxiety was reduced to a level characteristic of nonstuttering adults. Such findings may be leading to a shift in clinician perceptions of stuttering as involving characteristic personality traits such as anxiety or other negative affective states (Cooper & Cooper, 1996).

One of the more puzzling features of persistent stuttering is that speech can become completely fluent under certain circumstances. Let us consider the following case:

Mr. Tirai, age 27, was a graduate student who had come to this country to study three years earlier. Although he spoke two other languages with native proficiency, he had only rudimentary English at that time. He spent his first academic year in the United States studying primarily for his English language proficiency exam. He needed to pass this exam to continue his studies in engineering. An outgoing man, he also spent his time going to campus and community cultural events, through which he developed a number of American friends. Through his determined study, his circle of English-speaking friends, and a measure of talent for learning languages, he steadily gained proficiency in English over the next three years. Other than his accent, his English seemed largely unremarkable. He had long since acquired the common grammatical forms of English. His vocabulary had grown to a point where he rarely needed to search for words in conversation. However, in his final year of study, he was beginning to show occasional episodes of stuttering-like disfluencies. Although "stuttering" was not a word he had acquired in English, he managed to convey that he did indeed stutter in his two native languages. He had initially thought that he had escaped from stuttering through English, but that it appeared to have caught up with him just as he was feeling comfortable with this new language.

Mr. Tirai was fluent for an extended period of time during which he was learning English. Others have discovered that short-term fluency can be induced under a number of speaking conditions. Fluency may be achieved under conditions of delayed auditory feedback. This involves use of instrumentation that presents the speaker's own voice, through headphones, at a slight time delay. So, as the speaker is talking, what he or she hears lags behind what is currently being said. Choral reading or speaking, during which people speak in concert, also tends to promote fluency. Likewise, intentional changes in the rhythm of speech, as in chanting or singing, will produce fluency. All of these speaking conditions, from learning a foreign language to chanting, involve either an increase in effort or a change in the timing of speech production. It appears that such changes may "override" whatever mechanisms may lead to disfluent episodes in regular speech. Unfortunately, as Mr. Tirai found, as speakers grow proficient with these "unusual" speaking conditions, stuttering may reappear.

Stuttering in the Population

The **prevalence** of a disorder is the number of people in the population who have a particular problem at any given time. There have been several prevalence studies of stuttering over the years. The

National Institute of Deafness and Other Communication Disorders (NIDCD) of the National Institutes of Health (NIH) estimated that approximately 2 million Americans stutter (1992). This corresponds to a prevalence of approximately 0.8%. This figure is comparable to estimates of 0.8% derived by Hull, Mielke, Willeford, and Timmons (1976), 0.7 percent by Young (1975), and 0.8 percent by Morley (1952).

Although less than 1% of the population may be identified as stutterers at any given time, the percent of people who stutter varies across the life span. Morley (1972) followed approximately 1000 children in Newcastle-upon-Tyne for 15 years to examine various aspects of development. The incidence of stuttering, or the number of new cases identified during a period of time, in this particular study was about 4%, or 1 in 25 children. NIDCD estimates that 1 in 30 children will go through a period of disfluency that lasts a minimum of 6 months.

Stuttering is typically first identified before the age of 5 and many resolve to normal fluency before puberty (Morley, 1972; Wingate, 1976). Wingate (1976) summarized fourteen studies and concluded that approximately 80% of children recover from stuttering. Although there has been some dispute about the exact number, it appears that for the majority of children who stutter at an early age, stuttering will disappear before they graduate from high school. Curlee (1980) came to the following conclusion: ". . . if the incidence of stuttering among the general population does approximate 4%, a recovery rate of 80% would account for a 0.7% prevalence of stuttering" (p. 281).

In some respects, stuttering is an "equal opportunity" disorder. It affects people of all racial and socioeconomic backgrounds. However, it does appear that some individuals are at higher risk for developing the disorder than others. Stuttering affects more boys than girls. NIDCD (1992) estimated that four times as many boys stutter as girls. Others have placed the male:female ratio at the somewhat lower figures of 3:1 (Hull et al., 1976) or 2:1 (Morley, 1972; Yairi & Ambrose, 1992). These differences may reflect, in part, the different age groups examined in these studies. The male:female ratio tends to increase with older ages, which has lead some to suggest that girls may show higher rates of recovery with age than boys (Yairi, Ambrose, & Cox, 1996).

In addition to the surplus of males among individuals identified as stutterers, a family history of stuttering increases an individual's risk for the disorder. Although the population prevalence for stuttering is thought to hover around 0.7 to 0.8%, the prevalence among the relatives of an individual who stutters is much higher (Andrews & Harris, 1964; Howie, 1981; Kidd, 1980; Yairi & Ambrose, 1992, Yairi, Ambrose, & Cox, 1993). Yari and Ambrose reported that almost half (46.6%) of their sample of young children who stutter had parents or siblings who also stuttered at some time. If blood relatives in the extended family were considered, two-thirds (66.3%) of the children had a positive family history for stuttering. The pattern of family aggregation for stuttering may signal the presence of a single major gene that contributes to expression of the disorder (Yairi et al., 1993). However, the actual components that contribute to the development of stuttering may be more complex. Some have suggested that genetic factors may confer a risk for stuttering, but that certain environmental factors are needed to trigger the disorder (Andrews et al., 1983; Howie, 1981).

Family history for stuttering may account for some of the variability seen among individuals who stutter. Janssen, Kraaimaat, and Brutten (1990) examined a variety of traits in subjects who stuttered with reference to family history for stuttering. Compared with those who lacked any relatives who stuttered, those with a positive family history for stuttering had more sound prolongations and silent blocks in their speech. They also showed differences on measures of duration and variability in the acoustic stream than those without a positive family history. In contrast, the two stuttering groups did not differ on measures of reading, autonomic nervous system response, or responsiveness to therapy.

Janssen and colleagues suggest that these results indicate that familial or genetic contribution to stuttering may impact the motoric aspects of stuttering more than other associated features of the disorder.

Definitions

Definitions of stuttering are many and varied. Let us consider a few of the definitions that have appeared in the literature over the years.

1955, Johnson: "Stuttering is an anticipatory, apprehensive, hypertonic avoidance reaction" (p. 23). According to Johnson, stuttering is what speakers do when they expect stuttering to occur: dread it, tense in anticipation of it, and attempt to avoid doing it.

1977, World Health Organization: Stuttering includes "disorders in the rhythm of speech, in which the individual knows precisely what he wishes to say, but at the time is unable to say it because of an involuntary, repetitive prolongation or cessation of sound" (p. 227).

1978, Wingate: "Stuttering is characterized by audible or silent elemental repetitions and prolongations. These features reflect a temporary inability to move forward to the following sound" (p. 249).

1980, Perkins: "Stuttering is the abnormal timing of speech sound initiation."

1987, Speech Foundation of America: Stuttering is defined as "a communication disorder characterized by excessive involuntary disruptions or blockings in the flow of speech, particulary when such disruptions consist of repetitions or prolongations of a sound or syllable, and when they are accompanied by avoidance struggle behavior" (p. 183).

1991, Perkins, Kent, and Curlee: "Stuttering is a disruption of speech experienced by the speaker as a loss of control" (p. 734). They differentiate stuttering from non-stuttered forms of disfluencies by identifying the latter as "abnormal as well as normal sounding disfluency not experienced as loss of control" (p. 734).

1995, Cooper and Cooper: "Stuttering . . . is a clinical syndrome characterized by abnormal and persistent disfluencies in speech accompanied by characteristic affective, behavioral, and cognitive patterns" (p. 126).

There is no one definition of stuttering that is uniformly accepted by experts in the field. The differences among these and other definitions available in the literature reflect the fact that stuttering is a complex disorder that is not simply characterized. These definitions highlight the differences in perspective among stuttering experts. Several of the definitions are limited to the description of stuttering behaviors (e.g., prolongations, repetitions), from a listener-based perspective. Three include the perspective of the individual who stutters by including their perception of it (i.e., loss of control) or their reaction to it (e.g., apprehension, avoidance). The interpretation that disfluent episodes are involuntary in nature further reflects the perceptions of the person who stutters. A few definitions make inferences concerning the underlying cause of the disorder (e.g., psychological reaction to disfluency, timing disruptions). In all, the definitions reflect the changing trends within the field that have emphasized different aspects of the disorder at different times.

Consider how the components of these various definitions might apply to a particular case.

Laura's parents report that she has stuttered since she was 3 years old. At the time of her speech evaluation at age 7, she was found to repeat the first sounds and syllables of many words at the beginning of a phrase or sentence. At times, she seemed to posture her mouth and blink, and no sound could be heard. She made no attempt to avoid talking and had moments of normal fluency; suddenly the fluency would end, seemingly without warning. During her stuttering, she would often purse her lips, close her eyes, and appear as if she were trying to push out the word she was attempting to say. Laura's parents reported that she has expressed frustration at times over her inability to speak fluently.

In this brief case description, we recognize some of the common components of many definitions of stuttering:

1. Repetition and prolongation of sounds and syllables
2. Sudden or involuntary fluency interruptions
3. Often accompanied by physical signs of struggle
4. Often perceived negatively by the speaker

Therefore, despite the differences in definitions of stuttering, it is possible to observe the various components that these definitions present within a single case.

Theories of Stuttering

There is probably no clinical area in speech-language pathology that has generated more controversy than our understanding of the cause and nature of stuttering. The number of causative theories is astonishing and reflects an evolution in thought over the last century. At any given time, one theoretical position becomes more popular as research advances and changing social mores shift the clinical perspective on this disorder. As Van Riper indicated in 1971, the pendulum of popular and clinical opinion tends to swing between physical and psychological causes. Despite these shifts in theoretical perspective over time, we will clearly see the impact of these various theories reflected in approaches to intervention later in this chapter. Let us consider a few of the more prominent theoretical positions that have appeared over time.

Diagnosogenic Theory of Stuttering

Wendell Johnson is considered one of the founding fathers of the field of speech-language pathology. He spent his professional life studying the onset of stuttering. He concluded that the normal disfluencies experienced by many children were often labeled by their parents and other listeners as stuttering (Johnson, 1959). His **diagnosogenic theory of stuttering** was built on the belief that stuttering begins when normal disfluencies are labeled as stuttering. This theory recognized that normal children often pass through a period of nonfluent speech as they are in the process of language acquisition. Parents may hear their young children's normal episodes of disfluent speech and react negatively to them. They may call attention to their children's speech by telling them to "slow down" or to "take a deep breath and start over." Johnson suggested that these children are sensitive to their parents' reactions and become nervous or self-conscious about their speech. This leads them to become more disfluent in response, until stuttering becomes a learned behavior.

During his years of research at the University of Iowa, Johnson was never able to document any biological or psychological differences between those who do and do not stutter. However, his research occurred during a period that predated many more recent techniques for investigating potential biological correlates of the disorder. For many years, the lack of evidence to the contrary shaped the belief that people learned to stutter and that those who stutter were not otherwise different, as a group, from anyone else. For Johnson, the genesis of stuttering lay in the interactions between the listener and speaker. He believed that stuttering existed "in the ear of the listener." This causative idea is known as the *interaction theory of stuttering*.

As we saw earlier, Johnson (1955) defined stuttering as an "anticipatory, apprehensive, hypertonic avoidance reaction." In his view, the fear of stuttering is conditioned over time, and this fear becomes at least as great a problem as the actual stuttering. Sheehan (1970) considered the anticipatory fear of those who stutter and developed his *approach-avoidance theory*, so called because those who stutter were thought to be in a struggle over whether to speak. Feeling that they are going to stutter, they begin to use all kinds of avoidance behaviors (grimacing, eye blinking, and noise making) that they have learned instead of making an easy, open sound or syllable repetition. Sheehan suggested that without these distracting behaviors, "little stuttering would remain."

Psychological Aspects of Stuttering

As we saw earlier in the chapter, those who stutter can show physiological signs of stress and anxiety (Blood et al., 1994; Weber & Smith, 1990). These signs of anxiety associated with speaking led to the idea that stuttering might be a manifestation of an underlying emotional conflict (Blanton, 1965; Bryngelson, 1971; Glauber, 1958; Travis, 1971). Lee Travis (1971) was one of the strongest proponents of a psychological cause of stuttering. He developed the *repressed-need theory*. In his view, stuttering is the surface symptom of repressed needs, often disguised hostility. Children's primitive likes and wants, which may be socially unacceptable, are thwarted by those around them. "The parents not only induced in the child the drives of fear, guilt, and shame as checks on the child's primary drives, but they and their helpers in society perpetuated these checks" (p. 1020). Stuttering becomes a way to get around these societal checks.

In his classic chapter, "The Unspeakable Feelings of People with Special Reference to Stuttering" (Travis, 1971), Travis detailed what he considered to be the repressed needs and feelings of adults who stutter. Rather than working directly on stuttering, Travis and others (Barisara, 1962; Glauber, 1958) recommended psychotherapy with the intent of uncovering the hidden prohibitions that were at the root of an individual's stuttering. Travis concluded that "those stutterers who recovered and expressed what we have termed unspeakable feelings and thoughts did enjoy increased speech fluency and less anxiety over speech blocks" (p. 1032).

Psychotherapists commonly believe that most patients come for help when their personal misery is intense. The same is true for those who stutter. If they seek treatment because they are miserable about their stuttering, they may require counseling to develop some degree of perspective about their stuttering. In recognition of this, Bryngelson (1971) urged speech-language pathologists not to become so concerned with stuttering symptomatology that they neglect the "patient's need to be an acceptable human being." A counseling approach may reduce anxiety and negative self-image sufficiently to permit subsequent work on controlling fluency through behavioral techniques.

Neurological Theories of Stuttering

The idea that a physical, rather than psychological cause for stuttering existed was popular early in this century. One early organistic theory was the *cerebral dominance theory* of stuttering. The idea that a disturbance in the normal hemispheric specialization for and control of behaviors might underlie developmental disorders was made popular by Orton in the 1920s. Although Orton is best known for his work in dyslexia, the basic ideas of cerebral dominance were applied to stuttering as well. Likewise, Travis pursued the cerebral dominance theory before he embraced the repressed need theory of stuttering (see Van Riper, 1971, for a discussion).

The cerebral dominance theory recognized that one cerebral hemisphere (usually the left) plays a dominant role in speech and language. Although one hemisphere may lead in the sequencing of sounds and words, the actual execution of these sounds requires well-coordinated bilateral innervation. The paired muscles of speech production must receive their impulses at exactly the same time. The cerebral dominance theory hypothesized that the arrival of impulses at the peripheral muscles is poorly timed. This lack of precise timing is known as *dysphemia*. In the case of stuttering, the flow of nervous impulses to the paired speech musculature might break down with the slightest provocation. The bilateral coordination that is essential for normal speech would be compromised when one side received innervation before the other. As Van Riper (1971) put it, it is very difficult to lift "a wheelbarrow with one handle."

A number of early investigations seemed to support the cerebral dominance theory. Researchers used such techniques as dichotic listening, which involves simultaneous presentation of different auditory stimuli to each ear as a measure of brain lateralization. Others looked at the pattern of ongoing electrical activity measured from electrodes placed on the scalp. However, this early research failed to reveal robust differences between those who stutter and those who do not. In summarizing years of research on the topic, Andrews and colleagues (1983) concluded that there was no clear evidence that those who stutter have poorly lateralized speech or gross neurological abnormalities. Despite this history, biological investigations may yet enjoy rebirth with the advent of new biomedical technologies. For example, Ingham and colleagues used positron emission tomography (PET) to re-examine the issue of baseline physiological differences. They reported slight differences in bloodflow within the resting brain, which were localized to areas associated with speech and hearing functioning. However, the directionality (left vs. right hemisphere) of the effect was inconsistent (Ingham, Fox, Ingham, Zamarripa, Martin, Jerabek, & Cotton, 1996).

Recently, Perkins, Kent, and Curlee (1991) provided a paradigmatic shift away from the cerebral dominance theory with their *neuropsycholinguistic theory* of stuttering. This theory posits that disfluencies in general result from dyssynchronies in the timing and coordination of any one of the neural systems that support communication. This theory differentiates between disfluencies that are attritable to an identifiable interruption (e.g., a momentary distraction) and those unknown sources that interrupt or delay the neural systems that support communication. Stuttering only occurs when the speaker encounters a breakdown in fluency without apparent reason and tries to press through. The unknown nature of the breakdown accounts for the perception of a loss of control central to their definition of stuttering. The causes of these breakdowns may include biological factors (e.g., developmental, genetic, acquired factors) that predispose the nervous system to dyssynchronies, as well as environmental factors that may exacerbate processing problems. The complexity embraced by this theory gives it a great deal of flexibility in accounting for the range of symptoms that has made stuttering so difficult to characterize in any unified way.

Perkins and colleagues based their theory on a few fundamental premises. The first is that oral communication is a complex behavior that requires the coordination of multiple brain systems. For example, the linguistic and emotional components of communication appear to be served by different brain systems. Furthermore, there is evidence that different systems support different components of the linguistic aspects of communication (see Chapter 2). We can imagine that if the timing of just one of these components was delayed (e.g., retrieval of the specific sounds that make up the words), then the synchronization needed to bring sounds, grammar, and emotional content together into an utterance would be interrupted. Furthermore, the speaker would be unaware that phonemic retrieval was at heart of the processing breakdown, as this process happens without conscious awareness. From the perspective of this theory, it is easy to account for developmental disfluencies, which occur during that period when children are in the process of acquiring and coordinating the various components of oral language, and why they disappear as these systems mature. It would also account for why persistent stuttering sometimes seems to involve different linguistic components (e.g., sound repetitions, blocks at the beginning of syntactic clauses) during different stuttering episodes. This variation in the surface manifestation may relate to variation in the coordination of underlying neural systems involved in oral communication.

Motor Theories of Stuttering

The neurological theories of stuttering focused on the central nervous system as the source of fluency breakdown. With motor theories, we see a shift in focus to the peripheral nervous system control of speech. Schwartz (1976) was one of the leading supporters of the view that stuttering was caused by a disorder of the vocal mechanism. In 1976, he published a book with the relatively immodest title, *Stuttering Solved*, in which stuttering was attributed to an abnormal airway dilation reflex (ADR). Normally, the ADR is a rapid opening of the glottis during inspiration that occurs due to rising subglottal air pressure. It will occur reflexively if there is a subglottal obstruction and a need for a greater air supply. According to Schwartz, as the individual who stutters speaks, the vocal folds may reflexively open, creating a stuttering block. Phonation is suddenly out of synchrony for the speaker, whose mouth is already postured for the intended sound.

Work by others supported the idea of a laryngeal role in stuttering. Adams and Reis (1974) found less stuttering when individuals read a passage designed to have no voiceless sounds, thus maximizing time spent with the vocal folds together. Conture (1984) reported that the vocal folds, viewed fiberoptically, seemed to open and close inappropriately during stuttering. Furthermore, stutterers seem to need more neural response time for various verbal acts that require a quick reaction (Netsell & Daniel, 1974; Reich, Till, & Goldsmith, 1981; Till, Reich, Dickey, & Seiber, 1983). Although many investigations of motor functioning have focused on the speech mechanism, some have attempted to find evidence of a more generalized problem in motor functioning. However, these studies have not resulted in a clear consensus concerning peripheral motor movements.

Other investigators have suggested that the motor component of stuttering may involve both central and peripheral mechanisms. Neilson and Neilson (1991) proposed that the phenomenon of stuttering is the manifestation of inadequate or poorly functioning neural resources for speech production.

In their *Adaptive Model Theory*, they posited that speech production involves both systems involved in motor movements and feedback mechanisms that allow online, moment-to-moment monitoring of speech. However, the neural resources needed to accomplish these complex interactions may be limited or inefficient in those who stutter. They used an auditory tracking task during which subjects hear a tone and adjust the pitch of a second tone, by either hand or jaw movements, to match the first. This is parallel to hearing one's own speech and making motor adjustment to the vocal tract, based on the auditory feedback. Adults who stuttered were deficient at this task, even though they did well with a visual tracking task. Neilson and colleagues suggested that the source of this limitation may be in the cortical and subcortical components of the motor system (Neilson, Neilson, & O'Dwyer, 1992).

Evaluation of Developmental Stuttering

The broad goals of a fluency evaluation are to determine whether clinically significant disfluencies are present, to understand (to the extent possible) the nature and potential cause of these disfluencies, and to understand the impact of these disfluencies within the context of the client's life. As we have discussed throughout the chapter, everyone experiences disfluent speech from time to time, and many young children typically pass through a period of normal disfluency as they acquire language skills. One of the first jobs of the clinician is to assess the likelihood that the client's disfluencies fall outside the range of normal. Typically, the clinician will consider the types of disfluencies observed, their frequency and duration, associated nonspeech behaviors (e.g., struggle, avoidance), and the client's (or parents') attitudes toward the periods of disfluencies. The clinician may need to assess fluency in more than one context, because stuttering severity can change remarkably depending on the situation. School-based clinicians, for example, may observe a child in the classroom, out on the playground, or even request a taped speech sample from home. Different task demands, such as making a phone call or providing an explanation, often alters the frequency of disfluent speech as well.

As we will see later in this chapter, there are other forms of disfluent speech besides stuttering. Disorders such as cluttering can produce disruptions in fluency that are qualitatively different from stuttering. The clinician must also differentiate between the breakdowns in fluency that result from an expressive language disorder or that occur in conjunction with it. A sudden disruption of fluency, particularly in later childhood, may be the first sign of a neurological disorder, which would prompt referral to a neurologist. Formal and informal measures of speech and language, as well as a detailed case history, are invaluable in distinguishing among disorders that affect fluency. Failure to do so can lead to inappropriate attempts to manage these conditions.

Finally, the perceptions and attitudes of clients who stutter can have an enormous impact on the degree to which their lives are altered by stuttering and their readiness and motivation for change. Gaining this information is an ongoing process that starts with an initial interview and continues over the course of intervention. Clients may have very specific intervention goals ("I need to be able to conduct interviews for my job") or completely unrealistic ones ("I want my child to stop repeating himself all the time when he's excited"). A client's internal anxiety or lack of confidence about speaking may interfere with his or her ability to benefit from speech modifications. Unless we know what these attitudes and perceptions are, subsequent intervention may be fruitless or even offensive to the client.

Stuttering Therapy

Stuttering can be successfully treated. There are now numerous reports in the literature that show that clients can develop and maintain fluency over time (e.g., Blood, 1995; Hasbrouck, 1992; Onslow, Costa, Andrews, Harrison, & Packman, 1996; Packman, Onslow, & van Doorn, 1994). The primary questions in intervention are who should receive treatment, when it should begin, and what form it should take. For adults, the decision to seek treatment is a personal one. For children, a number of factors may influence parents' decisions to initiate treatment. Because many children who show early signs of stuttering will overcome this difficulty, some professionals have advocated vigilant waiting, with parent counseling, and regular monitoring of the child's speech (Zebrowski, 1995). In contrast, Starkweather (1990) noted a growing emphasis on early intervention for stuttering. He noted that a wait-and-see attitude is more risky than the cost of treatment for a child who would have recovered later on his or her own. In addition, he reported that recovery rates with treatment routinely exceed the rate of spontaneous recovery. Finally, there is some evidence to suggest that waiting to initiate treatment with the child who stutters is associated with more time spent in treatment. All these factors support the trend toward early intervention for children who show early signs of stuttering.

Parental Involvement

There are a number of components of fluency therapy. For children, one critical component may be the assessment of parent and family attitudes. Subsequent family involvement in the therapy process may be key to its success (e.g., Healey, Scott, & Ellis, 1995; Rustin & Cook, 1995). Kelly (1995) noted that mothers and fathers often differ in how they interact with their children and may require different advice and guidance in order to best improve their child's fluency. We can see the need to understand the parent's perspectives in the following case:

> Gerry and Anna had very different reactions to their 4-year-old son's periods of disfluency. Anna told of her anxiety whenever Gerry Jr. would stutter: "It hurts me to see him struggle. I don't want other kids teasing him, either." She went out of her way to "not call his attention to it." As a result, she would allow her son to interrupt her conversations with others, and often intervened when she thought his brothers and sisters might upset him and cause him to stutter. Gerry Sr. interpreted his wife's actions as "spoiling the boy." He didn't see his son's disfluencies as a problem. If anything, he thought that stuttering was one way that Gerry Jr. could get more attention in a household that included four other children. Needless to say, these differences in how each parent reacted to their son's disfluencies were a source of friction between them. It was apparent that intervention would have to include the parents' reactions to their child's disfluencies. This began with discussions to help the parents differentiate between the actual disfluent episodes and their reactions to it. The parents were provided with weekly "homework assignments" that were designed to help them develop workable and appropriate means of responding to specific situations that had been problematic from either a fluency or a social-interaction perspective (e.g., Should Gerry Jr. be allowed to interrupt at will?). For these parents, this approach allowed them to develop new perspectives on their son's disfluencies.

Parents may have many roles in the intervention process. They are often the ones to first seek help on behalf of their children and should be involved in setting long and short term goals for their child. As we saw in Gerry's case, parents may hold a range of attitudes and beliefs about stuttering. They may need information about what changes they can reasonably expect from therapy (Healey et al., 1995). They can also become invaluable assets in the intervention process. For example, Stephenson-Opsal & Bernstein-Ratner (1988) reported that slower parental speaking rates have been associated with positive outcome in therapy. Parents may be asked to reinforce the goals established for their children outside of the therapy session. Some intervention programs have used parents as the primary service provider with success (e.g. Craig, Hancock, Chang, McCreary, Shepley, Mccaul, Costello, Harding, Kehren, Masel, & Reilly, 1996).

Treatment Approaches

Speech therapy for stuttering in both children and adults may take different forms, depending primarily on the treatment philosophy of the speech-language pathologist. To simplify our discussion of the treatment of stuttering, let us identify three main approaches:

Psychological approach: Counseling and psychotherapy are given to improve the individual's attitude toward the problem, decrease avoidance, and create a better self-image.

Modifying speech: Therapy is given to facilitate speech that is free of stuttering by modifying rhythm, rate, and voicing.

Modifying the stuttering: Therapy is given to modify the stuttering behaviors, helping the individual to stutter more fluently.

Although these approaches can be thought of as philosophically and practically distinct, in practice, speech-language pathologists tend to combine and adapt these approaches to fit the needs of individual clients. Gregory (1995), for example, stated that therapy may emphasize a certain approach or component more than others at any given time. However, change for the client may involve behavioral and psychological components simultaneously. In order to understand the potential contributions of the individual approaches, we will consider them each separately.

Psychological Approach

You would not have to stutter for very long before you might develop negative feelings about speaking. Some go to great lengths to avoid speaking and begin to employ avoidance behaviors of various kinds (being silent, not using words they "know" will come out stuttered, and so on). Counseling or psychotherapy may help clients who stutter to see themselves as a whole, having a complete life that includes many different kinds of experiences, including stuttering. Such therapy is often helpful in giving clients who stutter a perspective on the problem, so that the stuttering does not loom larger than it should.

As mentioned earlier in this chapter, psychotherapy has been used as a treatment for stuttering, particularly as described by Travis (1971). From the psychotherapy view, stuttering is only a symptom of an underlying psychological conflict. To treat the symptom (stuttering) per se would not diminish the *need* for the stuttering. Thus, counseling and psychological therapy are needed to provide the client who stutters with a healthier mental perspective.

There is little documentation that a psychotherapeutic approach alone will give patients permanent fluency. However, clinicians frequently find that counseling can be a valuable support to programs that focus on the behavioral aspects of stuttering. Cooper and Cooper (1995) stated that stuttering can be thought of as having three components (the ABCs): *A*ffective (feelings), *B*ehaviors (moments of stuttering), and *C*ognitive (thoughts and attitudes). They expressed that "While the Bs (disfluencies) may be the most attention-getting aspect of the problem, the As and Cs are far more significant in assessing and treating stuttering syndromes" (p.127). Their intervention program includes specific goals to reinforce feelings, attitudes, and behaviors that enhance fluency. In some cases, a poor self-concept, which may result from constant struggles with fluency, may begin to taint reality, imposing itself on every dimension of the patient's life. For example, some who stutter blame stuttering for all their misfortunes. A woman who stuttered told us, "If I didn't stutter, I would have gone on to law school, but no one wants to go see a lawyer who can't even say, 'Your Honor,' don't you agree?" A poor self-image begins to taint reality, imposing itself on every dimension of the patient's life. Counseling and psychotherapy have been found to be most important in giving the stuttering client a better (more realistic) self-concept (Wingate, 1976).

Modifying Speech

In the treatment of stuttering during the mid-1970s, there was a shift away from its modification and toward the shaping of fluent speech. It remains an important component of many current intervention methods today (e.g., Cooper & Cooper, 1991; Healey & Scott, 1995; Ramig & Bennet, 1995). The fluency-shaping approach came directly out of learning theory, in which a baseline behavior (such as a baseline of fluency) is followed by shaping approaches designed to extend or refine that behavior. One of the early practitioners of fluency shaping was Webster (1974), who established fluency by primarily mastering five target behaviors: the stretched syllable, syllable transition, slow change, full breath, and gentle voicing onsets. Webster's patients were required to spend three weeks of intensive, daily training mastering the five target behaviors in sequence. Schwartz (1976) required massive therapy practice (as much as three months of three-times weekly therapy, two hours per day) to overcome the laryngeal airway problem (airway dilation reflex), which he felt precipitates the stuttering. Schwartz emphasized the preparation for speech, attempting to establish a passive flow of air to initiate easy-onset voicing. In fluency shaping, effort is made to find an easy, fluent way of speaking (easy onset, reduced rate, and prolonged speech). Massive practice is then used to establish this fluent speech as a method of talking. There is less need for a change of attitude through counseling because this change is "thought to occur secondary to improved speech control" (Guyette & Baumgartner, 1988, p. 646).

Wingate (1976) offered a fluency-shaping program that focused on the rate and prosodic flow of speech. In stuttering, these aspects are seriously interrupted. To establish more normal fluency, Wingate recommended the rate of speech be slowed down, primarily by prolonging the length of vowels. As he explained in his monograph, *Stuttering and Laryngeal Behavior: A Review*, Starkweather (1982) stated that although Wingate's vowel lengthening is effective in reducing stuttering, it is effective also because of the reduced rate of speaking and the regularity of rhythm that are induced. Adams (1974) shaped fluency by focusing on the timing and smoothness of voicing onsets, with some attention given to extending the duration and ease of expiratory airflow. Starkweather concluded that although some stuttering may be precipitated by laryngeal-system disfunction, some is also the result of an oral-system breakdown (poor coordination of lips, tongue, and jaw).

Techniques that facilitate fluency are highly individualized for each person who stutters. What works for one person may not be helpful for another. Among the battery of techniques used by the speech-language pathologist are prolonging speech (usually achieved by prolonging vowels), reducing speaking rate and maintaining fluency, increasing breathiness at the onset of speech, and otherwise reducing tension during speech (Perkins, 1984; Schwartz, 1976; Shames & Florence, 1980). Such symptomatic therapy for stuttering as fluency shaping is often aided by some counseling, designed to give the client who stutters a more positive perspective toward communication (Cheasman, 1983).

Modifying the Stuttering

At the turn of the century in the United States, the primary treatment for stuttering was to work on easy voicing onsets, developing a rhythm of some kind and maintaining speech fluency. Modifying the stuttering (instead of the fluent speech) developed as an opposite form of therapy and is still widely used as a treatment for stuttering. In modifying stuttering, the belief is "that the root of stuttering is in the struggle to be fluent," as described by Perkins (1980). Consequently, most such therapy is of a dual nature: improving the attitude toward speaking and learning to stutter with less effort and reduced tension.

After a lifetime's experience, both first hand and clinical, with the problem of stuttering, Van Riper (1990) concluded, "The stutterer already knows how to be fluent. What he doesn't know is how to stutter. He can be taught to stutter so easily and briefly that he can have very adequate communication skills. Moreover, when he discovers he can stutter without struggle or avoidance most of his frustration and other negative emotions will subside" (p. 318). Many clinicians agree with this position. In modifying the stuttering, the belief is "that the root of stuttering is in the struggle to be fluent," as described by Perkins (1980). Others (e.g., Healey & Scott, 1995) turned to stuttering modification techniques for clients whose stuttering included marked avoidance behaviors or who were unsuccessful with fluency enhancement techniques alone.

Clients can be taught to stutter with less tension, avoidance, and interruption to the flow of communication with specific techniques (Peters & Guitar, 1991). Treatment may include intentional stuttering that is relaxed in order to reduce the fear and embarrassment associated with involuntary stuttering episodes. A client's awareness of the difference between typical stuttering and the new, modified stuttering may be enhanced by practice that contrasts tense, struggle-prone stuttering with intentional, easy stuttering, and nonstuttered speech. Clients may learn to monitor their ongoing speech for instances of problematic disfluencies. These can be "cancelled" by pausing after the onset of a stuttered word and a fresh attempt at the word with easy, slower, struggle-free stuttering.

Other Disorders of Fluency

Cluttering

Clinical Signs

Another clinical disorder associated with altered fluency is **cluttering**. Like those who stutter, children who are described as clutterers have abnormally high frequencies of word and phrase repetitions. In contrast to stuttering, cluttering involves fewer sound or syllable-level disfluencies (e.g., prolongations, sound repetitions). In addition, cluttering usually occurs without signs of struggle, tension, or avoidance that occur in stuttering (St. Louis, Hinzman, & Hull, 1985). Although the prevalence of cluttering is unknown, speech-language pathologists in the United States tend to report familiarity with a few cases of cluttering in their practices. Children are more likely than adults to be seen by a speech-language pathologist for cluttering, and the prevalence in caseloads declines from grades 1 to 12.

Wood (1971) defined cluttering as "rapid, nervous speech marked by omissions of sounds and syllables" (p. 10). This definition gives equal prominence to the symptoms of rapid rate and articulatory errors and is thus is similar to that of Wingate (1978), who defined cluttering as "a fluency disorder of unknown origin characterized by sporadically excessive rate and incomplete and distorted articulation" (p. 268). In one of the few monographs written on the topic, Arnold (1966) reviewed a detailed European literature, which described cluttering as a disorder that included symptoms of rapid rate, faulty articulation, and related reading and writing problems. All three speech-language problems were often associated with "disorders of lateral dominance." Wall (1988) said that cluttering is characterized by rapid speed and disordered articulation but added this important part to the definition: "a lack of awareness of the problem on the part of the speaker" (p. 637). It would appear that most clutterers, unlike stutterers, are not upset by their continuing disfluency.

Clutterers speak much faster than stutterers; in fact, the word *tachyphemia*, which is sometimes used as a synonym for cluttering (although it is not), literally means "rapid speech." Clutterers may be differentiated from stutterers by the former's slurred and omitted phonemes, periods of unusually rapid rate of speech, lack of awareness of their poor speech, and the fact that they neither avoid nor feel tense about the act of speaking. In addition, clutterers are often observed to exhibit faulty thought processes, some problems in auditory language comprehension, and some problems in reading and writing (St. Louis et al., 1985). Such problems may lead services for language and learning disabilities during the school years (St. Louis & Hinzman, 1986). By combining the views of several writers, let us define cluttering:

> Cluttering is rapid speech characterized by fluency and articulation errors, sometimes accompanied by language difficulties, usually without the speaker's awareness or concern.

Treatment of Cluttering

Although both stuttering and cluttering involve disfluencies, the differences between the two disorders dictate very different treatment approaches. St. Louis and Meyers (1995) offered a series of working principles to guide treatment of cluttering. St. Louis and Meyers begin with a recognition that stuttering and cluttering are, in fact, independent disorders. For the child who clutters, disfluencies are a direct combination of fast speaking rate combined with a weak ability to handle the phonologic, syntactic, or semantic aspects of spoken language.

Children who clutter can increase their fluency by slowing their rate. However, as anyone who has tried to change their speaking rate knows (e.g., slowing down speech for a class presentation), maintaining a different speaking rate at the same time one is thinking about what to say is difficult. We can use direct methods to address rate. The speaker might pace his or her speaking rate to different rates of a metronome to raise awareness about his or her rate of speech. Later, a clinician might provide visual feedback, such as an arrow indicator of whether speech is too fast, just fine, or too slow. The following case provides an example of an indirect method of addressing rate, by having the speaker alter loudness (which later can be reduced to normal levels when rate has been reduced). This 17-year-old was asked to listen to a recording of himself followed by one of a normal male speaker near the client's age:

Clinician: You must talk twice as fast as that other kid. Did you hear that?

Client: He donna wanna go fatter than me.

Clinician: Maybe if we just had you talk a little louder, like this: "I'm going to speak loudly for a bit." That sure makes me sound better, doesn't it?

Client: Talin' loud is easy for me. I tal' loud at home and they all hear me.

Clinician: Well, let's make a recording of you talking louder, and we'll see how that sounds.

Rather than working on the components of rate and articulation, both of which were far from normal in this case, the clinician elected to work holistically on making the patient aware that he could speak better by changing his speaking habits. Given a tangible method of changing his speech, the patient could better monitor his speech when he spoke more loudly, which served to slow the rate of speech and improve his articulation.

Sometimes, indirect methods can be used to decrease rate, by concentrating on another element of speech or language. For example, if a child's poor articulation contributes to cluttering, exercises designed to remediate articulation may have the side effect of reducing speaking rate. Likewise, if fluency breakdowns are occurring because of linguistic deficits such as word finding problems or difficulty with syntactic constructions, then it makes sense to remediate these linguistic problems directly. In many cases, improved fluency is a side effect of a linguistic approach.

St. Louis and Meyers (1995) pointed out that a synergistic approach that focuses on improved communication may be best. Linguistic formulation problems may be aided when rate is slowed because the individual has more time to organize his ideas and give them linguistic structure. Improved self-monitoring may help the individual concentrate on correct articulation, which in turn, will tend to slow speaking rate. Word finding strategies may help prevent semantic breakdowns that reduce fluency. This dynamic approach may also include coordinated services with others (e.g., family members, teachers, psychologists) who can help to manage social and educational aspects associated with this disorder.

Acquired Disfluency

Most adults who stutter have a history of childhood stuttering. There are, however, numerous cases of previously fluent adults who have an abrupt onset of stuttering (Market, Montague, Buffalo, & Drummond, 1990). In most instances, acquired stuttering is associated with neurological damage from a stroke, head injury, progressive neurological disease, or exposure to toxins (Helm-Estabrooks, 1998; Ringo & Dietrich, 1995). Less frequently, acquired stuttering may have a psychological origin related to anxiety, depression, or other psychological disturbance (Baumgartner & Duffy, 1997). Although the symptoms of neurogenic and psychogenic stuttering may be difficult to distinguish from one another, a review of the patient's history is usually helpful in distinguishing its probable cause. We were asked recently to help interpret the disfluencies of 69-year-old man.

Mr. Nelson was referred by his neurologist following a series of transient ischemic attacks or possibly small strokes. The most recent episode was followed by what appeared to be stuttering. The disruption of speech was a concern to Mr. Nelson who was a highly educated, articulate man and a frequent public speaker as president of a volunteer organization. Despite his neurological history, the referral letter from the neurologist described Mr. Nelson's disfluency as "a functional acquired stuttering, possibly secondary to some sort of depression or anxiety."

Prior to his visit, Mr. Nelson was asked to write a narrative of his recent medical history to describe any changes in his speech or language. His description clarified that he had experienced two episodes that involved neurological signs that were about two years apart. The first episode included persistent numbness and tingling on the left side of his body that lasted for about a week. The second included a more dramatic onset of right-sided weakness and some problems speaking. Mr. Nelson was hospitalized following the second episode and put on blood thinning medication because of his risk for stroke. He wrote that he was recovering fully from the second episode but he began to have increasing difficulty talking within a month. He had some trouble coming up with the names of things, but his most vexing problem was stuttering which he described as having "a lot of hesitation" in his speech.

An evaluation of Mr. Nelson's speech revealed many disfluencies. For example, as he read a 100-word passage aloud, he was disfluent on 10 words: 5 were tense pauses, 3 were sound prolongations, and 2 were sound repetitions. His conversational speech was similarly disrupted by pauses—although his articulators were postured correctly to produce a word, he seemed unable to proceed. No secondary stuttering characteristics such as facial grimacing, hand clenching, or head movements were observed. In fact, Mr. Nelson appeared to be annoyed by his disfluencies, but not overly upset by them.

Mr. Nelson's disfluencies and his medical history suggested that he had acquired neurogenic stuttering. Although an MRI brain scan revealed some small areas of white matter changes, and it was not clear that Mr. Nelson had suffered a stroke, his medical history clearly indicated some compromise of his neurological functions. Neurogenic stuttering is not limited to damage to a particular region of the brain, but has been related to left and right hemisphere damage, cortical and subcortical damage, as well as damage to the cerebellum and brainstem. It co-occurs with aphasia about a third of the time (Baumgartner & Duffy, 1997). In Mr. Nelson's case, he evidenced some mild word finding problems (anomia), but his overall performance was excellent for spoken and written language.

Neurogenic versus Developmental Stuttering

Neurogenic stuttering refers to an acquired disruption of fluency that can be linked with an identifiable neurological event, such as a stroke or head injury. This is in contrast to developmental stuttering, which may also have an underlying neurological component as described earlier. The disruptions in normal speech production that are observed in neurogenic disfluency are similar in some ways to developmental stuttering, but there are some differences. Whereas instances of disfluency in developmental stuttering occur most often on words that start with consonants than with vowels, neurogenic stuttering occurs similarly often on words beginning with consonants and vowels (Ringo & Dietrich, 1995). Likewise neurogenic stuttering occurs equally often on substantive and function words, whereas content words are more likely to be stuttered by adults who have stuttered since childhood. As was true with Mr. Nelson, most individuals with neurogenic stuttering are notably free of anxiety about their speech and characteristics such as accessory behaviors and facial tension that are common in stuttering having a developmental origin.

Neurogenic versus Psychogenic Stuttering

Mr. Nelson's disfluencies differed from psychogenic stuttering in several ways. Although psychogenic stuttering can be similar to neurogenic stuttering, Baumgartner and Duffy (1997) found several distinguishing features. Unlike neurogenic stuttering, psychogenic stuttering may be intermittent and associated with specific speaking situations, struggle behaviors and other signs of anxiety are not uncommon, and unusual or bizarre speech patterns that are not observed in other speech or language disorders, such as using "me" for the pronoun "I," are often present. Moreover psychogenic stuttering usually responds quickly to behavioral treatment.

Intervention

After we determined that Mr. Nelson's disfluencies were consistent with those of a neurogenic origin, we needed to decide whether treatment was warranted. Cases reviewed in the literature indicated that neurogenic stuttering often resolves on its own without treatment within a month or two of onset. Therefore, we assured Mr. Nelson that his stuttering appeared to be related to the neurological episodes he had experienced and told him that we suspected his fluency would improve on its own. He was scheduled for a follow-up visit 6 weeks later, at which time he showed considerable improvement in fluency. Some brief pauses were still observed as he spoke, but they were relatively subtle, and he reported that they were not as bothersome to him. In fact, he said that he was most annoyed by his occasional word finding difficulty at that time, a problem he minimized during his initial visit.

Had Mr. Nelson's stuttering persisted and had he wanted treatment, we might have treated it behaviorally in much the same way as developmental stuttering. Approaches that enhance fluency such as slowed speaking rate and easy onset of voicing have been used with success in neurogenic stuttering (Market et al., 1990). Fluency can also be facilitated by pacing speech production so that it is not disrupted by hesitations, prolongations, or repetitions (Helm-Estabrooks, 1998). In some cases, medications have been shown to improve neurogenic disfluency, although some cases of acquired dysfluency appear to have been caused by medication (reviewed in Helm-Estabrooks, 1998). Thus, a careful a review of a patient's history and medications are essential in instances of adult-onset disfluency.

Clinical Problem Solving

Annette first came to the attention of the school speech-language pathologist through a phone call from the district director of Special Education. Annette's parents had been phoning both his office and home requesting that their daughter be treated for her stuttering. Annette's father was an adult stutterer, and both parents wanted Annette's speech to be "corrected before her stuttering became permanent." They also reported that Annette began speaking somewhat late, but they had no concerns about her speech or language other than the stuttering. Annette was enrolling in kindergarten that fall. After school began, the clinician was able to observe Annette on several occasions in the classroom, during which her speech was consistently fluent. The clinician reported her observations to the parent, advising them to allow Annette time to settle into the school routine. The parents were adamant that Annette stuttered frequently at home and were insistent that she be treated through the school. At the parents urging, the clinician set up a classroom monitoring program to permit the classroom teacher to systematically document Annette's speech. From September to December, only two disfluent episodes were noted. After receiving this news, the parents sent the clinician a taped sample of Annette's speech at home. The tape revealed frequent episodes of disfluent speech, including part word repetitions, sound prolongations, and silent episodes, which may well have reflected blocks.

1. Do you think that Annette does stutter? What makes you think so/not?
2. What risk factors for stuttering appear in Annette's history?
3. Select two theories and discuss how this case profile might relate to each theory.
4. Speculate on the reasons why Annette may stutter at home, but not in her new kindergarten.
5. Do you think that Annette should receive therapy for stuttering? If so, what factors would you consider in developing a plan of intervention for Annette?

References

Adams, M.R. (1974). A physiologic and aerodynamic interpretation of fluent and stuttered speech. *Journal of Fluency Disorders, 1*: 35–67.

Adams, M.R. (1978). Stuttering theory, research, and therapy: The present and future. *Journal of Fluency Disorders, 3*:139–147.

Adams, M.R., & Reis, R. (1974). Influence of the onset of phonation on the frequency stuttering, a replication and re-evaluation. *Journal of Speech and Hearing Research, 17*: 752–754.

Andrews, C., Craig, A., Feyer, A., Haddinott, S., Neilson, M., & Howle, P. (1983). Stuttering: A review of research findings and theories circa 1982. *Journal of Speech and Hearing Disorders, 48*: 226-245.

Andrews, C., & Harris, M. (1964). *The Syndrome of Stuttering.* London: Heinemann Dynamic Medical Books.

Arnold, C. (1966). *Studies in Tachyphemia: An Investigation of Cluttering and General Language Disability.* New York: Speech Rehabilitation Institute.

Baumgartner, J., & Duffy, J.R. (1997). Psychogenic stuttering in adults with and without neurologic disease. *Journal of Medical Speech-Language Pathology, 5*, 75–95.

Barisara, D. (1962). *The Psychotherapy of Stuttering.* Springfield, IL: Charles C. Thomas.

Blanton, S. (1965). Stuttering. In D. Barbara (Ed.), *New Directions in Stuttering.* Springfield, IL: Charles C. Thomas.

Blood, G.W. (1995). A behavioral-cognitive therapy program for adults who stutter: Computers and counseling. *Journal of Communication Disorders, 28*, 165–180.

Blood, G.W., Blood, I.M., Bennett, S., Simpson, K.C., & Susman, E.J. (1994). Subjective anxiety measurements and cortisol responses in adults who stutter. *Journal of Speech and Hearing Research, 37*: 760–768.

Bryngelson, B. (1971). Speech and personality. In L. Travis (Ed.), *Handbook of Speech Pathology and Audiology.* Englewood Cliffs, NJ: Prentice Hall.

Cheasman, C. (1983). Therapy for adults: An evaluation of current techniques for establishing fluency. In P. Dalton (Ed.), *Approaches to the Treatment of Stuttering.* London: Croom Helm.

Conture, E.C. (1984). Observing laryngeal movements of stuttering. In R.F. Curlee & W.H. Perkins (Eds.), *Nature and Treatment of Stuttering: New Directions.* San Diego: College-Hill Press.

Conture, E.G. (1990). Childhood stuttering: What is it and who does it? *ASHA Report Series, 18*: 2–14.

Conture, E.G., & Kelly, E.M. (1991). Young stutterers' nonspeech behaviors during stuttering. *Journal of Speech and Hearing Research, 34*: 1041–1056.

Cooper, E.B., & Cooper, C.S. (1991). *Personalized Fluency Control Therapy—Revised.* New York: DLM-Teaching Resources.

Cooper, E.B., & Cooper, C.S. (1995). Treating fluency disordered adolescents. *Journal of Communication Disorders, 28*: 125–142.

Cooper, E.B., & Cooper, C.S. (1996). Clinicians attitudes towards stuttering: Two decades of change. *Journal of Fluency Disorders, 21*: 119–135.

Craig, A. (1990). An investigation between anxiety and stuttering. *Journal of Speech and Hearing Disorders, 55*, 290-294.

Craig, A., Hancock, K., Chang, E., Mccreay, C., Shepley, A., Mccaul, A., Costello, D., Harding, S., Kehren, R., Masel, C., & Reilly, K. (1996). A controlled clinical trial for stuttering in persons age 9–14 years. *Journal of Speech and Hearing Research, 39*: 808–826.

Curlee, R. F. (1980). A case selection strategy for young disfluent children. *Seminars in Speech, Language, Hearing, 1*: 277-287.

Glauber, I.P.(1958). The psychoanalysis of stuttering. In J. Eisenson (Ed.), *Stuttering. A Symposium.* New York: Harper and Row.

Gregory, H. (1995). Analysis and commentary. *Language, Speech, and Hearing Services in Schools, 26*, 196-200.

Guyette, T.W., & Baumgartner, J.M. (1988). Stuttering in the adult. In N.J. Lass, L.V. McReynolds, J.L. Northern, & D.E. Yoder (Eds.), *Handbook of Speech-Language Pathology & Audiology.* Philadelphia: B.C. Decker.

Hasbrouck, J.M. (1992). FAMC intensive stuttering treatment program: Ten years of implementation. *Military Medicine, 157*: 244-247.

Healey, E.C., & Scott, L.A. (1995). Strategies for treating elementary school-age children who stutter: An integrative approach. *Language, Speech, and Hearing Services in Schools, 26*: 151–161.

Healey, E.C., Scott, L.A., & Ellis, G. (1995). Decision making in the treatment of school-age children who stutter. *Journal of Communciation Disorders, 28*: 107–124.

Helm-Estabrooks, N. (1998). Stuttering associated with acquired neurological disorders. In R. F. Curlee (Ed.), *Stuttering and Related Disorders of Fluency* (pp. 255–268). New York: Thieme Medical Publishers.

Howie, P.M. (1981). Concordance for stuttering in monozygotic and dizygotic twin pairs. *Journal of Speech and Hearing Research, 24*: 317–321.

Hull, F.M., Mielke, P.W., Willeford, J.A., & Timmons, R.J. (1976). *National Speech and Hearing Survey.* Final Report, Project 50978. Washington, DC: Office of Education, Bureau of Education for the Handicapped, Department of Health, Education, and Welfare.

Ingham, R.J., Fox, P.T., Ingham, J.C., Zamarripa, F., Martin, C., Jerabek, P., & Cotton, J. (1996). *Journal of Speech and Hearing Research, 39*: 1208–1227.

Janssen, P., Kraaimaat, F., & Brutten, G. (1990). Relationship between stutterers' genetic history and speech-as-sociated variables. *Journal of Fluency Disorders, 15*: 39–48.

Johnson, W. (1955). A study of the onset and development of stuttering. In W. Johnson & R.R. Leutenegger (Eds.), *Stuttering in Children and Adults.* Minneapolis: University of Minnesota Press.

Johnson, W. (1959). *The Onset of Stuttering.* Minneapolis: University of Minnesota Press.

Kalinowski, J., Lerman, J., & Watt, J. (1987). A preliminary examination of the perceptions of self and others in stutterers and nonstutterers. *Journal of Fluency Disorders, 12*: 317–331.

Kelly, E.M. (1995). Parents as partners: Including mothers and fathers in the treatment of children who stutter. *Journal of Communciation Disorders, 28*: 93–106.

Kidd, K.K. (1980). Genetic models of stutttering. *Journal of Fluency Disorders, 5*: 187-202.

Market, K.W., Montague, J.C., Buffalo, M.D. & Drummond, S.S. (1990). Acquired stuttering: Descriptive data and treatment outcome. *Journal of Fluency Disorders, 15*: 221-233.

Miller, S., & Watson, B.C. (1992). The relationship between communication attitude, anxiety and depression in stutterers and nonstutterers. *Journal of Speech and Hearing Research, 34*: 789–798.

Morley, M.E. (1952). A ten year survey of speech disorders among university students. *Journal of Speech and Hearing Disorders, 17*: 25–31.

Morley M.F. (1972). *The Development and Disorders of Speech in Childhood.* Edinburgh: Churchill Livingstone.

National Institutes of Deafness & Other Communication Disorders. (1992). Research in Human Communciation. (NIH Publication No. 93–3562.) Washington, DC: U.S. Governmental Printing Office.

Neilson, M.D., & Neilson, P.D. (1991). Adaptive model theory of speech motor control and stuttering. In H.F.M. Peters, W. Hulstijn, & C.W. Starkweather (Eds.), *Speech Motor Control and Stuttering.* New York: Excerpta Medica.

Neilson, P.D., Neilson, M.D., & O'Dwyer, N.J. (1992). Adaptive model theory: Application to disorders of motor control. In J.J. Summers (Ed.), *Approaches to the Study of Motor Control and Learning.* Amsterdam: Elsevier Science Publishers.

Netsell, R., & Daniel, B. (1974). Neural and mechanical response time for speech product ion. *Journal of Speech and Hearing Research, 17*: 608–618.

Onslow, M., Costa, L., Andrews, C., Harrison, E., & Packman, A. (1996). Speech outcomes of a prolonged-speech treatment of stuttering. *Journal of Speech and Hearing Research, 39*, 734–749.

Packman, A., Onslow, M., & van Doorn, J. (1994). Prolonged speech and modification of stuttering: Perceptual, acoustic, and electroglottographic data. *Journal of Speech and Hearing Research, 39*, 724–737.

Perkins, W. H. (1977). *Speech Pathology: An Applied Behavioral Science.* St. Louis: C. V. Mosby.

Perkins, W.H. (1980). Disorders of speech. In T. Hixon, L. Shriberg, & J. Saxman (Eds.), *Introduction to Communication Disorders.* Englewood Cliffs, NJ: Prentice Hall.

Perkins, W.H. (1984). Techniques for establishing fluency. In W.H. Perkins (Ed.), *Stuttering Disorders.* New York: Thieme Stratton.

Perkins, W.H., Kent, R.D., & Curlee, R.F. (1991). A theory of neuropsycholinguistic function in stuttering. *Journal of Speech and Hearing Research, 34*: 734–752.

Peters, T.J., & Guitar, B. (1991). *Stuttering: An Integrated Approach to its Nature and Treatment.* Baltimore, MD: Williams & Wilkins.

Ramig, P.R., & Bennett, E.M. (1995). Working with 7- to 12-year-old children who stutter: Ideas for intervention in the public schools. *Language, Speech, and Hearing Services in Schools, 26*: 138–150.

Reich, A., Till, J., & Goldsmith, H. (1981). Laryngeal and manual reaction times of stuttering and nonstuttering adults. *Journal of Speech and Hearing Research, 24*: 192–196.

Ringo, C.C., & Dientrich, S. (1995). Neurogenic stuttering: An analysis and critique. *Journal of Medical Speech-Language Pathology, 3*(2): 111–122.

Rustin, L., & Cook, F. (1995). Parental involvement in treatment of stuttering. *Language, Speech, and Hearing Services in Schools, 26*: 127–137.

Shcwartz, M.F. (1974). The core of the stuttering block. *Journal of Speech and Hearing Disorders, 39*: 169–177.

Schwartz, M. F. (1976). *Stuttering Solved.* Philadelphia: Lippincott.

Schwartz, H.D., Zebrowski, P.M., & Conture, E.G. (1991). Behaviors at the onset of stuttering. *Journal of Fluency Disorders, 15*: 77–86.

Shames, G.H., & Florence, C.L. (1980). *Stutter-free Speech: A Goal of Therapy.* Columbus, OH: Charles E. Merrill.

Sheehan, J.G. (1970). *Stuttering: Research and Therapy.* New York: Harper and Row.

Speech Foundation of America (1987). *Self-Therapy for the Stutterer* (6th ed.). Publication 12. Memphis, TN: Speech Foundation of America.

St. Louis, K.O., & Hinzman, A.R. (1986). Studies of cluttering: Perceptions of cluttering by speech-language pathologists and educators. *Journal of Fluency Disorders, 11*: 131–149.

St. Louis, K.O., Hinzman, A.R., & Hull, F.M. (1985). Studies of cluttering: Disfluency and language measures in young possible clutterers and stutterers. *Journal of Fluency Disorders, 10*: 151–172.

St. Louis, K.O., & Meyers, F.L. (1995). Clinical management of cluttering. *Language, Speech, and Hearing Services in Schools, 26*: 187–195.

Starkweather, C.W. (1982). *Stuttering and Laryngeal Behaviors: A Review* (ASHA Monograph 21). Rockville, MD: American Speech-Language-Hearing Association.

Starkweather, C.W. (1990). Current trends in therapy for stuttering children and suggestions for future resarch. *ASHA Report Series, 18*: 82–90.

Stephenson-Opsal, D., & Bernstein-Ratner, N. (1988). Maternal speech rate modification and childhood stuttering. *Journal of Fluency Disorders, 13*: 49–56.

Till, J., Reich, A., Dickey, 5., & Seiber, J. (1983). Phonatory and manual reaction times of stuttering and nonstuttering children. *Journal of Speech and Hearing Research, 26*: 171–180.

Travis, L.E. (1971). The unspeakable feelings of people with special reference to stuttering. In L.D. Travis (Ed.), *Handbook of Speech Pathology and Audiology* (2nd ed.). Englewood Cliffs, NJ: Prentice Hall.

Van Riper, C. (1971). *The Nature of Stuttering.* Englewood Cliffs, NJ: Prentice Hall.

Van Riper, C. (1973). *The Treatment of Stuttering.* Englewood Cliffs, NJ: Prentice Hall.

Van Riper, C. (1990). Final thoughts about stuttering. *Journal of Fluency Disorders, 15*: 317–318.

Wall, M.J. (1988). Disfluency in the child. In N.J. Lass, L.V. McReynolds, J.L. Northern, & D.E. Yoder (Eds.), *Handbook of Speech-Language Pathology and Audiology*. Philadelphia: B. C. Decker.

Weber, C.M., & Smith, A. (1990). Autonomic correlates of stuttering and speech assessed in a range of experimental tasks. *Journal of Speech and Hearing Research*, *33*: 690–706.

Webster, R. (1974). A behavioral analysis of stuttering: Treatment and theory. In K. Calhoun, H. Adams, & K. Mitchell (Eds.), *Innovative Treatment Methods in Psychopathology*. New York: Wiley.

West, R. (1958). An agnostic's speculations about stuttering. In J. Eisenson (Ed.), *Stuttering: A Symposium*. New York: Harper and Row.

Wingate, M.E. (1962). Personality needs of stutterers. *Logos*, *5*: 35–37.

Wingate, M.E. (1976). *Stuttering Theory and Treatment*. New York: Irvington.

Wingate, M.E. (1978). Disorders of fluency. In P. Skinner & R. Shelton (Eds.), *Speech, Language, Hearing, Normal Processes and Disorders*. Reading, MA: Addison-Wesley.

Wood, K.S. (1971). Definitions and terms. In L.D. Travis (Ed.), *Handbook of Speech Pathology and Audiology* (2nd ed.). Englewood Cliffs, NJ: Prentice Hall.

World Health Organization. (1977). *Manual of the International Statistical Classification of Diseases, Injuries, and Causes of Death*, Vol. I. Geneva: WHO.

Yairi, E. (1983). The onset of stuttering in two- and three-year-old children: A preliminary report. *Journal of Speech and Hearing Disorders*, *48*: 171–178.

Yairi, E., & Ambrose, N. (1992). Onset of stuttering in preschool children: Selected factors. *Journal of Speech and Hearing Research*, *35*: 782–788.

Yairi, E., Ambrose, N.G., & Cox, N. (1993). Genetic aspects of early childhood stuttering. *Journal of Speech and Hearing Research*, *36*: 701–706.

Yairi, E., Ambrose, N.G., & Cox, N. (1996). Genetics of stuttering: A critical review. *Journal of Speech and Hearing Research*, *39*: 771–784.

Yairi, E., Ambrose, N.G., Paden, E.P., & Throneburg, R.N. (1996) Predictive factors of persistence and recovery: Pathways of childhood stuttering. *Journal of Communication Disorders*, *29*: 51–77

Young, M. A. (1975). Onset, prevalence, and recovery from stuttering. *Journal of Speech and Hearing Disorders*, *40*: 49–58.

Zebrowski, P.M. (1995). The topology of a beginning stutterer. *Journal of Communication Disorders*, *28*: 75–92.

Disorders of the Voice and Swallowing Disorders

Julie Barkmeier

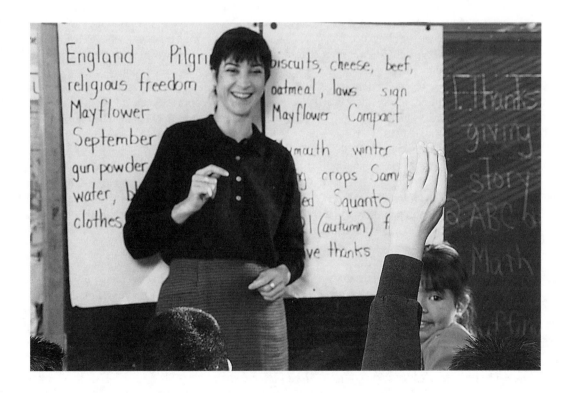

Preview

The larynx serves to protect the airway during swallowing and generates sound during speech production. Damage to the larynx or structures of the vocal tract may result in voice or swallowing problems. Most people experience problems with voice due to improper use of the vocal mechanism. Such voice disorders frequently can be treated or improved by therapy that identifies damaging behaviors and teaches better methods of voice production. Voice disorders related to physical damage to the vocal mechanism may be effectively treated with voice therapy, although, in some cases, medical intervention is warranted. Swallowing disorders can often be improved by adapting postures and food consistencies during eating or with exercises to strengthen oral and pharyngeal structures.

Voice Disorders

As described in Chapter 3, vocal fold vibrations produce sound, which is modified by the vocal tract. Individual differences in the vocal mechanism and its resonance characteristics contribute to the individual characteristics of each person's voice. Many temporary conditions, such as a stuffy nose or the effects of prolonged yelling, can change the voice. These types of problems tend to resolve on their own and typically do not require professional attention. However, permanent changes to the voice may occur with damage or disease that require professional intervention.

The exact number of individuals who experience voice disorders in the population is not known. For children, the incidence of voice disorders has been estimated to range from 3 (Hull, Mielke, Willeford & Timmons, 1976) to 23.4% (Silverman & Zimmer, 1975). The prevalence in adults has been estimated at 7.2% for men and 5% for women, based on voice screenings (LaGuaite, 1972). Occupations carrying the highest risk for developing voice problems include sales-related work (13%), teaching (4.2%), and other jobs for which workers were considered professional voice users (Titze, Lemke & Montequin, 1996). Of these occupations, teaching is estimated to have the highest incidence of voice disorders (Fritzell, 1995; Smith, Gray, Dove, Kirchner, & Heras, 1997). A majority of voice patients report that their voice problem had a negative impact on their career options, social interactions, and other aspects of their daily lives (Smith, Verdolini, Gray, Nichols, Lemke, Barkmeier, Dove, & Hoffman, 1996).

Voice disorders can be described as problems related to pitch, loudness, vocal quality, and resonance. Voice problems may stem from vocal misuse, disease, congenital defects, laryngeal trauma, aging affects on the voice, and neurological disorders. Emotional and psychological factors may also contribute to acquired voice disorders. Treatment of voice disorders usually requires the combined specialties of the ear-nose-throat doctor (otolaryngologist) and a speech-language pathologist with expertise in assessing and treating voice disorders.

Voice Disorders Related to Vocal Fold Tissue Changes

Most voice disorders arise from overuse or frequent improper use of the voice, which can result in tissue changes that disrupt normal fold vibration.

Susan, age 17, was a cheerleader for her high school varsity football team for 3 years. During her first 2 years as a cheerleader, she experienced temporary bouts of hoarseness following each game. These usually subsided in a couple of days. During her third year as a cheerleader, however, she began to experience longer periods of hoarseness that did not fully resolve before the next game. By the end of the football season, her voice almost always sounded hoarse and she had difficulty being heard in the football stands. Eventually, she was no longer able to cheer.

An otolaryngologist found bilateral nodules on her vocal folds (see Figure 11-1). The nodules prevented her vocal folds from coming together unless she increased her loudness. She was discouraged from participating in cheerleading until the vocal nodules diminished. She was also referred to a speech-language pathologist for voice therapy. The speech-language pathologist helped Susan identify additional habits that were contributing to physical damage, such as coughing, clearing her throat frequently, and yelling at her younger brother when he teased her. Susan reduced the frequency of these behaviors and learned better ways to produce her voice. After one month, the size of the vocal nodules had reduced dramatically, and Susan's voice was significantly improved.

Traumatic Laryngitis

In the early stages of her voice disorder, Susan experienced repeated bouts of **traumatic laryngitis**. This condition is characterized by swollen and red vocal folds resulting from excessive yelling, screaming, or other traumatic uses of the voice (see Figure 11-2). Traumatic laryngitis is common and usually resolves within days of its onset. It often results from continuous vocal misuse such as yelling,

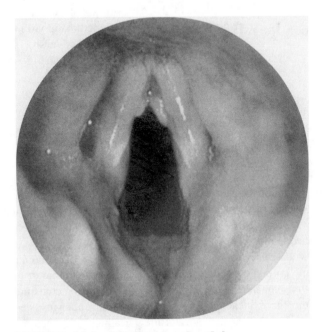

FIGURE 11-1   Bilateral vocal nodules.

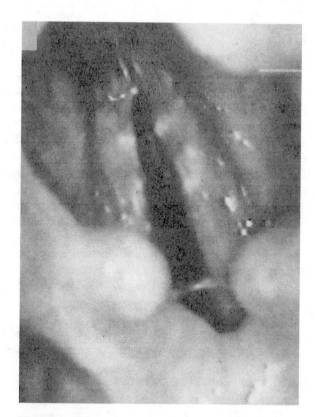

FIGURE 11-2   An example of the appearance of traumatic laryngitis obtained using video-endoscopy. (Courtesy of The University of Arizona, Department of Speech & Hearing Sciences)

or cheering throughout an exciting athletic event. In such situations, people yell at high intensity over loud environmental noise so that the vocal folds are slammed together at high velocities causing trauma to the tissue at the site of impact. As a result, the vocal folds become swollen and irritated. Tissue swelling along the length of the vocal folds disrupts normal vocal fold vibration, causing changes in voice quality. In severe cases, there may be a complete loss of voice (**aphonia**). The best treatment for traumatic laryngitis is to rest the voice, allowing the vocal folds to heal. After two to five days, depending on the extent of damage, vocal fold swelling and irritation typically resolve and the normal voice returns. In Susan's case, she experienced this pattern of recovery during her first 2 years of cheerleading.

If the vocal misuse continues, vocal fold irritation can become chronic. The mucosa that covers the vibrating portion of the vocal folds may thicken. Chronic irritation may result from attempts to talk over environmental noise (e.g., in a factory or during construction work) or talking for long periods of time. Once thickening of the mucosa occurs, changes need to be made in daily voice use to prevent further permanent damage and allow healing. Voice therapy may be necessary to identify poor vocal habits and to teach improved techniques for using the voice.

Vocal Nodules

Vocal nodules are small bumps that develop on the medial border of the vocal folds (see Figure 11-1). These bumps consist of fibrous tissue, much like calluses that develop on the hands or feet. Nodules occur along the anterior one-third of the membranous vocal folds as a result of persistent improper voicing patterns with prolonged periods of vocal fold inflammation. Vocal nodules can occur on one vocal fold, but most frequently develop on both vocal folds at the site of impact. In early stages, vocal nodules may appear as small swollen areas on the vocal folds. In later stages, the nodules become hard and impair normal vocal fold vibration. If the nodules become large enough, they can prevent the vocal folds from coming together completely, as occurred with Susan. She demonstrated signs of traumatic laryngitis that preceded the development of nodules. She could have prevented the development of vocal nodules with modification of her voice use. Instead, Susan's vocal fold tissue adjusted to the continual irritation and traumatic impact by developing vocal nodules. While vocal nodules certainly are not life-threatening, they can result in significant voice problems. The symptoms of vocal nodules arise gradually and manifest as increasing hoarseness and difficulty projecting the voice. This condition can be treated effectively by first identifying patterns of voice misuse. Intervention involves reducing poor vocal habits and learning better methods for producing and projecting the voice.

Vocal Polyps

Vocal polyps are small, fluid-filled sacks that develop on the vocal folds as a result of yelling, screaming, and other excessive uses of the voice. However, unlike the prolonged vocal misuse that leads to vocal nodules, it is believed that as little as a single event of vocal misuse can lead to development of a polyp. Compared to nodules, which are fibrous, polyps are soft and compliant. They may occur anywhere in the larynx such as on the vocal folds, or ventricular folds, or between the arytenoids. They usually occur on one side only. They are thought to be caused by a single intense event of harmful laryngeal behavior such as screaming or even intense coughing.

> Mrs. Delvechio, age 56, began to experience gradual onset of hoarseness after an upper respiratory infection with severe coughing episodes. She was seen by an otolaryngologist who identified a polyp located near the posterior segment of the vibrating portion of the left vocal fold. The physician suspected the polyp resulted from traumatic vocal fold impact during repeated episodes of severe coughing. The physician referred Mrs. Delvechio to a speech-language pathologist for counseling concerning excessive coughing and throat clearing. During counseling, Mrs. Delvechio mentioned that her husband was hard of hearing and she often tried to talk to him over the television or from another room in the house. She was encouraged to speak at comfortable loudness and not to speak over noise. In addition, she was instructed to talk to her husband only when they were in the same room. After 6 weeks, her polyp was reduced in size and her voice was almost completely normal.

A vocal polyp may result in significant voice problems that include breathiness or hoarseness. The polyp may also cause each vocal fold to vibrate at a different rate, causing a double voice or **diplophonia**. Frequently, treatment for a vocal polyp entails identification of the behaviors that led to the problem (e.g., yelling, throat clearing, coughing). In Mrs. Delvechio's case, once she became aware of the behaviors that were contributing to the voice problem, she could eliminate those habits.

Subsequently, the polyp reduced in size as the laryngeal tissues healed. In other cases, the individual may need specific therapeutic instruction by a speech-language pathologist to improve use of the voice.

Papilloma

Papillomas are wart-like growths found along the vocal tract and respiratory system. They are caused by a virus and are found predominantly in preschool children. Papilloma growths do not usually appear after puberty (Kleinsasser, 1979), so adults infrequently develop this disorder. The onset of this condition may be characterized by breathiness and hoarseness. If the papilloma grows large enough, a stridor or whistling sound may be heard during breathing. Papillomas may be treated with laser surgery, but unfortunately, they grow back quickly and multiple surgeries may be necessary. Frequent laser surgeries may result in vocal fold scarring that cannot be repaired. Eventually, the vocal folds may become so scarred that the voice cannot be produced due to the stiffness of the scarred vocal folds. Voice therapy can sometimes help these individuals make the best of their voice after surgery.

Carcinoma

Cancer, or **carcinoma**, of the larynx can be a life-threatening disease if not identified during its early stages. Persistent vocal hoarseness is the most common symptom associated with laryngeal cancer. Other warning signs include swallowing problems, swelling in the throat and neck region, and pain.

> Mr. Mahr, age 45, had smoked a pack of cigarettes per day for 25 years. He also enjoyed a cigarette along with a couple of drinks during cocktail hour every night before dinner. Over a period of 6 months, his voice became increasingly hoarse. He did not experience any illness during this time, although he noticed that he felt more fatigued than usual and sometimes felt as though he could not breathe in enough air. Mr. Mahr loved his work as an attorney and usually had a lot of energy. He finally went to see an otolaryngologist, who discovered that his vocal folds were covered with a whitish mass that impaired their normal movement. The physician scheduled surgery to remove a piece of the mass and determine its pathology. The biopsy revealed that it was cancer. Mr. Mahr was told that the cancer had invaded much of the larynx and that the entire larynx would need to be removed. After surgery, Mr. Mahr also needed to undergo a series of radiation treatments to reduce the risk that the cancer would reoccur. Fortunately, Mr. Mahr's laryngeal cancer was caught early enough that a positive outcome was likely. However, the treatment would cost him his voice. Mr. Mahr was referred to a speech-language pathologist who offered alternatives for creating a new voice after the laryngectomy.

As in Mr. Mahr's case, those who develop laryngeal cancer usually smoke and drink alcohol (McKenna, Fornataro-Clerici, McMenamin & Leonard, 1991). Caught in its early stages, laryngeal cancer can frequently be treated using conservative medical approaches. These include radiation, chemotherapy, and surgery to remove the cancer, leaving the larynx as intact as possible (Mendenhall, Parsons, Stringer, Cassisi & Million, 1988). In its later stages, laryngeal cancer is typically treated by surgical removal of the entire larynx.

When the larynx is removed, the trachea is attached to a permanent opening in the neck called a **tracheostomy** (see Figure 11-3). After his **laryngectomy**, Mr. Mahr will be able to breathe nor-

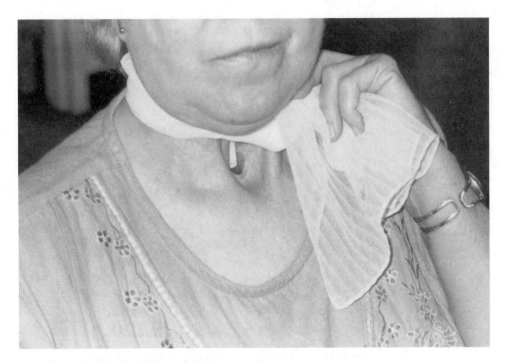

FIGURE 11-3   This woman is showing the location of the airway opening in her neck called a tracheostoma. She now breathes through the tracheostoma since undergoing a laryngectomy. The white tab attached to the tracheostoma secures the one-way valve used for shunting air into the esophagus.

mally except that the air will now come in and exit through an opening in his neck rather than the nose or mouth. Food and drink are still taken by mouth, although the sense of taste is diminished because air-borne odors no longer are breathed through the nose.

After surgery, a speech-language pathologist will work with Mr. Mahr to develop alternative ways of generating a sound source for speech. One method is esophageal speech. To use this method, Mr. Mahr must learn to trap air in his mouth and project it into the esophagus (McKenna et al., 1991). Once the air is trapped in the esophagus, it is belched back, creating sound by vibration of esophageal tissues. This sound source is transformed into words by the articulatory movements of the teeth, tongue, and lips, as with normal speech.

A second method of speech production involves an electronic device called an **electrolarynx**, or artificial larynx (Casper & Colton, 1993). The electrolarynx is a hand-held vibrator that makes a buzzing sound that substitutes for vocal fold vibration. The device is placed onto the neck so that the sound travels through the skin into the vocal tract, providing a "voice" that is modified into speech by mouthing words (see Figure 11-4). The speech-language pathologist provides therapy to help improve intelligibility using the electrolarynx.

A popular surgical method to provide voice is a tracheo-esophageal puncture (TEP). This surgical procedure involves creating a hole for the placement of a small tube into the tissue that divides the trachea from the esophagus (see Figure 11-3). The tube has a one-way air valve that shunts air

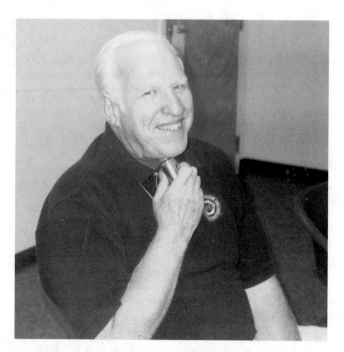

FIGURE 11-4   This gentleman is holding an electro-larynx securely against the front side of his neck to pro-vide his "voice" for speech.

from the trachea into the esophagus when the tracheostoma is covered by the individual's thumb or finger. The shunted air vibrates the esophageal tissue in the same way as the belching in esophageal speech, resulting in a voice.

Whichever method Mr. Mahr uses to communicate, training and practice will be necessary to maximize speech intelligibility. Many individuals such as Mr. Mahr are grateful that they have another chance at life and resume their activities with great enthusiasm. Others may fall into depression and need professional care to help them deal with the psychological and social issues that arise.

Neurological Voice Disorders

Mrs. Finley, age 45, developed a voice problem after undergoing surgery to remove her thyroid gland. She awoke after the surgery with a breathy voice and choked whenever she drank liquids too quickly. She was evaluated by an otolaryngologist who diagnosed paralysis of the right vocal fold. The doctor suggested that the nerve innervating the vocal fold was probably injured during thyroid surgery. Because this nerve may recover from such damage, the physician decided to wait for 6 months before considering surgical intervention for the condition. In the meantime, Mrs. Finley was referred to a speech-language pathologist to learn techniques to stimulate the functioning left vocal fold to vibrate against the paralyzed right vocal fold. In addition, the speech-language pathologist needed to address Mrs. Finley's swallowing problem. She was able to avoid choking by taking small sips of liquid while tilting her chin toward her chest. This position protected her airway during swallowing.

Through voice exercises, Mrs. Finley learned to produce a soft voice instead of a breathy one. By 5 months post-surgery, her voice had become stronger and closer to normal, indicating that nerve innervation was returning. By six months, her voice was clear and strong. The otolaryngologist re-examined her larynx at that time and determined that her right vocal fold had regained mobility.

Vocal Fold Paralysis

The recurrent laryngeal nerve is a branch of cranial nerve X (the vagus nerve). It provides neural input to muscles that move the vocal folds during voicing and swallowing (see Chapter 2). Vocal fold paralysis may result from damage to one or both recurrent laryngeal nerves on either side of the larynx. Unilateral vocal fold paralysis is most common. As in Mrs. Finley's case, damage to the nerve can occur when it is cut or compressed during surgery. Nerve damage can also result from a tumor or viral infection. In some cases, there is no known cause for nerve damage. Once the nerve to the laryngeal muscles is damaged, the vocal fold on the same side as the nerve is immobilized. Because the vocal folds cannot close completely, the voice is breathy and patients often choke on liquids. In many cases, the impaired nerve recovers or regenerates within 6 months resulting in recovery of the voice (Hockauf & Sailer, 1982; Mu & Yang, 1991).

To compensate for the paralyzed vocal fold, patients are taught to use greater effort to help increase the movement of the working vocal fold. With increased exertion, the healthy vocal fold may be able to vibrate against the paralyzed vocal fold to produce voicing. If the impaired nerve does not recover within 6 months, several surgical procedures are available to improve voice production. The surgical procedures all move the immobile vocal fold medially so that the working vocal fold can vibrate against it. This was not necessary in Mrs. Finley's case because her vocal fold function recovered over time.

Paralysis of both vocal folds is a more serious problem than one-sided vocal fold paralysis. This disorder is typically caused by an impairment to the central nervous system such as a tumor or stroke that interferes with the generation of the neural signals that control movement of the vocal folds. Bilateral paralysis may result in difficulty breathing when the vocal folds are paralyzed in the closed (or nearly closed) position. Surgical intervention is usually necessary to create an open airway adequate for breathing.

Spasmodic Dysphonia

Spasmodic **dysphonia** is a rare voice disorder characterized by a strained-strangled voice quality. The cause of this disorder was once thought to be related to psychological dysfunction (Arnold, 1959). It is currently thought to result from a dysfunction involving the neural signals that control the vocal folds during speaking (Ludlow, 1995b). There are two types of spasmodic dysphonia: *ABductor* and *ADductor* type. The ADductor type occurs when the vocal folds close together too tightly during voiced speech sounds resulting in a strained-strangled voice quality, or voice stoppage. The ABductor type occurs when the vocal folds spasm apart during production of unvoiced speech sounds resulting in excessive breathiness. Thus, the difference between the two types of spasmodic dyspho-nia can be remembered by these two rules:

1. The "AD" part of ADductor means that the vocal folds spasm together.
2. The "AB" part of ABductor means that the vocal folds spasm apart.

ADductor spasmodic dysphonia is characterized by intermittent onset of the strained-strangled voice quality, or voice stoppage. The additional muscular force needed to move the folds results in effortful voice production. The ABductor type of spasmodic dysphonia is less frequent than the AD-ductor type and is characterized by intermittent bursts of breathy voice quality. The breathiness re-sults from vocal fold spasms that keep the vocal folds apart during speech. Thus, these individuals may complain that they cannot make their voice loud enough to be heard.

Mr. Sparks, age 42, began to experience a catch in his voice while giving business reports to his employer. When this first began, he thought it was related to being nervous. How-ever, he noticed the catches in his throat occurred more frequently over time. They also oc-curred at times when he was not nervous, such as after a church service or at home. Over the course of a year, the condition worsened. He put such effort into forcing his voice to func-tion that he often became exhausted after a short period of talking. As the voice problem increased, his employer became displeased with Mr. Sparks's productivity and inability to provide regular business presentations. In desperation and frustration, Mr. Sparks went to see his doctor.

Mr. Sparks's primary care physician thought the problem was related to stress, but agreed to refer him to a speech-language pathologist specializing in voice disorders. The speech-language pathologist recognized Mr. Sparks problem as spasmodic dysphonia. Voice therapy was initiated to modify some of the problematic voice patterns he had de-veloped to compensate for his uncooperative larynx. The speech-language pathologist also recommended consultation with an otolaryngologist for further evaluation. The otolaryn-gologist diagnosed Mr. Sparks with ADductor-type spasmodic dysphonia and recom-mended medical treatment that consisted of injections of a toxin (Botox®) into the muscles of the vocal folds to reduce spasms during talking.

The injection of toxin into the vocal folds is the current treatment of choice for ADductor-type spasmodic dysphonia. The toxin is Botulinum Type A, most often referred to as Botox®. Botox im-pairs the ability of nerve endings to cause contraction of the vocal fold muscles. This results in weak-ened vocal fold muscles that cannot spasm closed during talking. However, the vocal folds are so weak that they cannot come together to create a strong voice or protect the airway during swallowing. After a few weeks, the Botox is absorbed by the body and new nerve endings grow. At this point, the vocal folds begin to move more normally, resulting in an improved voice quality. After three to six months, the Botox wears off and the symptoms of spasmodic dysphonia typically return, requiring reinjection of Botox to maintain an improved voice.

In some individuals, Botox does not effectively weaken the vocal fold muscles. In those cases, an alternative is surgery to cut one of the recurrent laryngeal nerves to create unilateral vocal fold paral-ysis (Dedo & Behlau, 1991; Dedo & Izdebski, 1983; Weed, Jewett, Rainey, Zealear, Stone, Ossoff, & Netterville, 1996). Although the resulting voice is slightly breathy, it allows the individual to function more normally in daily communication. In approximately 20% of individuals who undergo surgical cutting of the recurrent laryngeal nerve, the nerve regrows and the symptoms of ADductor spasmodic dysphonia return within 1 to 3 years after the surgery (Dedo & Behlau, 1991). Although it is a treatment of last resort, newer methods of cutting the recurrent laryngeal nerve show promise for more successful long-term benefits for those who do not respond well to Botox treatment (Weed et al., 1996).

Despite its success in the treatment of ADductor-type spasmodic dysphonia, Botox injections are not as effective with ABductor spasmodic dysphonia. Botox treatment is typically attempted in those with ABductor spasmodic dysphonia to see if it will effectively weaken the laryngeal muscles that pull the vocal folds apart during a spasm. However, the improvement following Botox treatment for ABductor spasmodic dysphonia is typically minimal and lasts only two to four weeks. These individuals often experience an extremely breathy voice for several weeks after treatment before their voice improves (Ludlow, 1995a). Presently, there is no known effective way to treat ABductor spasmodic dysphonia.

Voice Assessment and Management

The goal of a voice evaluation is to determine the nature of the problem, its probable cause, and the options available to treat the problem. Some people go to their primary care physician first, who then refers them to an otolaryngologist or a speech-language pathologist. Others seek help on their own and go directly to the otolaryngologist. Otolaryngologists with specialized interest in voice disorders often work with a speech-language pathologist with similar interests. Thus, medical evaluation and treatment may be augmented by voice therapy from a speech-language pathologist. Depending on the setting and equipment available to those assessing the voice problem, various methods of evaluation may be undertaken.

Voice evaluations begin with gathering information about the history of the problem and the symptoms present at the time of the examination. This information influences the evaluation procedures as well as the treatment plan.

Ms. Norwood worked as a real estate agent for the past 6 years and was one of the top salespeople in her company. Her company relocated to a new building 2 years ago. Since the relocation, numerous renovation projects were necessary such as putting in new carpet and paint. She noticed that whenever she worked in her new office, her voice became increasingly hoarse over the course of the day. When her productivity dropped significantly and she felt increasingly anxious about her work, she sought medical help from an otolaryngologist.

The otolaryngologist looked at Ms. Norwood's larynx and noted that both vocal folds were swollen and red and did not vibrate normally during phonation. Thinking that she probably developed improper voicing patterns that led to changes in the vocal folds, the otolaryngologist referred her to a speech-language pathologist for voice therapy. The speech-language pathologist thoroughly documented events leading to Ms. Norwood's voice disorder and discovered her problems began after her office was relocated to the new building. More specifically, her voice problems coincided with the new carpet and paint in her office. The speech-language pathologist suspected that Ms. Norwood was sensitive to chemicals in the air from the renovations. Ms. Norwood also had begun to cough frequently and clear her throat to try to get her voice to improve. Furthermore, she reported drinking a lot of coffee and only small amounts of water each day. The caffeine from the coffee and the low amount of other fluids may have caused dehydration that exacerbated her voice disorder. The speech-language pathologist helped Ms. Norwood monitor and eliminate the daily habits that were irritating her voice and taught her techniques to improve the sound of her voice. In addition, she was instructed to avoid the office for 2 weeks to determine if the chemicals from the new carpet and paint were irritating her vocal folds.

Ms. Norwood's voice improved dramatically over the 2 weeks she was away from her office. Upon her return, the voice problem returned despite her efforts to speak using the techniques she was taught by the speech-language pathologist. Thus, it appeared that Ms. Norwood's voice problem was caused by her sensitivity to the chemicals in her office. She decided not to work in her office to avoid exposure to the chemical fumes until the renovation was completed.

In the example above, the true source of Ms. Norwood's voice problem was uncovered after all the information related to the onset of her voice disorder was obtained. The physical appearance of her larynx was similar to that associated with chronic improper and effortful use of the voice. However, the following case history guidelines helped to determine the probable causes of a voice problem and, consequently, influenced the course of treatment:

1. Obtain the client's description of the voice problem.
2. Determine whether the onset of the voice problem was associated with an illness, accident, or other significant circumstance.
3. Note the duration and consistency of the symptoms of the voice problem.
4. Note patterns or variability in the reported symptoms or severity of the voice problem on a daily, weekly, monthly, and seasonal basis.
5. Obtain a description of the client's daily voice use.
6. Obtain a description of the client's work, home, and social activities.
7. Note whether the client's voice changes across different environments, speaking situations, or times of the day.

The case history provides information concerning development and impact of the voice disorder on the client's life. It also provides an opportunity for the speech-language pathologist to get to know the client as an individual. As in Ms. Norwood's case, an examination of the circumstances leading to the voice problem helped reveal the true cause of the voice problem, resulting in an effective voice treatment plan.

In addition to the case history, a voice evaluation also includes examination of the vocal mechanism. In Ms. Norwood's case, the otolaryngologist examined the larynx to determine whether vocal pathology was present. To observe the pharynx and larynx, the physician may need to use a tongue depressor, a light to illuminate the structures, and a laryngeal mirror to reflect their image. Other ways of viewing the soft palate and throat utilize fiberoptic equipment to obtain a picture of the soft palate or throat. This procedure is called videoendoscopy. Videoendoscopy can be done using a scope placed through the mouth or nose. The scope that is placed through the nose (i.e., **nasoendoscope**) is a small tube with fiberoptic cables that illuminates and allows viewing of the nasal passages, soft palate, pharynx, and larynx (see Figure 11-5). Another type of scope that can be used to view the larynx is a rigid scope. This scope looks like a steel rod with a lens on the end. It acts like a periscope in that it is placed over the tongue and provides a view of the larynx as it is placed just beyond the back of the tongue. The image obtained by either scope is displayed on a television monitor and can be recorded onto a videotape. The rigid scope obtains a closer view of the vocal folds than the flexible scope. However, the client cannot talk with the rigid scope in his or her mouth. The flexible scope is a good way to obtain a recording of the structures in the throat while someone is talking. The lighting used for both scopes can be changed into a strobe light while the client sustains a vowel sound such as *ee*. The strobe light illuminates only a fraction of the vocal fold vibrations so that they appear to occur in slow motion.

The voice evaluation may also assess the facial muscles, lips, teeth, soft and hard palate, tonsils, and pharynx because these structures may be affected when a voice disorder is present. Other components of a voice evaluation include respiration testing, acoustic measurements of the voice (e.g., pitch and loudness), and descriptions of the voice quality (e.g., breathy, hoarse) as perceived during different speaking tasks. The combined information from observation and measurements help the speech-language pathologist to determine the best approach for treating the client's voice problem and can be compared to findings after therapy.

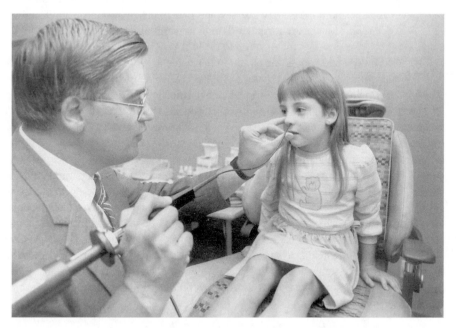

FIGURE 11-5   A flexible endoscope is being placed into the left nasal passageway of this young girl. Once inserted, it can be advanced to obtain views of the soft palate, pharynx, and larynx. (Used with permission of S. C. McFarlene, University of Nevada Medical School, Reno.)

Ms. Alvarez worked as a kindergarten teacher. During the first 6 months of her job, she began experiencing increased hoarseness that worsened from morning to night. By the end of each week, she could barely make herself heard in the classroom. Ms. Alvarez became frightened that she may have laryngeal cancer, so she went to see an otolaryngologist. The otolaryngologist looked at Ms. Alvarez's larynx and noted the development of two small bumps on her vocal folds, called vocal nodules. In addition, her vocal folds were red and swollen. Ms. Alvarez was referred to a speech-language pathologist for further evaluation of her voice and voice therapy.

The speech-language pathologist performed videoendoscopy on Ms. Alvarez using the rigid scope and a strobe light to assess vocal fold vibration. The speech-language pathologist also tape recorded Miss Alvarez's voice during sustained phonation of *ah* and *ee* and while reading. The speech-language pathologist asked Ms. Alvarez about her work, family, and social life to obtain a better idea of how she uses her voice in different environments. From this information, the speech-language pathologist determined that Ms. Alvarezs problems were primarily related to how she used her voice at work. She often needed to shout above noise to get the children's attention. The speech-language pathologist suggested using a microphone system so that Ms. Alvarez could project her voice above the noise without using much effort. In addition, they developed instructional strategies such as using a whistle to get attention and using more visual aids that helped preserve her voice. Finally, the speech-language pathologist taught Ms. Alvarez how to project her voice without straining. After one month, Ms. Alvarez's voice had improved noticeably. On re-examination, the vocal nodules appeared smaller than they were initially.

In Ms. Alvarez's case, the strain on her voice at work led to the development of vocal nodules. The speech-language pathologist was able to determine the likely cause of the voice problem by getting information surrounding the onset of her voice problem. In addition, the speech-language pathologist knew that vocal nodules usually occurred with chronic misuse of the voice. The type of therapy done with Ms. Alvarez could be described in two ways:

1. Elimination of harmful daily vocal habits.
2. Learning new techniques to effectively use the voice without strain.

These are the two primary approaches used to treat voice disorders resulting from harmful vocal habits. In severe cases, surgical removal of a growth may be necessary; however, more frequently, voice therapy is successful in treating clients such as Ms. Alvarez and Ms. Norwood. Medical intervention (e.g., surgery, medication) is provided by a physician such as an otolaryngologist. When medical interventions are used, the speech-language pathologist often provides voice therapy prior to and afterwards to help the client improve vocal techniques and to eliminate or prevent the use of harmful vocal habits.

Swallowing Disorders

Eating is vital to maintaining life and providing the energy for basic bodily functions. The process of ingestion begins with chewing and swallowing food, a complex process that we do not often give much thought. However, when swallowing is impaired, we become more aware of how large a role eating plays in our daily living. In addition to nutrition, eating is the focus of many social functions. Impaired swallowing, called **dysphagia**, may create such difficulties during eating that social occasions are avoided and eating may become an unpleasant activity.

Most individuals diagnosed with dysphagia are over 55 years of age. In that age group, the prevalence is estimated to range between 16 to 22% (Bloem, Lagaay, van Beek, Haan, Roos, & Wintzen, 1990; Kjellen & Tibbling, 1981). This includes a wide range of swallowing problems related to stroke, neuromuscular problems, traumatic brain injury, progressive neurological diseases, surgery to structures involved in ingestion and digestion, head and neck cancer, and cognitive problems such as dementia. Although older individuals more frequently experience symptoms of dysphagia, infants, children, and young adults may also have dysphagia. In young people, dysphagia may be due to illness, surgeries of the head and neck, or congenital deformations.

In order to understand dysphagia, one must appreciate the components of the normal swallow. There are four stages of the swallow, any of which may be impaired in someone with dysphagia. These can be seen in Figure 11-6.

Stage One

The first stage of the swallow is referred to as the *oral preparatory stage* (see Figure 11-6A). This stage is important for preparing food placed in the mouth for transport to the stomach. During this stage, the lips, tongue, and soft palate play a major role in holding the food within the oral cavity. The tongue moves the food around so that it can be chewed and, finally, gathered into a central groove formed by the tongue prior to swallowing. The collection of food held together by the tongue is referred to as a food **bolus**. During this stage of the swallow, saliva produced by glands in the mouth begins the digestion process. Saliva coats the food so that it is moist, and the digestive chemicals soften the food prior to swallowing. Problems with the oral preparatory stage may arise because of changes in the oral structures from congenital malformations, age-related changes, surgery, trauma, and neurological problems.

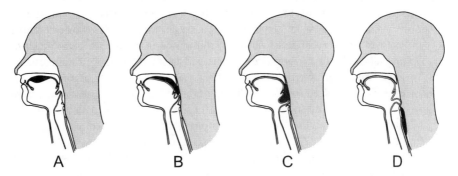

A   B   C   D

FIGURE 11-6   **The four stages of the swallow are shown. (A) The oral preparatory stage. (B) The oral transport stage. (C) The pharyngeal stage. (D) The esophageal stage.**

Mrs. Baker, age 71, lost her teeth and could not afford dentures to replace them. As a consequence, she was unable to eat any food that required chewing such as meat, popcorn, salad, or fruit. Her self-imposed diet was restricted to soups, applesauce, oatmeal, and fluids. After 6 months, Mrs. Baker lost considerable weight and became malnourished. She sought help from her doctor who recognized the difficulties related to her diet and chewing problems. Mrs. Baker was admitted to the hospital where she was given intravenous fluids to rehydrate and rebalance her body chemistry. She was seen by a dietician who recommended the addition of a nutritional drink to supplement her meals. It was also recommended that Mrs. Baker obtain dentures to allow her to eat more normally. Once Mrs. Baker regained weight and was healthy, she was released from the hospital and instructed to check back with her doctor and dietician periodically to monitor her health and diet.

In this example, Mrs. Baker's lack of teeth resulted in difficulties chewing that limited her food options. She did not make wise food choices to ensure adequate nutritional and caloric intake. As a consequence, she lost weight and jeopardized her health due to poor nourishment. Mrs. Baker's situation was easily remedied by obtaining dentures. However, if dentures were not an option for her, Mrs. Baker would need to continue using nutritional supplements to make sure her diet was well-balanced and to ensure adequate caloric intake.

Stage Two

Once food is chewed and ready to be swallowed, the tongue gathers it into a cohesive bolus held between the tongue and hard and soft palate. The tongue propels the bolus posteriorly into the pharynx by pressing up against the hard palate and pushing the bolus backwards. This stage of transporting the bolus from the oral cavity into the pharynx is called the *oral transport stage* of the swallow (see Figure 11-6B).

Mr. Roswell, age 85 years, suffered a stroke that impaired his ability to control tongue and lip movements. As a consequence, it was difficult to control the food in his mouth while chewing. Food and fluids often spilled out of his mouth because his lips were too weak to keep them in his oral cavity. Mr. Roswell also had difficulty collecting the food in his mouth into a cohesive bolus for swallowing. After swallowing, food remained in his mouth.

The speech-language pathologist assessed Mr. Roswell while he ate and determined that his primary difficulty was controlling food in the mouth. A *F*lexible *E*ndoscopic *Ex*-amination of *S*wallowing (FEES) was performed to visualize the pharynx while he swallowed measured amounts of milk and then applesauce. It was observed that after a teaspoon of milk was placed in his mouth, the milk ran back into the pharynx before he initiated a swallow. Milk also spilled through his lips. Mr. Roswell was able to control applesauce so that it did not spill into the pharynx or out through his lips. He was also able to swallow all of the applesauce so that none remained in his mouth.

The speech-language pathologist recommended that Mr. Roswell's wife try thickening liquids and soups using cornstarch or a food thickening product. This allowed Mr. Roswell to place a spoonful of food with a consistency similar to applesauce on his tongue and immediately swallow without having to chew first. Adding thickener to liquids also allowed

Mr. Roswell improved oral control so that liquids did not spill out of his mouth or into his throat before initiating a swallow. The speech-language pathologist recommended that Mr. Roswell receive therapy that included exercises to strengthen his tongue, lips, and jaw and improve the range of motion and control of oral structures to improve his ability to control food in his mouth. The combination of strengthening exercises and increased successful swallowing using specific food consistencies helped Mr. Roswell recover most of his oral control during swallowing so that he could eat a wider variety of food consistencies.

As seen in the example of Mr. Roswell, difficulty with the oral transport stage can prevent an individual from moving food out of the oral cavity. However, simple measures can be taken to help compensate for this problem by restricting foods to those the client can best swallow. In addition, weakness of the oral musculature may be improved by strengthening and range-of-motion exercises with the tongue, lips, and jaw (Logemann, 1983).

Stage Three

The *pharyngeal stage* of the swallow is characterized by movement of the bolus of food through the pharynx and into the esophagus (see Figure 11-6C). The bolus is propelled into the pharynx and, as it passes the back of the tongue, muscles of the pharynx contract to continue the propulsive action initiated by the tongue. As the superior portion of the pharynx contracts, the airway opens and closes and the larynx elevates. This raised position during the swallow maximizes protection from **aspiration** of food into the airway. After the bolus enters the esophagus, the pharyngeal structures return to their resting positions. This stage is less than 1 second in duration.

Mrs. Lasser, age 65 years, began having difficulty getting food to clear from her throat when she swallowed. She felt as though there was something caught in her throat and she needed to drink lots of fluids to clear the food that was stuck. In addition, she began choking on the fluids she drank to clear food stuck in her throat. Her swallowing difficulties required so much time and effort that she was embarrassed to eat in front of her friends and stopped enjoying meals. Thus, she reduced the amount of food eaten and declined invitations to join friends for meals. After losing weight and becoming malnourished, Mrs. Lasser went to see her doctor.

Mrs. Lasser's doctor, in turn, referred her for a swallowing examination, which was performed jointly by a radiologist and speech-language pathologist. During the test, Mrs. Lasser experienced all of the swallowing difficulties described earlier. The examination revealed that Mrs. Lasser's pharyngeal muscles appeared weak and her larynx was not elevating completely during swallowing. Not all food swallowed was cleared completely from her throat. The speech-language pathologist showed Mrs. Lasser a way to swallow while tilting her chin downward. Mrs. Lasser used this posture while eating and found it less difficult to swallow. However, she still needed to follow each bite of food with water or juice to clear her throat.

As shown in this case, impairment of the pharyngeal stage of the swallow can often be compensated for by simple posturing changes while swallowing. When food does not clear the throat during this stage of the swallow, the individual risks aspiration of food into the airway. This can lead to inflamation of the lungs, which is a potentially serious illness called aspiration pneumonia. A team assessment by the radiologist and speech-language pathologist is the best way to assess the pharyngeal stage of swallowing. A procedure called a modified barium swallow (MBS) is performed in which the patient is given food or liquid mixed with a radiocontrast material, barium, which is detected using an x-ray procedure called **videofluoroscopy**. This allows visualization of the pharyngeal structures and their movement during the pharyngeal stage of the swallow. Videofluoroscopy also allows identification and estimation of the amount of food aspirated into the airway before, during, and after the swallow. The MBS method allows assessment of changes in posture to improve the swallow and clearing of food from the mouth and throat. The effects of different food consistencies (e.g., fluid, paste, solids) can also be determined using the MBS.

Stage Four

The fourth stage of the swallow is the *esophageal stage* that includes transportation of the bolus to the stomach by the esophagus (see Figure 11-6D). The esophagus pushes the bolus toward the stomach using muscle contractions that squeeze each portion of the esophagus from the top to the bottom, called **peristaltic contractions**. This contraction is similar to that which propels a worm as it moves along the ground. That is, each muscle segment surrounding the esophagus contracts in sequence from the upper esophageal sphincter to the stomach so that the bolus is squeezed through the esophagus into the stomach.

> Mr. Gilford, age 56, started experiencing problems with food that had been eaten during meals coming back up. This regurgitation, or **reflux**, became increasingly worse over a 6-month period before he sought medical assistance. His physician examined his throat and noticed that the pharyngeal tissues appeared red and irritated. Given Mr. Gilford's symptoms, his physician suspected reflux or some type of swallowing abnormality. Mr. Gilford was referred to a gastroenterology specialist who determined that Mr. Gilford had an adequate swallow to clear food from the mouth and throat; however, undigested food appeared to come back up rather than continue through the esophagus toward the stomach. The gastroenterologist requested a barium swallow examination to assess Mr. Gilford's esophagus and digestive tract. The radiologic test entailed swallowing cupfuls of barium contrast while a videofluoroscopic image was monitored to follow the path of the barium. This test revealed that Mr. Gilford's esophagus was not contracting strongly enough to push the barium into the stomach. As a result, most of what Mr. Gilford drank during the test remained in the esophagus and some of it squeezed back into the pharynx as reflux. The gastroenterologist prescribed a medication that increased the contraction of the esophageal muscle to improve propulsion of food toward the stomach. The medication helped reduce Mr. Gilford's symptoms dramatically.

As all of the above examples demonstrate, dysphagia occurs when there is a problem with any or all of the four stages of the swallow. Common signs of dysphagia include:

- Difficulty initiating a swallow
- Difficulty chewing food due to poor dentition (as in Mrs. Baker's case)

- Difficulty controlling food in the oral cavity so that it spills out of the mouth or spills into the airway before the larynx closes to protect the airway (as in Mr. Roswell's case)
- Choking when swallowing food, and food sticking in the throat (as Mrs. Lasser experienced)

Various methods exist for assessing the swallow, as demonstrated by the above examples. Imaging techniques are most frequently used to visualize the oral and pharyngeal structures such as the FEES method (Langmore, Schatz & Olsen, 1988) and the MBS (Logemann, 1993). While the speech-language pathologist can perform the FEES method if properly trained, an otolaryngologist may also obtain FEES images while the speech-language pathologist administers the test food substances. During a MBS, the radiologist or radiology technician performs the videofluorographic imaging while the speech-language pathologist administers the barium contrast substances and determines which postures or consistencies appear to be successfully swallowed during testing. The gastroenterologist and radiologist are best trained to assess esophageal and other digestive organs during the barium swallow.

Many professionals may be involved in assessing and providing care to someone with dysphagia, including a speech-language pathologist, radiologist, gastroenterologist, otolaryngologist, neurologist, dentist, nurse, social worker, dietician, occupational therapist, and psychologist. The speech-language pathologist plays a major role in the assessment of swallowing, making recommendations to compensate for the dysphagia, and referring the individual for further assessment by other dysphagia team members. Treatment of dysphagia most frequently entails simple measures such as changing the posture of the head and body during swallowing, the consistency of the types of foods eaten, changing the temperature of foods eaten to improve initiation of the swallow, and performing exercises to improve strength and range of motion of oral structures. Other treatment methods provided by physician specialists entail use of medications to improve smooth muscle contraction, non-oral (called **parenteral**) feedings using a nasogastric tube (NG tube) or gastric tube (G tube) and surgical methods.

Clinical Problem Solving

Mrs. Hepple, age 65 years, underwent surgery to remove a portion of her esophagus that was cancerous. After surgery, her voice was breathy and she choked every time she drank water. In addition, the food she swallowed came back up. She was sent to an otolaryngologist who examined her vocal folds and noted that the left vocal fold was not moving during voicing. She was referred to a speech-language pathologist who further evaluated her voice. Rigid videoendoscopy using a strobe light was used to assess vocal fold vibration. However, Mrs. Hepple's vocal folds did not come together completely when vibrating. The speech-language pathologist was concerned about Mrs. Hepple's difficulties with swallowing and suggested a modified barium swallow (MBS). During MBS testing, the speech-language pathologist noted that liquids entered Mrs. Hepple's trachea during the pharyngeal stage of the swallow. Subsequently, she choked and coughed to clear the liquid from her airway.

1. Why does Mrs. Hepple have a breathy voice quality?
2. What do you think caused her left vocal fold to stop moving?
3. How might the speech-language pathologist try to help her improve her voice quality?
4. Might the voice problem go away with voice therapy?
5. What stage of the swallow is impaired?

References

Arnold, G.E. (1959). Spastic dysphonia: I. Changing interpretations of a persistent affliction. *Logos, 2*: 3–14.

Bloem, B.R., Lagaay, A.M., van Beek, W., Haan, J., Roos, R.A.C., & Wintzen, A.R. (1990). Prevalence of subjective dysphagia in community residents aged over 87. *British Medical Journal, 300*: 721–722.

Casper, J.K., & Colton, R.H. (1993). *Clinical Manual for Laryngectomy and Head and Neck Cancer Rehabilitation*. San Diego, CA: Singular Publishing Group.

Dedo, H.H., & Behlau, M.S. (1991). Recurrent laryngeal nerve section for spastic dysphonia: 5- to 14-year preliminary results in the first 300 patients. *Annals of Otology, Rhinology, & Laryngology, 100*(4): 274–279.

Dedo, H.H., & Izdebski, K. (1983). Intermediate results of 306 recurrent laryngeal nerve sections for spastic dysphonia. *Laryngoscope, 93*: 9–16.

Fritzell, B. (1995). *Occupation and Voice Problems*. Paper presented at the Proceedings from XXIII World Congress of IALP [abstract].

Hockauf, H., & Sailer, R. (1982). Postoperative recurrent nerve palsy. *Head and Neck Surgery, 4*: 380–384.

Hull, F.M., Mielke, P.W., Willeford, J.A., & Timmons, R.J. (1976). *National Speech and Hearing Survey* (Final Report Project 50978). Washington, DC: Bureau of Education for the Handicapped, Office of Education, Department of Health, Education, and Welfare.

Kjellen, G., & Tibbling, L. (1981). Manometric oesophageal function, acid perfusion test and symptomatology in a 55-year-old general population. *Clinical Physiology, 1*: 405–415.

Kleinsasser, O. (1979). *Microlaryngoscopy and Endolaryngeal Microsurgery: Technique and Typical Findings*. Baltimore: University Park Press.

LaGuaite, J. (1972). Adult voice screening. *Journal of Speech and Hearing Disorders, 37*: 147–151.

Langmore, S.E., Schatz, K., & Olsen, N. (1988). Fiberoptic endoscopic examination of swallowing safety: A new procedure. *Dysphagia, 2*: 216–219.

Logemann, J.A. (1993). *Manual for the Videofluorographic Study of Swallowing*. (2nd ed.). Austin, TX: Pro-Ed.

Logemann, J.A. (1983). *Evaluation and Treatment of Swallowing Disorders*. Austin, TX: Pro Ed.

Ludlow, C. (1995a). Treating the spasmodic dysphonias with botulinum toxin: A comparison of results with adductor and abductor spasmodic dysphonia and vocal tremor. In J. Tsui, & D. Calne (Ed.), *The Dystonias*. New York: Dekker.

Ludlow, C.L. (1995b). Management of the Spasmodic Dysphonias. In J.S. Rubin, R.T. Sataloff, & G.S. Korovin (Eds.), *Diagnosis and Treatment of Voice Disorders* (pp. 436–434). New York: Igaku-Shoin.

McKenna, J.P., Fornataro-Clerici, L. M., McMenamin, P.G., & Leonard, R.J. (1991). Laryngeal cancer: Diagnosis, treatment and speech rehabilitation. *American Family Physician, 44*(1): 123–129.

Mendenhall, W.M., Parsons, J.T., Stringer, S.P., Cassisi, N.J., & Million, R.R. (1988). T1-T2 vocal cord carcinoma: A basis for comparing the results of radiotherapy and surgery. *Head and Neck Surgery, 12*: 204–209.

Mu, L., & Yang, S. (1991). An experimental study on the laryngeal electromyography and visual observations in varying types of surgical injuries to the unilateral recurrent laryngeal nerve in the neck. *Laryngoscope, 101*: 699–708.

Silverman, E., & Zimmer, C. (1975). Incidence of chronic hoarseness among school-age children. *Journal of Speech and Hearing Disorders, 40*: 211–215.

Smith, E., Gray, S., Dove, H., Kirchner, L., & Heras, H. (1997). Frequency and effects of voice problems in teachers. *Journal of Voice, 11*: 81–87.

Smith, E., Verdolini, K., Gray, S., Nichols, S., Lemke, J., Barkmeier, J., Dove, H., & Hoffman, H. (1996). Effect of voice disorders on quality of life. *Journal of Medical Speech-Language Pathology, 4*(4): 223–244.

Titze, I.R., Lemke, J., & Montequin, D. (1996). Populations in the U.S. workforce who rely on voice as a primary tool of trade. *NCVS Status and Progress Report, 10*: 127–132.

Weed, D.T., Jewett, B.S., Rainey, C., Zealear, D.L., Stone, R.E., Ossoff, R.H., & Netterville, J.L. (1996). Long-term follow-up of recurrent laryngeal nerve avulsion for the treatment of spasmodic dysphonia. *Annals of Otology, Rhinology, Laryngology, 105*(8): 592–601.

_C h a p t e r_ _12_

Professional Issues

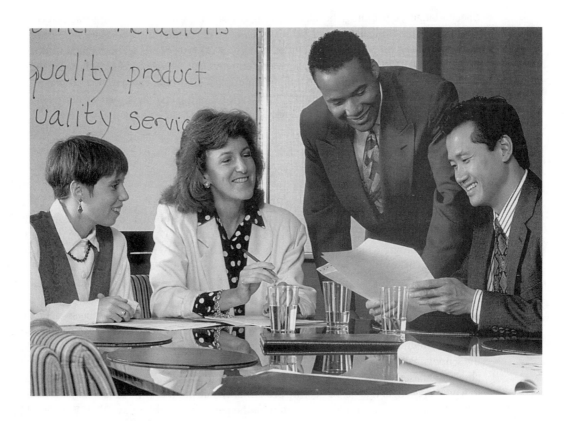

> ### Preview
>
> *In this book we have reviewed normal communication processes and disorders of communication that require the professional services of speech-language pathologists and audiologists. Along the way, we have introduced various aspects of clinical practice. In this final chapter we will provide an overview of professional work settings, discuss interdisciplinary interactions, and address some professional issues such as standards, ethics, and certification requirements. Future advances in the understanding of communication processes and disorders will influence approaches to evaluation and treatment. In addition, professional practice patterns are likely to undergo change in response to social, political, and economic influences. We will touch on some forseeable future trends.*

Speech-language pathologists and audiologists work in a variety of settings. Each work environment is shaped by the clinical caseload, professional colleagues, administrative and support personnel, and the physical and procedural characteristics of the work site. A change in clinical setting can mean a drastic change in the characteristics of one's employment. Some professionals enjoy the opportunity to shift the nature of their work by changing clinical environments over the course of their career. Even those who appreciate remaining in one type of setting are likely to experience considerable variety in their professional activities from day-to-day and year-to-year.

Clinical Settings

Public Schools

The public schools employ 53% of all speech-language pathologists, and 11% of all audiologists, making it the most common work setting for ASHA members (ASHA, 1998). The initiation of speech and hearing programs in the schools dates as far back as 1910 in the Chicago public school system (Paden, 1970). Programs developed because educators recognized that speech and hearing problems affected performance in the classroom and deemed it appropriate to provide services onsite. The scope of public school services has expanded over the years to include any child who has a communication disorder that negatively affects his or her education. Services for "educationally handicapped children" became nationwide with the passage of Public Law 94-142, The Education for All Handicapped Children Act, in 1975. Other public laws were passed that govern services for children within the schools. Public Law 95-561 expanded remedial services by providing federal support to improve children's basic educational skills, including listening and speaking. Preschool children who appear to have a speech, language, or hearing problem became eligible for assessment and remediation services through their local school system with the passage of Public Law 99-457. The public schools also conduct hearing screening programs at specified intervals that may involve the direct or indirect participation of the audiologist.

Speech-language pathologists in the public schools may work with children individually, in small groups, or in an entire classroom. The caseload can vary from multiply handicapped children to those with specific speech or language difficulties. Some professionals serve children in only one school, whereas others are itinerant, traveling to several schools. Audiologists provide a range of services to public school children that include screening, diagnostic, and aural habilitation programs. They also assist students with the wide variety of personal and classroom amplification systems. One notable feature of work in the public school setting is the academic calendar, which holds appeal for some professionals, particularly if their own children are of school age.

Medical Settings

Medical settings are second to schools as the most common employment site for speech, language, and hearing professionals. In 1997, 72% of audiologists and 39% of speech-language pathologists worked in medical settings (ASHA, 1998). These worksites include a broad spectrum of health care delivery environments including hospital-based acute care and rehabilitation units, in- and out-patient rehabilitation facilities, nursing homes, and medical clinics. Even within one hospital, there are a variety of settings where speech-language pathologists and audiologists work. In the past it was common for audiology and speech-language pathology to comprise their own department, but that is no longer standard practice. In relatively large hospitals, speech-language pathologists and audiologists tend to be members of various teams throughout the hospital. For example, audiologists may be associated with otolaryngology or physical medicine and rehabilitation. Speech-language pathologists may be allied, for example, with in-patient neurology or neurosurgery, pediatrics, or the dysphagia team. The particular demands of medical settings have been addressed in some excellent resources for medical speech-language pathology (Golper, 1992; Johnson & Jacobson, 1998).

Just as clinical practice in the public schools has been influenced by public laws, service delivery in medical settings is greatly influenced by forces such as health care legislation, managed care, and health insurance policies. Hospital stays have shortened considerably in recent years, and there has been an increase in service delivery in the home provided through home health care agencies. Patients tend to receive therapy for shorter durations than in the past, and clinicians must clearly justify their patients' need and benefits of their services. These changes have been accompanied by an emphasis on the functional outcomes of treatment, so that clinicians focus on very practical aspects of the patient's needs and how treatment will make a difference in their everyday life (Frattali, 1998).

Academic and Clinical Training Programs

Clinical training in the evaluation and treatment of communication disorders is conducted in many colleges and universities. The departments that provide coursework and professional preparation in speech-language pathology and audiology have various names, such as Speech and Hearing Sciences, Audiology and Speech-Language Pathology, and Communication Disorders. Clinical training involves academic coursework at the undergraduate and graduate levels and supervised clinical training. Most university programs include an on-campus clinic that offers student training opportunities and practicum training with cooperating clinical placement sites in the community. University clinics typically serve both children and adults who have hearing, language, articulation, voice, and fluency problems. The clinics may offer students the opportunity to observe evaluation and treatment procedures in communication disorders prior to beginning direct clinical work and provide supervised clinical training for graduate students. Many training programs confer both bachelor's and master's degrees, the latter being the entry level for employment for audiologists and speech-language pathologists.

University programs also contribute to the knowledge base of the professions through the conduct of basic and applied research. The research endeavors within a particular department reflect the areas of interest to the faculty. Students may become involved in research in a variety of informal and formal ways through work-study programs, volunteering, independent study, and thesis options. Most doctoral degree programs are research-oriented and require completion of original research in the form of a dissertation. There are also doctoral programs that focus on the clinical aspects of the professions.

Community Speech and Hearing Centers

Many of the first speech and hearing services in the United States that were outside of the public schools were provided in community speech and hearing centers. Such clinics are often housed in free-standing buildings rather than within an educational or medical facility. Community clinics are not as common as they once were, but those that exist often derive some of their financial support from supplemental sources. For example, they may be funded by agencies such as United Way or county public health programs, philanthropic groups such as Scottish Rite, or national organizations such as the Easter Seal Society. The clientele may be specific to certain disorders, such as children with cerebral palsy, or may include a wide variety of disorders that affect individuals of all ages.

Private Practice

An increasing number of audiologists and speech-language pathologists are choosing careers in private practice. In 1997, almost 8% of certified speech-language pathologists were in full-time private practice, and another 18% worked part-time. In audiology, 24% of the certified professionals were in full-time private practice and 13% worked in part-time private practice (ASHA, 1998). These individuals may provide services in their own office setting or through contractual arrangements with other care providers (e.g., hospitals, schools, nursing facilities). Practitioners who do part-time private work may spend the rest of the day in another clinical setting (such as a public school). Private practitioners treat a wide variety of disorders. Adults may seek a private practice speech-language pathologist to continue treatment for a chronic condition, such as aphasia or a motor speech disorder. Parents may contact a private practitioner to supplement the services their child receives through the schools or to treat conditions not otherwise covered in school-based programs (e.g., tongue thrust). Schools, hospitals, and other agencies may contract with private practitioners in order to relieve personnel shortages. In such cases, the private practitioner operates as an independent contractor to these businesses and organizations rather than as one of their employees. It is this autonomy that appeals to clinicians who choose to maintain a private practice.

Interdisciplinary Interactions

Almost all speech-language pathologists and audiologists work in conjunction with other professionals to some degree. Some of the cases presented earlier in this text provide examples of interdisciplinary interactions in the treatment of communication disorders. We can find out more about the nature of these interactions by reading about the experiences of clinicians who work on interdisciplinary teams. We will also consider the professions that comprise these teams and work with speech-language pathologists and audiologists in a variety of settings.

Team Approach in Public Schools

We begin with professionals who work with children in a public school setting. These individuals are jointly involved at all levels of case management, from the initial referral through the implementation of therapy goals on a daily basis.

Patty is a speech-language pathologist with 10 years experience in the public school setting. She currently works with Cheryl, an occupational therapist, and Jean, a physical therapist, along with psychologists and several regular preschool and special education teachers. "An obvious motor impairment or speech-language problem is usually the cause for referral at our center. But often, with years of experience, you can just watch a kid and know that this kid needs to be seen by other professionals," Cheryl reported. The initial screening team in this school consisted of the classroom teacher, the speech-language pathologist, and the psychologist, with additional professions brought in as needed.

Each of the team members participate in joint evaluation of the child. However, their participation fluctuates as activities are more or less appropriate for providing each of them with relevant information. For example, Patty may do some formal language testing and come back to the evaluation during assessment of gross motor activities, because she knows that children are likely to use the most spontaneous language during that time. Cheryl reported that the group has come to work smoothly by getting to know what each other does. "Initially, it was intimidating, not knowing when it was my turn to do something. Then [over time] it just kind of smoothed out." "We pretty much follow the child's lead," added Patty. "When I'm preparing my next set of materials, Cheryl is already in there doing her next thing. The nice thing is it really speeds up the evaluation so the child doesn't really get bored."

The group pointed to several factors that made their work as an evaluation team effective. "First, it really helped that we all had experience with this population. Then, it was a matter of picking up on each other's pace," reported Jean. Patty added, "It's also a matter of knowing which activities of the others are going to provide me with language information. Or when I'm presenting information, Cheryl might say 'You want to hold that at an angle because you can tell he's got low vision,' which helps me get optimal performance." The group agreed that teams work well when there is a respect for other professions and some knowledge of what each can contribute. The members must understand that the domains represented by each profession really do affect each other. As Cheryl put it, "I think that if you go in thinking that your own profession is the only one that is going to make the difference for that child, you're missing out on an integrated picture of the whole child."

This group offered many examples of how the goals of different therapists interrelate for a particular child. For example, the positioning guidelines from the physical therapist may also be used by the occupational therapist and speech-language pathologist to provide the stability a child needs before learning can occur. To maximize their joint efforts, they often develop methods to address multiple goals at the same time.

Patty related, "If I am working on increasing requests by a child, I can have the child ask for materials during an art project. When the request is made, I hand the crayon or straw to the child. I can do that in a way that reinforces the reaching or grasping behaviors I know Cheryl is working on as well." Often, motor activities can serve as the reinforcement for training speech goals. One popular activity is an obstacle course that primarily serves OT and PT goals. Children are "allowed" to run the course after producing three correct articulation targets. Jean remarked that she often watches Patty to see at what level she is presenting language to the child. "It doesn't do me any good if a child can't perform a movement because he didn't understand my directions." In return, Patty has "borrowed" techniques from both Cheryl and Jean because she has noticed their effectiveness in helping children maintain their attention during various activities.

In the school setting, the speech-language pathologist may find himself or herself interacting with a variety of other professionals. In the example above, we have seen how some of these professionals may work together with preschool children. Let us now take a closer look at the professions a school-based speech-language pathologist commonly encounters.

Team Approach in a Pediatric Clinic

Lora is a speech-language pathologist who serves as the coordinator of her hospital's cleft palate team (see Chapter 9 for a discussion of this condition). This team consists of an audiologist, geneticist, nurse, otolaryngologist (ENT), pediatrician, plastic surgeon, dentist, orthodontist, prosthodontist, and social worker, who interact as a full team or as individuals with the parents and child.

"We get notified [that a child has been born with a cleft palate] from the birthing clinic. If it's feasible, we try to do a hospital visit within that first 24 to 48 hours," Lora reports. This visit usually involves a speech-language pathologist, a social worker, or a nurse. These individuals provide the parents with initial information concerning their child's condition, what can be done and what to expect as the child develops. Lora also provides important information about feeding their child during this early visit. Lora commented, "We feel that this early visit provides a valuable service."

Soon afterwards, the audiologist will see the child to evaluate hearing status and to counsel the parents about possible concerns with hearing health as their child develops. Other early appointments will be with the geneticist, ear-nose-throat doctor, and the plastic surgeon. "As the child grows," related Lora, "he will be seeing the ENT, plastic surgeon, and some of the other team members on a regular basis. Then our program requires that the child visit the entire team, which meets once a month, for certain procedures to be approved. They want [the treatment] to be a team consensus to be sure that it is the appropriate treatment for the child." Procedures that routinely involve team discussion are things like pharyngeal flap, bone graphs, and lip and nose revisions. The team may brainstorm ideas about the timing and course of treatment that takes into consideration the various aspects of each child's condition.

The team meeting starts with a pre-conference. "I type a summary of what surgeries have already been done, the diagnosis, presenting concerns and [histories of all other services] ahead of time," reported Lora. "One of the physicians will act as the 'presenting or attending physician' who will say what the main concerns are. If any questions come up right then, we will discuss them." Then the parents come into the meeting and the team members have an opportunity to examine the child. This is also an opportunity for the parents to provide all the professionals with input on treatment decisions and to ask questions about possible future intervention. "We really try to encourage the parents to consider themselves a member of the team," said Lora, "and I know that it can sometimes be a bit intimidating for some of them."

The team meeting is an opportunity for the parents and professionals to see how all the components of intervention that they each contribute are coming together for the child. Through these meetings, Lora has learned about state-of-the-art techniques for the management of cleft palate from the other professionals. In addition, she has provided the team with valued contributions. She provides this example: "I've had to sell the team on the usefulness of videoendoscopy (see Chapter 11), and they've pretty much bought into it now. We've had a couple of cases where we discovered that the child didn't need surgery [based on the videoendoscopy results]. I feel really good about how that has developed." Lora concludes with this thought, "I know that I have grown tremendously being in this role professionally. I used to be so intimidated. I would dread that day and I would know inside 'Oh, it's three days away,' and now I've been doing it for six years. I've grown much more confident. Over time, I've earned the other team members' respect. And I had to earn it."

Team Approach in a Medical Setting

Tom is a speech-language pathologist with 12 years of professional experience. Most of his work has been in medical settings with adults with acquired communication disorders, typically related to stroke or head injury. Tom currently works in a hospital in a skilled nursing unit, which provides subacute care. The patients in the subacute program are medically stable, but in need of rehabilitation and nursing care. Many of them were transferred to the unit after a stay in the acute care unit of the hospital, where they were admitted following a medically significant event, such as a stroke. Other patients were admitted directly to the subacute unit for a period of diagnostic and rehabilitative care to improve their independent living skills. Although Tom works in a hospital setting, many skilled nursing facilities are not located on a hospital campus.

Tom is part of a multidisciplinary rehabilitation team that includes a physical therapist, occupational therapist, dietician, nurse, and medical director. His workspace is part of a common rehabilitation area where the physical therapist and occupational therapist also work with patients. Interdisciplinary interaction is completely natural and occurs in both planned and spontaneous ways. For example, Tom had a patient who fatigued easily and had a limited amount of time when he was awake, alert, and able to participate in therapy. In order to maximize the patient's optimal treatment time, Tom conducted speech and language therapy at the same time that the PT was working with the patient on balance. The simultaneous attention to two tasks, balance and speech, offered an additional challenge to the patient that was more representative of real life than treating each in isolation. In other cases, therapy goals may be common across several disciplines and may be referred to as *conjoint treatment goals*. Tom told of a patient with a hip fracture who could not remember the precautions he was given by the physical therapist to protect his healing hip; therefore, part of the cognitive training that Tom implemented with this patient included strategies to assist him in learning the hip precautions. In this case, all of the therapies had common treatment goals that related to safety and achieving independent living.

Team interaction is a big part of what Tom enjoys about his current job. In fact, he selected his current worksite because the team approach appealed to him. He said that "it is important to go beyond what you have been taught" to be successful in a given setting. Working side-by-side with other professionals is one important way to continually expand and integrate professional knowledge.

The Professional Association: The American Speech-Language-Hearing Association

History and Purpose

The professions of speech-language pathology and audiology emerged and grew over the course of the twentieth century. In the early 1900s the focus was on speech disorders, particularly articulation and stuttering. In 1925, a group of professionals devoted to the treatment of communication disorders started an association called the American Academy for Speech Correction (Paden, 1970). The profession of audiology developed after World War II, owing to the needs of many soldiers who returned home with acquired hearing loss (Cherry & Giolas, 1997). As the audiology profession was established, they were included among the ranks of professionals dealing with communication disorders. In 1948, the professional organization became the American Speech and Hearing Association (ASHA). As clinical attention to language impairments was increasingly evident in both children and adults, the profession changed the name again in 1978 to the American Speech-Language-Hearing Association, although the ASHA acronym was retained. In 1998, over 93,000 speech-language pathologists, audiologists, and speech, language, and hearing scientists belong to the organization. Information about this organization can be found at the ASHA website at www.asha.org. Additional discussion concerning professional issues is found in Lubinski and Frattali (1994).

ASHA is the primary professional organization for speech, language, and hearing professionals, although there are other related professional organizations to which audiologists and speech-language pathologists belong. The mission of ASHA is to promote the interests of the professions and to advocate for people with communication disabilities. The purposes are reflected in the Association bylaws (ASHA, 1997), which are paraphrased here:

1. To encourage basic research and scientific study of human communication and its disorders;
2. To promote appropriate academic and clinical preparation for individuals preparing to enter the professions, and to promote continuing education within the discipline;
3. To promote investigation and prevention of communication disorders;
4. To foster improvement of clinical procedures used in treating disorders of communication;
5. To stimulate exchange of information pertinent to communication and communication disorders;
6. To advocate for individuals with communication disorders; and
7. To promote the interests of members of the Association.

ASHA is an organization that is intended to serve the interests of the membership. There are two bodies that govern and establish the policies of the Association: the Legislative Council and the Executive Board. The Legislative Council establishes the policies of the organization and is composed of elected representatives from every state, and the Executive Board consists of officers who are elected by the ASHA membership, as well as the Executive Director of the Association. Many of the ASHA policies have significant impact on members of the Association, such as defining the scope of practice of the professions, and therefore are of great interest to speech-language pathologists and audiologists. The Executive Board also manages the affairs of the Association and often serves as official representatives of the Association. The committees, task forces, and boards that operate within the ASHA structure provide opportunities for the membership to significantly contribute to the professions.

Certification and Accreditation

Most practitioners in speech-language pathology and audiology in the United States are members of ASHA and have received the Certificate of Clinical Competence (CCC) in either audiology or speech-language pathology, or both, from ASHA. To be eligible to obtain the CCC, ASHA requires the completion of graduate coursework and graduate clinical practicum from a program that is accredited by ASHA (ASHA, 1997b). Academic coursework includes basic sciences and professional coursework that meets the ASHA standards. Clinical observation and supervised practicum must be completed across a range of ages and disorders as specified by the ASHA standards (ASHA, 1997c). Following the completion of the graduate degree, the CCC applicant must spend a Clinical Fellowship Year (CFY) working in an approved clinical setting, under the direct supervision of a clinically certified clinician. The applicant also must pass a certification examination. ASHA membership is not required for certification by the organization, but the percentage of nonmembers holding certification is small. Most states require a license to practice, although those requirements are often consistent with the standards set forth by ASHA for the CCC. Evidence of continuing education also may be required for periodic state licensure renewal.

Continuing Education

ASHA is devoted to continuing education and advancement of scientific and clinical knowledge in the professions. The Association publishes several scholarly journals that are available to members and are carried in many libraries: *American Journal of Audiology*; *American Journal of Speech-Language Pathology*; *Journal of Speech and Hearing Research*; and *Language, Speech, and Hearing Services in Schools*. These journals contain research articles that have been reviewed by experts in the professions (a process called peer review) and have been deemed worthy of publication. A bi-weekly newspaper called *ASHA Leader* helps keep the membership abreast of current events of interest to the profession, and a quarterly *Asha* magazine covers timely professional issues. Another continuing education opportunity is provided by the annual ASHA Convention. This convention often draws more than 10,000 participants, who have the opportunity to listen to professional presentations, view new books and clinical materials, and meet for a variety of formal and informal gatherings. Although the ASHA Convention is the largest educational event each year, there are many other activities such as workshops, telephone seminars, and videoconferences available throughout the year that are sponsored by ASHA, state and local organizations, academic programs, and private groups.

Ethical Conduct

A primary concern of ASHA is for certified speech-language pathologists and audiologists to practice their professions ethically. Consequently, all certified audiologists or speech-language pathologists (regardless of ASHA membership) must adhere to the Association's Code of Ethics (ASHA, 1994). The Code of Ethics provides guidelines for professional practice and is a helpful resource when ethical questions arise (Figure 12-1). A timely example of the value of the Code of Ethics pertains to the discussion of clinical cases via electronic mail and listserv discussion groups. There are many opportunities for clinicians to solicit the opinions and advice of other professionals regarding the diagnosis or treatment of a particularly difficult or unusual case by internet and electronic mail interactions. When seeking information, common sense would suggest that it would be inappropriate for a clinician to reveal the name or other identifying information about a specific patient in the context of a listserv discussion (Principle I in Figure 12-1). However, it might not be so obvious that it is unethical to conduct evaluation or treatment solely by correspondence, as indicated by Principle G (Figure 12-1). That principle should caution clinicians who seek and offer advice about specific patients. Whereas it is appropriate for clinicians to discuss clinical practice in the electronic mail venue, there are potential problems when diagnostic and treatment suggestions are given by someone

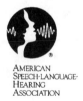

AMERICAN
SPEECH-LANGUAGE-
HEARING
ASSOCIATION

Code of Ethics

Last Revised January 1, 1994

Preamble

The preservation of the highest standards of integrity and ethical principles is vital to the responsible discharge of obligations in the professions of speech-language pathology and audiology. This Code of Ethics sets forth the fundamental principles and rules considered essential to this purpose.

Every individual who is (a) a member of the American Speech-Language-Hearing Association, whether certified or not, (b) a nonmember holding the Certificate of Clinical Competence from the Association, (c) an applicant for membership or certification, or (d) a Clinical Fellow seeking to fulfill standards for certification shall abide by this Code of Ethics.

Any action that violates the spirit and purpose of this Code shall be considered unethical. Failure to specify any particular responsibility or practice in this Code of Ethics shall not be construed as denial of the existence of such responsibilities or practices.

The fundamentals of ethical conduct are described by Principles of Ethics and by Rules of Ethics as they relate to responsibility to persons served, to the public, and to the professions of speech-language pathology and audiology.

Principles of Ethics, aspirational and inspirational in nature, form the underlying moral basis for the Code of Ethics. Individuals shall observe these principles as affirmative obligations under all conditions of professional activity.

Rules of Ethics are specific statements of minimally acceptable professional conduct or of prohibitions and are applicable to all individuals.

Reference this material as: American Speech-Language-Hearing Association (1994). Code of ethics. *Asha, 36* (March, Suppl. 13) pp. 1-2.

Index terms: Ethics, code of ethics, issues in ethics

Principle of Ethics I

Individuals shall honor their responsibility to hold paramount the welfare of persons they serve professionally.

Rules of Ethics

A. Individuals shall provide all services competently.

B. Individuals shall use every resource, including referral when appropriate, to ensure that high-quality service is provided.

C. Individuals shall not discriminate in the delivery of professional services on the basis of race or ethnicity, gender, age, religion, national origin, sexual orientation, or disability.

D. Individuals shall fully inform the persons they serve of the nature and possible effects of services rendered and products dispensed.

E. Individuals shall evaluate the effectiveness of services rendered and of products dispensed and shall provide services or dispense products only when benefit can reasonably be expected.

F. Individuals shall not guarantee the results of any treatment or procedure, directly or by implication; however, they may make a reasonable statement of prognosis.

G. Individuals shall not evaluate or treat speech, language, or hearing disorders solely by correspondence.

H. Individuals shall maintain adequate records of professional services rendered and products dispensed and shall allow access to these records when appropriately authorized.

I. Individuals shall not reveal, without authorization, any professional or personal information about the person served professionally, unless required by law to do so, or unless doing so is necessary to protect the welfare of the person or of the community.

FIGURE 12-1   ASHA Code of Ethics. (Reprinted with permission from the American Speech-Language-Hearing Association)

J. Individuals shall not charge for services not rendered, nor shall they misrepresent,[1] in any fashion, services rendered or products dispensed.

K. Individuals shall use persons in research or as subjects of teaching demonstrations only with their informed consent.

L. Individuals whose professional services are adversely affected by substance abuse or other health-related conditions shall seek professional assistance and, where appropriate, withdraw from the affected areas of practice.

Principle of Ethics II

Individuals shall honor their responsibility to achieve and maintain the highest level of professional competence.

Rules of Ethics

A. Individuals shall engage in the provision of clinical services only when they hold the appropriate Certificate of Clinical Competence or when they are in the certification process and are supervised by an individual who holds the appropriate Certificate of Clinical Competence.

B. Individuals shall engage in only those aspects of the professions that are within the scope of their competence, considering their level of education, training, and experience.

C. Individuals shall continue their professional development throughout their careers.

D. Individuals shall delegate the provision of clinical services only to persons who are certified or to persons in the education or certification process who are appropriately supervised. The provision of support services may be delegated to persons who are neither certified nor in the certification process only when a certificate holder provides appropriate supervision.

E. Individuals shall prohibit any of their professional staff from providing services that exceed the staff member's competence, considering the staff member's level of education, training, and experience.

F. Individuals shall ensure that all equipment used in the provision of services is in proper working order and is properly calibrated.

---

[1] For purposes of this Code of Ethics, misrepresentation includes any untrue statements or statements that are likely to mislead. Misrepresentation also includes the failure to state any information that is material and that ought, in fairness, to be considered.

Principle of Ethics III

Individuals shall honor their responsibility to the public by promoting public understanding of the professions, by supporting the development of services designed to fulfill the unmet needs of the public, and by providing accurate information in all communications involving any aspect of the professions.

Rules of Ethics

A. Individuals shall not misrepresent their credentials, competence, education, training, or experience.

B. Individuals shall not participate in professional activities that constitute a conflict of interest.

C. Individuals shall not misrepresent diagnostic information, services rendered, or products dispensed or engage in any scheme or artifice to defraud in connection with obtaining payment or reimbursement for such services or products.

D. Individuals' statements to the public shall provide accurate information about the nature and management of communication disorders, about the professions, and about professional services.

E. Individuals' statements to the public — advertising, announcing, and marketing their professional services, reporting research results, and promoting products — shall adhere to prevailing professional standards and shall not contain misrepresentations.

Principle of Ethics IV

Individuals shall honor their responsibilities to the professions and their relationships with colleagues, students, and members of allied professions. Individuals shall uphold the dignity and autonomy of the professions, maintain harmonious interprofessional and intraprofessional relationships, and accept the professions' self-imposed standards.

Rules of Ethics

A. Individuals shall prohibit anyone under their supervision from engaging in any practice that violates the Code of Ethics.

B. Individuals shall not engage in dishonesty, fraud, deceit, misrepresentation, or any form of conduct that adversely reflects on the professions or on the individual's fitness to serve persons professionally.

C. Individuals shall assign credit only to those who have contributed to a publication, presentation, or product. Credit shall be assigned in proportion to the contribution and only with the contributor's consent.

FIGURE 12-1   Continued

D. Individuals' statements to colleagues about professional services, research results, and products shall adhere to prevailing professional standards and shall contain no misrepresentations.

E. Individuals shall not provide professional services without exercising independent professional judgment, regardless of referral source or prescription.

F. Individuals shall not discriminate in their relationships with colleagues, students, and members of allied professions on the basis of race or ethnicity, gender, age, religion, national origin, sexual orientation, or disability.

G. Individuals who have reason to believe that the Code of Ethics has been violated shall inform the Ethical Practice Board.

H. Individuals shall cooperate fully with the Ethical Practice Board in its investigation and adjudication of matters related to this Code of Ethics.

FIGURE 12-1   Continued

who has not actually seen the patient. Therefore, advice proffered by mail (electronic or otherwise) should be taken as suggestions rather than prescriptions for treatment.

Student Membership

There is a student organization, the National Student Speech Language Hearing Association (NSSLHA), that undergraduate and graduate students may join as they pursue preprofessional education in speech-language pathology, audiology, and the associated sciences. Many colleges and universities have NSSLHA chapters. NSSLHA membership offers students the opportunity to receive professional journals, participate in educational activities, and even become involved in association governance activities.

Special Interest Divisions

Although members of ASHA are generally trained to manage a broad array of communication disorders, many members have special interests in particular disorders or aspects of the profession. In 1988, special interest divisions were established to allow ASHA members with common interests to identify themselves and affiliate with one another. The divisions have varied objectives but common purposes are to advance the education of their affiliates and to represent their special interests within ASHA. In 1998, there were fifteen special interest divisions, which are listed in Table 12-1. In addition to ASHA members and international affiliates, members of NSSLHA may choose to affiliate with one or more of the divisions, which may provide them with insight into current issues in prospective areas of interest. Affiliation with special interest divisions is optional; affiliate dues may be paid at the same time that ASHA or NSSLHA dues are paid.

Trends in the Profession

Specialty Recognition

Professional preparation in speech-language pathology and audiology is relatively broad-based so that there are many clinical populations and settings from which to choose. However, many professionals find that over time they tend to specialize in a particular area (or areas) of clinical practice.

TABLE 12-1   Special Interest Divisions of the American Speech-Language-Hearing Association

Division 1:   Language Learning and Education
Division 2:   Neurophysiology and Neurogenic Speech and Language Disorders
Division 3:   Voice and Voice Disorders
Division 4:   Fluency and Fluency Disorders
Division 5:   Speech Science and Orofacial Disorders
Division 6:   Hearing and Hearing Disorders: Research and Diagnostics
Division 7:   Aural Rehabilitation and Its Instrumentation
Division 8:   Hearing Conservation and Occupational Audiology
Division 9:   Hearing and Hearing Disorders in Childhood
Division 10:   Issues in Higher Education
Division 11:   Administration and Supervision
Division 12:   Augmentative and Alternative Communication
Division 13:   Swallowing and Swallowing Disorders (Dysphagia)
Division 14:   Communication Disorders and Sciences in Culturally and Linguistically Diverse Populations
Division 15:   Gerontology

Until recently, there was no way for professionals to establish or document that they had gained advanced knowledge and clinical expertise in a particular clinical specialty. In 1994, the Legislative Council of ASHA approved a program for specialty recognition within the professions of speech pathology and audiology. This voluntary program allows practitioners within a given specialty to petition for the establishment of specialty recognition in their area of expertise. The Clinical Specialty Board established by ASHA oversees the application process as groups within the profession take the responsibility to institute specialty recognition. The Clinical Specialty Board does not initiate the establishment of specialty recognition; the initiative comes from a group of practitioners in a given specialty. So in effect, speech-language pathologists and audiologists who have become specialists in a particular area take the responsibility to establish the criteria for such specialization. In some cases, the Special Interest Division may choose to petition for specialty recognition, in other cases, the petitioner may be a related professional organization. The specialty recognition process is in its infancy. Students and new professionals in speech, language, and hearing may be interested in researching the status of specialty recognition as they prepare to enter the profession.

Use of Support Personnel

The use of support personnel is an emerging trend within the professions. These individuals are sometimes referred to as speech-language assistants or aides, audiometric technicians, or audiology assistants. They work in a variety of settings under the supervision of an ASHA-certified speech-language pathologist or audiologist. Unlike the requirements for clinical certification of master's level clinicians, there is no widely accepted training standard for support personnel. However, ASHA has provided guidelines for the training, credentialing, use, and supervision of these individuals in clinical and educational settings (ASHA, 1995c; 1998). The use of support personnel is intended to occur as an adjunct to and under the supervision of clinically certified personnel. When managed properly, a program that includes both certified personnel and support personnel can be effective. Let's take a look at one such team.

Kendall, an ASHA certified speech-language pathologist, "inherited" a speech aide when she took a part-time job at a state residential facility for adults with severe developmental disorders. Her aide, Julie, had been working at this center for 20 years, the last 6 as a speech aide. She has a high school education and received on-the-job training for her current position. They have been working together for 3 years.

Kendall is responsible for initial assessments of the center's residents. She interviews the center staff concerning the resident's level of functioning, and develops programs designed to increase their functional communication. She discusses a new program with Julie to get her insights on how it might be integrated into the daily activities at the center. It is Julie, who is at the center on a daily basis, who oversees the implementation of those programs. She works with the center staff to explain the communication goals and provides them with materials for training those communication behaviors during the day. She also collects and compiles data on the frequency with which goals were addressed by the staff and how effective the program has been for a resident.

Julie's duties are fairly typical of support personnel. These duties may include clerical work, making materials for intervention programs, and implementing the programs planned by the certified clinician (Kimbarow, 1997). Julie's contribution on a daily basis increases frequency of services to the residents beyond what Kendall could provide on her own. Effective use of support personnel may mean that the certified clinician may have to rethink the components of his or her job and how to best carry them out.

"One of the things that has been very important for me in working with my assistant was learning to prioritize," said Kendall. "I had to decide which tasks were critical for me to complete, and let Julie do the rest."

As Kendall's experience shows, support personnel can make a positive contribution to the professions. However, the use of support personnel in clinical settings is not without controversy. Some clinicians are concerned that bureaucratic decisions will be made that increase the use of support personnel beyond their training and abilities, eroding the quality of services. Those who have had experience working with support personnel offered guidance for those who might have the opportunity to work with support personnel (Kimbarow, 1997). Their advice includes:

- Establish clear guidelines for use of support personnel.
- Establish minimum competencies for work setting.
- Learn how to supervise and train support personnel.
- Allow for a training period for developing competencies before working with patients.
- Explain the rationale behind therapy procedures so that they are implemented correctly.
- Do not assign support personnel to work with new clients or with certain types of complex disorders.
- Establish a plan of supervision and feedback.

Employment Outlook

Speech-language pathology and audiology are relatively young professions that continue to grow. In fact, they have been listed in *Money* magazine among the fastest growing professions in the

United States (Marable, 1995). The outlook is good for the professions, given factors such as increased awareness of communication disorders; early detection of hearing, speech, and language disorders in children; the aging of the population and associated increased prevalence of age-related communication impairments; and increased concern over occupationally related hearing disorders (ASHA, 1998). These trends suggest continued growth of the professions well into the future. While work settings and models of service delivery are likely to change over time, the professions will remain devoted to increased understanding of the nature and treatment of communication disorders.

References

American Speech-Language-Hearing Association. (1994). Code of ethics. *Asha*, 36 (March Suppl. 13): 1–2.

American Speech-Language-Hearing Association. (1995). Position statement for the training, credentialing, use, and supervision of support personnel in speech-language pathology. *Asha*, 37 (Suppl. 14): 21.

American Speech-Language-Hearing Association. (1997a). Bylaws and policies associated with the bylaws of the American Speech-Language-Hearing Association. *ASHA Desk Reference*, Vol. 1. Rockville, MD: Author.

American Speech-Language-Hearing Association. (1997b). Standards for accreditation of educational programs in speech-language pathology and audiology. *ASHA Desk Reference*, Vol. 1 (pp. 113–144). Rockville, MD: Author.

American Speech-Language-Hearing Association. (1997c). *Membership Certification Handbook*. Rockville, MD: Author.

American Speech-Language-Hearing Association. (1998). Position statement and guidelines on support personnel in audiology. *Asha*, 40 (Spring Suppl. 18).

American Speech-Language-Hearing Association. ASHA website: www.asha.org.

Cherry, R., & Giolas, T.G. (1997). Preface to aural rehabilitation with adults. *Seminars in Hearing, 18*: 75.

Frattali, C.M. (1998). Outcomes assessment in speech-language pathology. In A.F. Johnson & B.H. Jacobson (eds.), *Medical Speech-Language Pathology: A Practitioner's Guide*. New York: Thieme.

Golper, L.C. (1992). *Sourcebook for Medical Speech Pathology*. San Diego: Singular.

Johnson, A.F., & Jacobson, B.H. (1998). *Medical Speech-Language Pathology: A Practitioner's Guide*. New York: Thieme.

Kimbarow, M.L. (1997). Ahead of the curve: Improving services with speech-language pathology assistants. *Asha, 39*: 41–44

Lubinski, R. & Frattali, C. (1994). *Professional Issues in Speech-Language Pathology and Audiology: A Textbook*. San Diego: Singular.

Marable, L.M. (1995, March). The fifty hottest jobs in America. *Money, 24*(3): 114–117.

Paden, E. (1970). *A History of the American Speech and Hearing Association, 1925–1958*. Bethesda, MD: American Speech and Hearing Association.

Glossary

addition error   A type of speech articulation error characterized by adding a sound to the target phoneme or word; for example, for the word, *blue*, a child pronounces it *bolu*.

acoustic neuroma   A nonmalignant tumor that involves the myelin sheath of the VIIIth nerve.

affricate   A consonant that begins with a plosive phoneme and ends with a fricative, such as *ch*, written phonetically as /tʃ/.

agraphia   An acquired impairment of writing caused by brain damage.

air conduction audiometry   Testing hearing by introducing the tone into the ear canal, with the sound waves then traveling to the drum membrane at the end of the canal (as opposed to bone conduction).

alexia   An acquired impairment of reading caused by brain damage.

alexia with agraphia   An acquired impairment of reading and writing due to brain damage without other language impairments.

alexia without agraphia   An acquired impairment of reading that is not accompanied by a writing impairment; also called pure alexia.

allophone   One of the variant forms of a phoneme that is still recognized by the listener as the target phoneme.

Alzheimer's disease   The most common form of dementing illness; a chronic, progressive disease that results in intellectual decline affecting language, memory, and cognition.

anarthria   A severe impairment of motor control for speech resulting in complete lack of articulate speech.

anomia   The inability to name objects or retrieve desired words.

anomic aphasia   A fluent aphasia that is characterized by relatively good verbal expression and auditory comprehension, but notable difficulty coming up with the names of things.

APGAR   A five-point evaluation system for identifying the status of newborns.

aphasia   An acquired impairment of language due to damage to the language-dominant hemisphere, typically the left. *See* fluent aphasia and nonfluent aphasia.

aphonia   Attempts to produce a voice result in a whisper-like sound. This usually occurs with voice disorders that prevent the vocal folds from vibrating to produce sound.

apraxia of speech   An impairment of motor planning for the movements for speech so that voluntary control for speech is disrupted.

arcuate fasciculus   A bundle of nerve fibers (white matter) that originate in cell bodies in the superior temporal gyrus and project anteriorly to the frontal lobe.

articulation   Production of speech sounds.

articulation index   A theoretical construct that attempts to quantify the contribution of different frequency bands to the intelligibility of speech.

arytenoid cartilage   The paired, pyramid-shaped cartilages that sit on the signet portion of the cricoid cartilage and aid in abduction and adduction of vocal folds.

aspiration   Occurs when food penetrates below the vocal folds into the trachea and, possibly, into the lungs.

assimilation   A speech phenomenon in which the sounds that precede or follow a particular sound influence the production of that sound.

assistive listening device (*ALD*)   Any device designed to reduce the effects of distance, background noise, and reverberation on the perception of speech.

ataxia   A motor disorder characterized by marked loss of coordination, often associated with cerebellar disease.

athetosis   A form of cerebral palsy characterized by twisting and flailing of the extremities, neck, and trunk.

audiogram   A graphic representation of the results of a hearing test with axes for hearing level and frequency.

audiologist   A professional who is concerned with the prevention, evaluation, and rehabilitation of auditory, balance, and related disorders.

audiology   The study of normal and disordered hearing.

audiometer   An electronic instrument used to evaluate the auditory system.

auditory brainstem response   An electrophysiological response to sounds that results in 5 to 7 peaks that appear within 10 ms after the presentation of a signal (usually a click).

auditory stimulation   Sounds used given in training children with hearing impairments.

auditory training   The training of a hearing-impaired individual to make use of residual hearing abilities.

auricle   The external ear, also known as pinna.

axon   The nerve fiber that carries impulses away from the neuron body.

basal ganglia   A collection of subcortical gray matter structures, including the putamen, globus pallidus, and caudate, that contribute to control of motor behavior.

basilar membrane   A thin tissue layer found within the cochlea on which rests the organ of Corti.

bolus   Refers to a cohesive mass of some substance such as food.

bone conduction audiometry   In hearing testing, introducing the sound waves directly into the cochlea via the bones of the skull.

brainstem   The brain structures at the base of the brain excluding the hemispheres above, the cerebellum, and the spinal cord below.

Broca's aphasia   A nonfluent aphasia associated with damage to the inferior portions of the left frontal lobe.

canonical babbling   Consonant-vowel or consonant-vowel-consonant-vowel combinations produced by babies.

carcinoma   A cancer or malignancy.

***central auditory processing disorder* (*CAPD*)**　Difficulties understanding speech as a result of structural changes in the central auditory nervous system. The difficulties are most pronounced in background noise and other difficult listening situations (e.g., reverberation).

central nervous system　The brain and spinal cord, exclusive of the cranial and peripheral nerves.

cerebellum　A brain structure that sits below the cerebral hemispheres and above the pons, playing an important role in muscular coordination.

cerebral localization　A theory of brain function that associates particular functions and behaviors to particular sites of the brain.

cerebral palsy　A developmental motor disorder related to brain injury; the most common forms are spasticity, athetosis, and ataxia.

cerebrum　The largest division of the brain, containing the cerebral hemispheres and corpus callosum.

cerumen　Ear wax produced by glands that lie within the skin of the ear canal.

chromosome　A structure containing genes that transmit genetic information.

circumlocution　Talking with an excess number of words; or talking around the topic rather than being direct because of a failure to retrieve desired words, as in anomia.

cleft lip and cleft palate　A congenital fissure or absence of tissue of the lip, premaxilla, hard palate, and/or velum.

closed caption decoder　An electronic device that decodes the caption signals that are often broadcast with television programs. It causes captions to appear on the television screen and helps hearing-impaired individuals to understand the dialogue of television programs and movies.

cluttering　A disorder of fluency characterized by rapid speech, breaks in fluency, and faulty articulation.

coarticulation　The simultaneous production of two or more consonants or vowels in normal speech production of a word, such as the word *tram*—The first three phones (/t/ /r/ /æ/) might overlap in production.

cochlea　The snail-shaped part of the inner ear containing the sensory organs of hearing.

cochlear implant　A coil and electrodes surgically placed in the inner ear and connected to an external transmitter/signal processor. It is intended to produce sensations of sound for those with profound hearing impairments.

code switching　Shifting by speakers among one or more dialects or languages to accommodate social rules or situational demands.

cognate　A pair of sounds, such as /p/ and /b/, produced similarly except that one (/p/) is unvoiced and one (/b/) voiced.

communication　An interaction or exchange of one's feelings, ideas, thoughts, and wants among two or more people by such modes as speech, writing, facial expression, gesture, or touch.

conduction aphasia　A fluent aphasia characterized by relatively good auditory comprehension and poor verbal repetition.

conductive hearing loss　A loss of hearing related to obstruction or disease in the outer or middle ear in which sound transmission fails to reach the cochlea in the inner ear.

congenital　Present at birth.

consanguineous　Between blood relatives.

consistency effect　An observation among stutterers that certain words are more likely to be stuttered.

content　The elements of language that carry meaning; also called semantics.

continuant　A speech sound that can be continued or prolonged, such as /m/ or /s/.

cerebrovascular accident   *See* stroke.

corpus callosum   A large band of fibers that joins the two hemispheres of the brain.

cortex   The surface layer of the brain that contains the bodies of neurons.

cranial nerves   Twelve paired peripheral nerves that derive from or come into the cranial cavity, such as cranial nerves I, olfactory, or II, optic.

Creutzfeldt-Jakob disease   A dementing disease thought to be associated with a slow virus causing rapid onset of profound dementia.

cricoid cartilage   The ring of cartilage that forms the base of the larynx.

cricothyroid muscles   The paired laryngeal muscles that are involved with changing the pitch of the voice.

criterion-referenced test   A type of measure that is used to compare a child's performance against a standard, or criterion, for behavior.

decibel   A logarithmic unit of measurement of sound intensity.

dementia   A behavioral syndrome of generalized intellectual deficit that results from a number of diseases.

denasality   Insufficient nasal resonance; hyponasality.

dendrites   The receptors attached to each neuron in the central nervous system.

developmental language disorder   A condition involving poor language skills that appears during childhood.

diacritics   Markings that modify phonetic symbols, indicating slight change in the sound of the phoneme.

diadochokinesis   The rapid, alternating movements of a body part, such as in the lips and tongue rapidly saying *pataka*.

diagnosogenic theory of stuttering   Theory that posits stuttering begins when normal disfluencies are labeled as stuttering.

diaphragm   The muscular-tendonous partition that separates the thorax from the abdomen, serving as the primary muscle of respiration.

diphthong   A blending together of two vowels in the same syllable, such as heard as /aɪ/ in the word *right*.

diplophonia   This describes a voice that has two pitches occurring at the same time.

disfluency   A breakdown in the prosodic flow or fluency of speech.

distinctive features   Particular elements that are characteristic of a phoneme such as its duration and voicing elements.

distortion error   The production of a target phoneme utilizing a sound that is not in the language, such as in a lateral lisp.

dyadic communication   Two people communicating with each other.

dysarthria   An impairment of motor control for speech caused by weakness, paralysis, slowness, incoordination, or sensory loss in the muscle groups responsible for speech.

dyslexia   An impairment of reading to developmental brain damage or dysfunction.

dysphagia   An impairment of the ability to swallow.

dysphonia   A disorder of voice, such as hoarseness, breathiness, or harshness.

ear canal   The external opening into the ear.

effusion   Fluid that has exuded into the middle ear space.

electrolarynx   An electronic device that creates sound that can be used as a substitute for the voice (usually because the larynx has been surgically removed).

endogenous   Caused by genetic factors

endolymph   The fluid within the membranous labyrinth of the inner ear.

eustachian tube   The air tube that connects the middle ear with the nasopharynx.

exogenous   Acquired or caused by factors outside the genes.

expressive language   A coded system of communication that uses the modalities of speaking, writing, or signing.

fluency   The rhythm and flow of spoken (or signed) language.

fluent aphasia   An aphasia profile that is characterized by spoken output of relatively normal utterance length, ease of production, and prosodic variation.

FM system   A device that uses a transmitter to send the desired signal to a receiver using a radio wave. The receiver is coupled to the listener via earphones or a hearing aid.

form   The phonological, syntactic, and morphological elements of language.

four kilohertz (4k) notch   An increase in hearing impairment in the 3000–6000 Hz region with recovery of hearing at 8000 Hz. This pattern is associated with noise-induced hearing impairment.

frequency   The number of cycles per second of a sound wave; perceived as pitch.

fricative   A speech sound produced by the airstream passing between or through a constricted opening, such as /f/ and /v/.

frontal lobe   The anterior part of each cerebral hemisphere, from the Rolandic fissure forward.

functional dysphonia   A voice problem that has no physical or structural cause.

functional gain   The difference in dB between aided and unaided threshold measures obtained in a soundfield.

glossectomy   The surgical removal of the tongue.

glottis   The opening between the vocal folds.

granuloma   Hard, granulated tissue, sometimes found along the glottal rim in the larynx; sometimes seen following intubation during surgery or from continuous esophageal reflux.

habitual pitch   The modal or most frequently occurring voice pitch.

habituation   Gradual decrease in responsiveness following repeated exposure to a stimulus.

handicap   A disadvantage resulting from an impairment or disability that limits the fulfillment of a role that is normal for an individual.

hearing   The perception of sound.

hearing disability   The auditory difficulties that result from a hearing impairment.

hearing impairment   Any loss or abnormality of structure or function of the auditory system.

hearing loss   The term used when specific reference is made to a hearing impairment of a particular magnitude.

hemianopsia   A visual field defect in which half of the vision of each eye is lost, resulting in loss of visual input from the left or right visual field.

hemiparesis   Weakness of one side of the body.

hemiplegia   A unilateral weakness or paralysis of one side of the body.

hemisphere   Literally, half circle. In reference to brain anatomy, hemisphere indicates the half of the cerebrum or cerebellum to each side of midline.

Hertz   Unit of measure that reflects cycles per second.

hypernasality   Excessive nasal resonance.

impedance audiometry   Air-pressure and air-volume differences measured in the external and middle ear as a method of detecting conductive hearing loss.

incidence   The number of new cases that appear in a population over a set period of time.

intensity   A measure of the magnitude or pressure of a sound wave; perceived as loudness.

intercostals   The muscles (internal and external) between the ribs.

involuntary repetitions   A form of stuttering characterized by unexpected syllable or word repetitions.

jargon aphasia   An acquired impairment of language characterized by meaningless utterances.

language   The coding of meaning into a system of arbitrary symbols that are recognized by members of the community. Language may be spoken, written, or manual (signed).

laryngeal trauma   A direct, external blow to the larynx.

laryngeal web   A membranous growth across the laryngeal glottis, usually in an anterior to posterior direction.

laryngectomy   Surgical removal of the larynx (usually because of cancer).

laryngoscopy   Viewing the internal structure of the larynx by mirror (indirect) or at the actual site (direct).

learning disability   Educational difficulties in reading, writing, listening, speaking, or arithmetic, believed to be related to some kind of central brain dysfunction.

left neglect   Reduced awareness or responsiveness to sensory input from the left side of the body (intrapersonal space) or left half of the environment (extrapersonal space) that cannot be attributed to sensory or motor defects.

lesion   Damage to the nervous system.

lexicon   The terms and words of one's vocabulary.

mandible   The lower jaw.

maxilla   The upper jaw.

Ménière's disease   A disease of the inner ear thought to be associated with an overproduction of endolymph. Symptoms include tinnitus, vertigo, and hearing loss.

mental retardation   Reduced cognitive abilities, confirmed by measured intelligence quotients of 70 or below and poor adaptive abilities.

middle ear   The air-filled space located in the temporal bone containing the three small middle-ear bones, incus, malleus, and stapes.

misarticulations   Speech-articulation errors of omission, addition, substitution, or distortion.

mixed hearing loss   A hearing loss caused by both conductive and sensorineural problems.

mixed hearing impairment   Hearing impairment produced by abnormalities in the conductive and sensorineural hearing mechanisms.

mixed transcortical aphasia   A rare aphasia type characterized by severe language impairment with preserved ability to repeat sentences due to a relatively spared perisylvian region.

morpheme   Words or the smallest unit of a word that has meaning. For example, the word *cat* is one morpheme; in the plural form *cats*, the *s* is an added morpheme.

morphology   The study of words and word forms; the study of morphemes.

multi-infarct dementia   A form of dementia related to many small strokes (or infarcts).

myofunctional therapy   Muscle training of the tongue to reduce tongue pressures on dentition, that is, therapy for reverse swallow and tongue thrust.

nasoendoscope   A scope used during a videoendoscopy examination of the larynx. This scope is shaped like a long thin tube that is flexible. It is placed through the nose to view the soft palate and can also be positioned in the pharynx to view the larynx.

nasoendoscopy   Inserting a flexible viewing scope through the nose and positioning it in the pharynx, to view the nasopharynx, hypopharynx, and larynx below.

neologism A nonword, or literally "new word," produced by an individual with aphasia.

neonate Newborn.

neuron Cell within the brain that supports activity through the conduction of chemical-electrical signals.

nonfluent aphasia An aphasia profile that is characterized by effortful speech production, reduced grammatical complexity, and short utterance length.

normative sample A representative sample of individuals whose performance on a test or measure serves as a reference against which a single individual's performance can be compared.

norm-referenced test Test designed to allow comparisons between an individual's performance and a group of individuals of similar age.

occipital lobe The posterior part of each cerebral hemisphere.

omission error One of the four types of articulatory errors, in which the sound is totally omitted.

oral-peripheral examination An examination of the structure and function of the face, mouth, and oral cavity, intended to assess the integrity of the articulatory mechanisms of speech.

orbicularis oris The circular, sphincteric muscles that circle the lips.

organ of Corti Area within the cochlea containing the tectorial membrane and hair cells.

organogenesis The development of organs, which in humans occurs during the fetal period.

ossicles The three small bones (incus, malleus, stapes) that form the ossicular chain in the middle ear.

otitis media Inflammation of the middle ear.

otoacoustic emissions Sounds produced by the inner ear.

otosclerosis The formation of new spongy bone growth in the middle ear, most often near the footplate of the stapes. It produces a progressive, conductive hearing loss when it interferes with the movement of the stapes.

otoscope A lighted device with a speculum on the end used to visualize the tympanic membrane.

ototoxicity The capacity to damage the mechanisms of hearing.

oval window A membrane-covered opening of the vestibule of the cochlea that is attached to the footplate of the stapes. Vibration of the stapes footplate sets the oval window in vibration.

palatal lift A dental appliance designed to raise a paralyzed or weakened velum to the pharyngeal wall to produce closure of the velopharyngeal port.

palate The roof of the mouth. Anteriorly, the hard palate is bone, covered with a membrane; posteriorly, the soft palate (velum) is muscle covered with a membrane. The palate separates the oral and nasal cavities.

papilloma A wartlike tumor that can grow in the airway and larynx of primarily young children, possibly causing airway obstruction and severe dysphonia.

paraphasia An erroneous word or a nonword that reflects disorders of word choice (e.g., *man* for *woman*) or sound substitution errors (e.g., *tike* for *bike*).

parenteral This refers to non-oral ways of eating when someone has dysphagia and cannot eat enough food to maintain nutritional needs. One example of a parenteral method of feeding someone is a nasogastric tube (i.e., NG tube) that goes through the nose down into the stomach.

parietal lobe One of the four lobes of the cerebral hemisphere, extending posteriorly from the Rolandic fissure to the occipital lobe.

perinatal The period surrounding birth; between the twenty-ninth week of gestation to one to four weeks after birth.

peripheral nervous system   The nervous system that extends beyond the brain and the spinal cord, including peripheral sensory nerves that send impulses to the central nervous system and motor nerves that carry effector impulses to peripheral structures.

peristaltic contractions   In the esophagus, this term describes how the muscles squeeze together starting at the top and moving downward. Each neighboring segment squeezes together to push food toward the stomach.

perisylvian region   The region of the brain that surrounds the Sylvian fissure, which is the primary horizontal fissure for each cerebral hemisphere.

phone   A speech sound.

perseveration   Involuntary repetition of a word, phrase, sentence, or idea.

phoneme   The smallest sound unit of speech represented by a symbol of the International Phonetic Alphabet.

phonemic regression   Poor auditory comprehension often associated with advanced age.

phonetics   The study of the perception and the production of speech sounds.

phonologic process   The systematic simplification by children of the production of adult-modeled articulation, such as deleting the final consonant of words or deleting a syllable within a word.

phonology   The study of the sounds of spoken language, including the rules of phoneme use, phonemes, phonetic production, and voicing characteristics of prosody and suprasegmentals.

Pick's disease   A dementing disease that is associated with atrophy of the frontal and temporal lobes.

plosive   A speech sound produced by impounding air behind an articulator and suddenly releasing it, as in /p/ or /b/.

positive predictive validity   The calculated accuracy with which a test identifies impairment in the population. This metric differs from test *sensitivity* in that it takes into account the prevalence of a disorder in the population.

postnatal   Occurring after birth.

prenatal   Preceding birth.

presbycusis   Hearing impairment associated with the aging process.

prevalence   The total number of cases present in a population in a given period of time.

primary progressive aphasia   An acquired impairment of language that follows a slowly progressive, rather than abrupt, onset and is not associated with dementia.

prolongation   A form of disfluency often observed in stuttering, when a speech sound or syllable has increased in duration.

prosody   The melody, flow, and rhythm of a spoken language; melodic changes in syllable stress, pitch, loudness, and duration.

protoword   Early form of an actual word that usually contains some of the sounds of the target word.

pure tone   A periodic sound wave of a particular frequency that is generated in the audiometric testing of hearing.

real ear insertion response (REIR)   The amount of gain for various frequencies that a client gets from wearing a hearing aid. It is the difference between an aided and unaided measure made using a small probe microphone placed close to the eardrum.

recruitment   A large increase in the loudness of a sound produced by a small increase in the intensity above its threshold.

reflux   Refers to backward movement of food during swallowing. Often, reflux refers to acid from the stomach spilling upward into the throat, causing irritation to the tissues.

reliability   Quality of providing consistent information.

right hemiparesis   Weakness on the right side of the body.

Rolandic fissure   The central fissue that divides the posterior frontal lobe from the anterior parietal lobe.

rollover   A phenomenon in which word recognition scores decrease as intensity increases.

round window   An opening in the vestibule of the cochlea beneath the oval window on the cochlea, permitting the displacement or movement of fluid within the cochlea.

screening   The detection of individuals at risk for a condition (e.g., hearing loss, language disorder).

seizures   The convulsions of an epileptic attack; epilepsy.

semantics   The study of the history and meaning of words.

sensitivity   The rate at which a test correctly identifies individuals with the disorder the test is designed to detect.

sensorineural hearing loss   A hearing loss caused by disease of the inner ear or eighth cranial nerve.

sequelae   Conditions that follow or occur as a consequence of another condition (e.g., illness) or event (e.g., trauma).

spasticity   A paralysis characterized by extreme tension and hypercontraction of muscles with hyperactive tendon reflexes.

specific language impairment   A diagnosis of a child who demonstrates impairment in understanding spoken language, speaking, reading, and writing with no other demonstrable impairment.

specificity   The rate at which a test correctly identifies individuals with normal skills as having normal skills.

spectrogram   A visual display of the sound frequencies of a spoken utterance.

speech   Sound production via changes in the vocal mechanism and oral structures to form words and sentences in auditory-oral communication.

speech-language pathologist   A professional who specializes in the diagnosis and treatment of communication and swallowing disorders.

speech-language pathology   A profession that specializes in the diagnosis and treatment of communication disorders related to problems of hearing, articulation, language, voice, fluency, and swallowing.

speechreading   The use of visual cues from a talker's face to identify their spoken words.

speech-reception threshold   The amplification level or threshold at which the subject is able to repeat correctly after the examiner 50% of the words presented on a spondee list.

spinal cord   The lower portion of the central nervous system, originating at the medulla and extending down within the spinal vertebra.

spinal nerves   Thirty-one pairs of nerves that enter or exit the spinal cord.

spondaic words   Two-syllable words pronounced with equal stress on each syllable.

stapedectomy   An operation in which the stapes is removed and replaced with a prosthesis in an attempt to improve a hearing impairment that was caused by otosclerosis.

stimulability testing   In testing articulation, a determination of how well the client can produce the target sound when the sound has been repeatedly presented (visually and auditorially).

STORCH   Acronym for syphillis, toxoplasmosis, other, rubella, cytomegalovirus, and herpes simplex infections.

stroke   Sudden onset of disturbed neurological functioning caused by disruption of blood flow. Also called a cerebrovascular accident (CVA), usually one of three types: thrombosis, embolus, or hemorrhage.

stuttering   The involuntary repetition, interruption, and prolongation of speech sounds and syllables, which the individual struggles to end.

subglottal pressure   The air pressure within the airway below the vocal folds; outgoing air moves between the vocal folds when pressure below the folds is greater than air pressure above them.

substitution error   A type of articulation error characterized by an incorrect phoneme used in place of a target phoneme, such as /w/ said for /r/.

successive approximation   A technique used in articulation therapy in which the client experiences step-by-step success of moving from the incorrect sound to production of the target phoneme.

Sylvian fissure   The horizontal fissure that divides the inferior border of the frontal and parietal lobes from the superior temporal lobe.

syndrome   A collection of physical features that co-occur and characterize a disorder or condition.

syntax   The grammatical structure and word order of a language.

target sound   The correct model; the phoneme selected for articulation therapy.

telecommunication device for the deaf (*TDD*)   A keyboard that attaches to a telephone to allow typewritten communication with other TDDs. It enables individuals with hearing difficulties to communicate using the telephone.

telegraphic speech   Spoken communication that consists primarily of content words and is lacking functor words, such as pronouns, auxilary verbs, and articles.

temporal lobe   One of the four lobes of a cerebral hemisphere, lying below the Sylvian fissure.

thalamus   A large gray mass of sensory nuclei deep within the hemisphere, bordering the third ventricle.

thorax   The region of the body's trunk from below the neck to just above the diaphram.

thyroarytenoid muscles   The paired vocal folds in the larynx.

thyroid cartilage   The shield-shaped outer cartilage protecting the larynx; popularly called the Adam's apple.

tinnitus   Noises in the ear(s) usually described as ringing, hissing, or roaring.

tongue thrust   Abnormal tongue positioning, particularly during swallowing, which may have an adverse effect on the anterior dental bite.

tracheostoma   A permanent opening in the neck that is surgically created. This is usually done because the larynx has been surgically removed or is not able to open enough to allow breathing such as with bilateral vocal fold paralysis or injury to the larynx.

transcortical aphasia   See transcortical motor aphasia, transcortical sensory aphasia, and mixed transcortical aphasia.

transcortical motor aphasia   A nonfluent aphasia characterized by relatively preserved ability to repeat sentences because of a relatively intact perisylvian region.

transcortical sensory aphasia   A fluent aphasia characterized by relatively preserved ability to repeat sentences because of a relatively intact perisylvian region.

traumatic laryngitis   A dysphonia related to excessive use of harmful voicing behaviors such as yelling and screaming.

use   The rules for communicative interactions, including the social-interactive aspects of language, sometimes called pragmatics.

validity   The quality of providing accurate or true information.

velopharyngeal port   The closing site where the elevated velum makes contact with the pharyngeal wall, separating the oral and nasal cavities; a depressed (relaxed) velum allows continuity of the two cavities at the site of the port.

velum   The soft palate.

videoendoscopy   This procedure uses special fiber-optic equipment to obtain views of the internal structure of the larynx.

videofluorography   A motion picture x-ray that can be recorded on videotape.

vital capacity   The total volume one is able to expire after maximum inhalation; a maximum expiration.

vocalization   Voicing or phonation.

vocal nodules   Benign growths on the vocal folds, usually bilateral, which are typically the result of laryngeal abuse and voice misuse.

voice   The production of sound by vibration of the vocal folds.

vocal polyps   Benign growths on the vocal folds that usually occur unilaterally and are soft and compliant fluid-filled bags. These occur as a result of excessive use of harmful vocal habits such as yelling and screaming.

Wernicke's aphasia   A fluent aphasia characterized by poor auditory comprehension and paraphasic utterances.

Index